THE
DIABETES
DTOUR
DIET™

THE DIABETES

DTOUR

DIET™

THE REVOLUTIONARY
NEW FOOD CURE

BARBARA QUINN, MS, RD, CDE,
AND THE EDITORS OF
Prevention.

With Medical Advisor
Francine R. Kaufman, MD

RODALE

Prevention is a registered trademark of Rodale Inc.
Diabetes DTOUR Diet is a trademark of Rodale Inc.

Printed in the United States of America
Rodale Inc. makes every effort to use acid-free ♾, recycled paper ♻.

Recipe Photos by Marcus Nilsson; Prop Styling by Pamela Duncan Silver
for Big Leo Productions; Food Styling by Stephana Bottom
Before & After Photos by Jonathan Pozniak; Styling by Karen Schaupeter;
Hair and Makeup by Coleen Kobrick-Kuehne
Workout Photos by Jonathan Pozniak; Styling by Marie Bloomquist
and Hair and Makeup by Lynn Lamorte, both for Vivian Artists

Book design by Jill Armus

Library of Congress Cataloging-in-Publication Data

The diabetes dtour diet : the revolutionary new food cure / Barbara Quinn and the editors of Prevention ; with medical advisor, Francine R. Kaufman.
     p.   cm.
   Includes index.
   ISBN-13 978–1–60529–843–6 hardcover
   ISBN-10 1-60529-843-3 hardcover
   1. Diabetes—Diet therapy.   I. Quinn, Barbara, 1952- II. Prevention (Washington, D.C.)
RC662.D523 2009
616.4'620654—dc22   2009003502

6 8 10 9 7 5   hardcover

LIVE YOUR WHOLE LIFE™

We inspire and enable people to improve their lives and the world around them
For more of our products visit **rodalestore.com** or call 800-848-4735

To our fabulous DTOUR test panelists
for blazing a new trail to weight-loss success;
and to all those who will follow
in their footsteps

CONT

PART

1

PART

2

PART

3

OFF THE BLOOD SUGAR EXPRESS

THE DTOUR FAT-FIGHTING 4

HIT THE ROAD: START LOSING

ENTS:

INTRODUCTION

Welcome to the Diabetes DTOUR Diet; we're so glad you've joined us! It shows your determination and commitment to changing your health for the better. We're here to help you every step of the way.

We've designed DTOUR especially for people with blood sugar issues who need to lose weight. Slimming down can seem daunting under any circumstances; high blood sugar makes it that much trickier by prompting your body to store fat, among other things. Yet many experts agree that losing weight is the single most potent strategy for stabilizing blood sugar and effectively managing diabetes if not avoiding the disease altogether.

Which brings us to DTOUR. On our plan, you're going to learn a way of eating that can help you achieve the duel goals of weight loss and blood sugar control. We believe this sort of approach is important because too often food is portrayed as the bad guy in the battle of the bulge (and blood sugar).

DTOUR teaches you how to think about food in an entirely different and empowering way. You'll develop a new understanding of the relationship between nutrition and health—and how eating the right foods in the right portions at the right times of day can help melt away pounds and balance blood sugar. This is important whether you already have diabetes or you're at risk for it.

We call it the Diabetes DTOUR Diet precisely for this reason. By following our plan, you may be able to steer clear of diabetes altogether. If you've already been diagnosed with the disease, DTOUR can help you, too. With your weight and blood sugar in check, you may be able to delay or avoid using medication—and reduce your chances of developing complications down the road.

DTOUR consists of two stages. The first, the 2-Week Fast Start, is all about eating DTOUR-style. We want you to become familiar with the food choices and the portion sizes, as well as eating at regular intervals throughout the day. The second stage, the 4-Week Total Transformation, introduces a trio of lifestyle measures—exercise, sleep, and stress reduction—that can help melt away pounds even faster while maintaining blood sugar in a tighter range. You will get results on DTOUR without these tools. But if they can improve your progress on the plan, why not give them a try?

Along the way, you'll read about all the amazing studies that provide the scientific backbone for DTOUR. In fact, they're what set us on the path to our plan. As we talked with experts and reviewed the latest research, we began to realize how certain key findings from the diabetes and obesity fields have gone largely untapped.

Our Fat-Fighting 4 are a great example of this. A number of studies point to intriguing connections between this quartet of nutrients—fiber, calcium, vitamin D, and omega-3s—and improved weight loss and blood sugar control. Scientists are exploring just how these nutrients might work their magic. But since the Fat-Fighting 4 come from superbly nutritious foods, and since most of us don't get enough of these nutrients in our diets anyway, nothing but good can come from making them the stars of DTOUR. That's what we've done!

You'll also meet some truly wonderful people in the pages ahead. They're our DTOUR test panelists—eight volunteers who followed the plan for the full 6 weeks. Each of them had his or her own reasons for wanting to try DTOUR. Jean, for example, only recently found out that she has a family history of diabetes. Her partner, Tom, already has the disease but hopes to reduce his reliance on medications. For another of our panelists, Kris, motivation comes in the form of a red dress. Their willingness to put DTOUR through its paces helped us to fine-tune the plan. We're their biggest fans. We hope that their stories will inspire you, too.

Our panelists lost as much as 25 pounds and 10 inches over the 6 weeks of DTOUR. Their blood sugar stabilized or fell, often dramatically. They reported other benefits, too—like more energy, fewer headaches, and a brighter mood.

Of course, your results on DTOUR will depend on where you're starting from and how much you want to lose. Especially if you already have diabetes, we encourage you to consult your doctor or dietitian before starting our plan, to make sure it's right for you.

Once you're on DTOUR, you can expect to make safe and steady progress toward your goal weight, all while practicing a way of eating and living that will become habit before long. Then diabetes won't stand a chance!

–The Editors of *Prevention*

PART 1

OFF THE BLOOD SUGAR EXPRESS

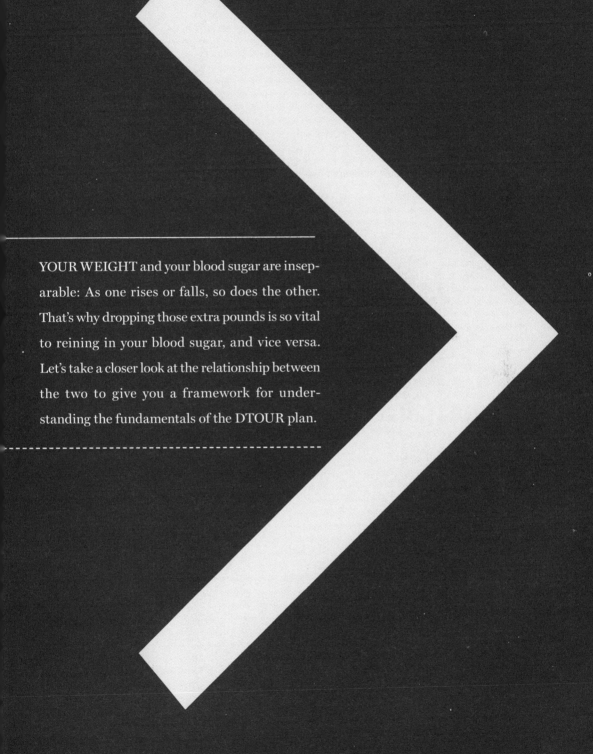

YOUR WEIGHT and your blood sugar are insep-
arable: As one rises or falls, so does the other.
That's why dropping those extra pounds is so vital
to reining in your blood sugar, and vice versa.
Let's take a closer look at the relationship between
the two to give you a framework for understanding the fundamentals of the DTOUR plan.

CHAPTER 1

YES, YOU CAN

BYPASS

DIABETES!

Right now, we're thinking, you probably want to be anywhere but here. Being here means diabetes is touching your life—whether you've been diagnosed with it or you're at risk for developing it because of high blood sugar. Whatever your story is, you realize that getting rid of those extra pounds can help you take a detour around diabetes, and you can be out loving your life instead of worrying about your blood sugar level.

So you're all set to do what you know you have to do. Except . . . you love to eat. (Who doesn't?) You can't bear the thought of giving up your favorite foods. (Who could?) And you really, really don't want to feel hungry all the time. (That's why so many diets fail in the first place!)

We hear you. And we promise, the Diabetes DTOUR Diet is going to be different—much different from any diet you may have tried in the past. You will lose weight. You will stabilize your blood sugar. And you'll do it with food.

What we've found, through analysis of the scientific research as well as interviews with experts in diabetes and weight loss, is that certain foods—or, more precisely, certain nutrients in foods—can help melt away pounds, lower blood sugar, and reduce insulin resistance, one of the hallmarks of prediabetes (high blood sugar) and diabetes. We call these supernutrients our Fat-Fighting 4, and you're going to be reading a lot about them in the pages ahead. For now, just know that they are the foundation of the Diabetes DTOUR Diet; collectively, they can help you achieve significant and sustainable results—*without ever going hungry or feeling deprived!*

In fact, on DTOUR, you will:

1. Eat more foods more often. We're talking three meals and two snacks every day. Though you may be taking in fewer calories, you'll never notice that they're missing. The secret is choosing the foods that pack the

Stop Here

GET ON YOUR FEET!
University of Missouri researchers discovered that 4 hours or more of inactivity causes a near shutdown of an enzyme that controls fat and cholesterol metabolism. Result: You store more fat, rather than using it for energy, all day long. To keep this enzyme active and increase your fat burn, break up long periods of downtime by standing up—for example, while talking on the phone.

most nutrients—including our fabulous Fat-Fighting 4—into the fewest calories.

2. Enjoy all your favorites. French toast for breakfast? Pizza for lunch? Ice cream with chocolate syrup for a snack? Yes, yes, and yes! Food is truly your friend on DTOUR, from familiar comfort foods to intriguing new creations that tempt your taste buds. (Pesto Pizza, anyone?)

3. Develop a new food 'tude. When you're dealing with extra pounds around the middle or blood sugar that has a mind of its own, food just seems like nothing but trouble. After all, it's what got you in a bind in the first place, right? But here's the thing: *You need to eat—* so celebrate it! The trick is to choose the right foods in the right portions. We'll show you how to do just that, because we know you're not looking for a temporary fix. On DTOUR, you'll learn how to eat for life.

FYI

CURRENTLY, THERE ARE 1.6 billion overweight and 400 million obese adults on the planet, according to the World Health Organization. By 2015, those numbers will grow to 2.3 billion and 700 million, respectively.

As we go along, we'll get into other factors that are important to achieving your weight and blood sugar goals—things like ramping up your physical activity, managing your stress, and getting enough sleep. Watch for the road signs directing you to tips and tools that break these and other parts of the DTOUR plan into easy, manageable steps. Remember, though, that DTOUR is all about making great food your partner in good health. We're absolutely convinced that when it comes to losing weight and controlling blood sugar, food isn't the problem—*it's the solution.*

WHY DIABETES, WHY NOW?

Before we get into the how of the Diabetes DTOUR Diet, let's take a moment to consider the why—as in, why this diet? And why now?

Diabetes is on the rise in the United States, and it shows no sign of letting up anytime soon. The latest data from the Centers for Disease Control and Prevention (CDC) suggest that as many as 24 million Americans—a number equal to the population of Texas—have some form of diabetes, the vast majority with type 2. According to the same report, another 57 million have prediabetes, which raises the risk for the full-blown disease. So wherever you are on the diabetes spectrum, you have plenty of company.

The good news—really!—is that type 2 diabetes is largely a lifestyle disease. Yes, genetics plays a role, as do environmental factors. (We'll say more about this in Chapter 2.) But lifestyle is what tips the scale in one direction or the other— toward disease or toward health. For example, overweight and obesity are powerful predictors of type 2. So is excess belly fat (as we'll discuss in Chapter 3).

What's good about the fact that lifestyle plays such a big role? It means you're in charge! You can stop high blood sugar or prediabetes before it advances to full-blown diabetes. If you already have type 2, losing weight may help you avoid or delay the use of diabetes medications, not to mention reduce your risk of complications. If you're in the prediabetic stage, you may be able to head off diabetes altogether.

Both type 2 diabetes and prediabetes involve *insulin resistance*. As the name suggests, insulin resistance means that the muscle, liver, and fat cells don't properly use insulin, the hormone that helps usher glucose (sugar) from the bloodstream into cells. Once there, glucose is converted to energy. When cells are insulin resistant, glucose builds up in the bloodstream. Meanwhile, cells aren't getting the fuel they need to carry out their basic functions.

In prediabetes, the pancreas secretes more insulin to try to sweep the extra glucose out of the bloodstream. Eventually, though, it just can't keep up. This marks the onset of type 2, which doctors diagnose at or above a fasting blood glucose level of 126 mg/dl.

If type 2 diabetes is the big show, then prediabetes is the dress rehearsal. It refers to higher-than-normal fasting blood glucose, in the range of 100 to 125 mg/dl.

Stop Here

MAKE A LIST! If you have diabetes, do this now: Create a list of your support team's telephone numbers and e-mail addresses—primary-care physician, nutritionist, pharmacist—so you'll be able to reach them quickly and easily if you have a question. Place a copy in your wallet and another by your home telephone. If you don't have a support team, talk to your doctor about assembling one.

Though it isn't the full-blown disease, it can lay the groundwork for complications later on. All the more reason to take action now, before it has a chance to do harm.

Whether you have prediabetes or diabetes, your primary goal is to achieve what experts call good control. In other words, you want to get as close to a normal, nondiabetic blood glucose level as you safely can. You and your doctor should work together to determine what that level is for you. As a general guideline, those with diabetes should maintain their blood sugar level between 70 and 130 mg/dl before meals and below 180 mg/dl 2 hours after. For everyone else, a healthy goal is less than 140 mg/dl.

NEW RECOMMENDATIONS FOR PREDIABETES

Until recently, formal guidelines for treating people with prediabetes didn't exist. That changed in 2008, when diabetes experts—hoping to put the brakes on the runaway diabetes epidemic—created the first comprehensive treatment regimen for prediabetes.

Developed by an American College of Endocrinology task force, the guidelines note that blood sugar testing doesn't go far enough to diagnose prediabetes. Furthermore, lifestyle changes—and not necessarily medication—should be the first line of treatment.

So if you have prediabetes, here are the new guidelines, developed especially for you.

◆ Lose 5 to 10 percent of your body weight. Setting realistic goals and seeking social support, along with other changes in thinking and behavior, can help.

◆ Engage in moderate-intensity physical activity for 30 to 60 minutes a day, at least 5 days a week.

◆ Limit your intake of total fat, saturated fat, and trans fats, and eat a fiber-rich diet.

◆ To lower your blood pressure, ease up on sodium and alcoholic beverages.

◆ Take a low-dose aspirin daily, unless you have a medical reason not to (ask your doctor first).

◆ Lower your blood pressure and cholesterol to the levels recommended for people with diabetes.

◆ If lifestyle isn't enough to reduce your risk of diabetes and heart disease, medications may be necessary—but you'll still need to lead a healthy lifestyle.

By the way, there's another number you'll want to keep an eye on, and that's your A1c. It's a measure of your average blood glucose over the previous several months. Current guidelines recommend keeping your A1c at less than 7 percent.

BLOOD SUGAR CONTROL: HOW LOW SHOULD YOU GO?

The Diabetes DTOUR Diet will shave points off your blood sugar reading, both directly and indirectly—in the latter case, by helping to trim your waistline. As your blood sugar stabilizes at a healthy level, you'll notice other changes, too.

NEAR MENOPAUSE, THE RISK OF "SYNDROME X" RISES

As women enter perimenopause, the transitional years before menstruation ends, their chances of developing metabolic syndrome rise. The good news, according to a 2008 study: Living *la vida* healthy may reduce that risk.

Researchers at Rush University Medical Center in Chicago tracked 949 women, all between the ages of 42 and 52, for 9 years. When the study began, none had metabolic syndrome, a cluster of conditions that includes high blood sugar, abdominal obesity, high "bad" LDL cholesterol, and high blood pressure. Also called syndrome X, metabolic syndrome can set the stage for type 2 diabetes.

Over the course of the study, 13.7 percent of the women developed metabolic syndrome by the time they had their last periods. In fact, the incidence of metabolic syndrome rose progressively from 6 years before to 6 years after a woman's final period—and neither age nor other known cardiovascular risk factors appeared to have much to do with it. Rather, the researchers say, the increase in risk may have been related to the male sex hormone testosterone, which becomes more influential in a woman's health as estrogen—the female sex hormone—declines.

The best way to counteract this hormonal shift: Watch your diet, move your body, and generally live healthfully—in other words, all the good stuff that DTOUR recommends! Together, these lifestyle changes can help keep metabolic syndrome and diabetes at bay.

You'll feel more energized, you'll concentrate better, your mood will be brighter, and your food cravings should all but disappear.

Maybe these benefits will provide a little motivation to be extravigilant about your blood sugar. We can't overstate the importance of maintaining good blood sugar control, especially in terms of the long-term health implications of type 2 diabetes. There's excellent research to illustrate how your risk of diabetes complications can rise and fall along with your blood sugar level.

A number of high-profile studies have explored the effects of what's known as *intensive therapy*, in which blood sugar is kept as close to normal as possible through a combination of oral medication, injected insulin, healthy lifestyle changes, and frequent interaction with health-care providers. One landmark study, known as the Diabetes Control and Complications Trial (DCCT), found that intensive blood sugar control reduced the risk of kidney disease by 34 percent, of diabetic neuropathy (nerve disease) by 60 percent, and of diabetic retinopathy (eye disease) by a phenomenal 76 percent. In the ADVANCE trial, a large-scale, multicountry study conducted by Australian researchers, participants with type 2 diabetes who practiced intensive blood sugar control lowered their risk of kidney disease by a respectable 21 percent.

A third study, the Veterans Affairs Diabetes Trial (VADT), involved 1,791 US veterans (mostly male, average age 60) who were assigned to standard- or intensive-treatment groups, both with a goal A1c reading of less than 7 percent. The participants started the trial with an average A1c of 9.5 percent; within 6 months, the average dropped to 6.9 percent among those receiving intensive treatment, compared with 8.4 percent among those getting standard treatment. Both groups were able to maintain their A1c levels for the duration of the trial.

FYI

OVERWEIGHT OR INSULIN-RESISTANT women are 50 percent more likely to be diagnosed with advanced-stage breast cancer, according to a 20-year study of more than 60,000 Swedish women. In the study, published in 2008 in the journal *Breast Cancer Research and Treatment*, researchers theorize that hormones linked with overweight or insulin resistance might cause tumors to grow faster. Additional studies are needed to confirm the connection.

Interestingly, though, neither the VADT nor the ADVANCE trial established that intensive blood sugar control protects against heart problems, which commonly occur in tandem with type 2 diabetes. In fact, another major study—the Action to Control Cardiovascular Risk in Diabetes (ACCORD) Trial, conducted by the National Heart, Lung, and Blood Institute—stopped 18 months ahead of schedule after 5 percent of the participants receiving intensive treatment to lower their A1c readings died within the first 3½ years of the trial. What's more, heart-related deaths were more prevalent in the intensive-treatment group (2.6 percent versus 1.8 percent).

The researchers involved in the ACCORD study are still trying to decipher what happened. They've speculated that medication combinations may have been a factor, in addition to weight gain—a common by-product of diabetes medications. It's also possible that participants simply lowered their blood sugar too quickly.

For now, though, these study outcomes have prompted diabetes experts to rethink the conventional wisdom on the use of intensive therapy as a means of preventing heart problems in those with diabetes. The consensus is that ultra-aggressive treatment to lower blood sugar simply isn't necessary, and neither are changes in the treatment guidelines.

Stop Here

LEARN YOUR DIABETES ABCs. *A* is for the A1c test, which tells you how effective your blood sugar control has been over the past 3 months. For most people with diabetes, the A1c goal is less than 7 percent. *B* is for blood pressure—shoot for 130/80 mm Hg or lower. *C* is for cholesterol—aim for a "bad" LDL cholesterol reading of less than 100 mg/dl.

BOTTOM LINE: STAY THE COURSE

What does all this research mean for you? First and foremost, it's vital to maintain good blood sugar control, regardless of whether you have diabetes or pre-diabetes. Losing weight, eating healthfully, exercising regularly—these factors will make a huge difference in how effectively you keep your blood sugar in check. It's no coincidence that all three are central to our Diabetes DTOUR Diet.

Second, medication isn't the only answer to blood sugar trouble *in most cases*. This last caveat is important, because we know that some people simply can't stabilize their blood sugar without meds. If you're in this group, you should know that following DTOUR might help reduce the amount of medication you require on a daily basis. (Please note, though, that you should never change your dosage or stop taking medication without consulting your doctor.) And what if you aren't using diabetes drugs yet? Well, you may be able to avoid them altogether, especially if you're prediabetic. (We'll say more about this in Chapter 4.)

Third, don't let your blood sugar control you. Too often, people with diabetes or prediabetes are so vigilant about managing their blood sugar that it becomes an all-consuming task. It is important, but it shouldn't drain the enjoyment and pleasure out of life. That's why we made a point of designing DTOUR to offer its share of treats and surprises. You'll dance. You'll relax. You'll eat ice cream! We want you to love this diet, because in our view, it isn't a diet at all. It's a way of life.

FROM THE DTOUR DIETITIAN

One of my most successful patients was a woman I'll call Madeline, who was referred to me for uncontrolled diabetes. She was almost 50 pounds overweight when we first met. Although she wasn't able to follow a complicated diet plan because of some mental challenges, she understood the importance of controlling her diabetes.

She also understood the concept of portion sizes. I suggested that she eat more vegetables and cut her portions of sugar- and starch-containing foods in half. She took this advice to heart.

At a follow-up visit, I noted that she was thinner and her blood sugar was coming down. She told me that she was ordering more vegetable-based meals in restaurants. Although she still enjoyed her favorite bran muffin at the coffee shop each morning, she ate only half at breakfast and saved the rest for a snack later in the day.

In 6 months, Madeline lost 38 pounds, and her blood sugar returned to a normal range. When a diabetes support group that she attended asked her to explain the secret of her success, Madeline said simply, "I'm on the diabetes diet. I eat more vegetables and half portions of everything else."

That's pretty much it. People with diabetes do not have to give up "normal" food. In fact, all of us should be eating "the diabetes diet"—balanced meals that include reasonable portions of fruits, veggies, whole grains, low-fat dairy, and sources of healthful fats such as fish and nuts. It's the diet that really works.

DTOUR WINNER!

Kris Sumey, 41
POUNDS LOST: 24
INCHES LOST: 10
BLOOD SUGAR: DROPPED
17 POINTS

BEFORE   **AFTER**

Despite the hundreds of diets we tried over the years, my husband, Randy, and I remained out of control with food. (See Randy's story on page 34.) We ate out every night, and our portions were gargantuan.

When Randy was diagnosed with type 2 diabetes, this was no longer an option. His life depended on learning a new lifestyle regardless of our unhealthy habits. But I didn't know how I was going to plan a healthy menu while juggling my hectic schedule. I found DTOUR at the perfect time.

As I reviewed the program, my brain chanted a mantra of defeat: *I can't do this. I can't eat these small portions. I don't have time to cook.* But 3 days into the program, the doubts were squashed. I felt lighter, more alert, and healthier. I found that we *could* eat from the menus provided, *could* measure our portions, and *could* shop for healthy food. It was just a matter of doing it!

It was a challenge to adapt to smaller portion sizes at first, but I did it. Eventually, I knew that another meal or snack would arrive in just a few hours. The menus are designed in a way that keeps me from being hungry throughout the day. The proof is in the reading on the scale and in the way my clothes fit today—way too loose.

The biggest change with DTOUR is planning and shopping for new foods. I had numerous food conversions. Before the program, for example, I hated hummus and beans. Now I love them. There's a new world of enjoyable and satisfying food adventures that we're exploring.

It feels incredible to lose 24 pounds in only a month. This started out to be about helping my husband and his blood sugar. Yet less than 18 months ago, my cholesterol was 320. I worked hard over the past few months, and it crept down to 261. But it was at 203 after 6 weeks on DTOUR–down 58 points. Now, that's exhilarating.

Losing 10 inches off my waist was a miracle. A dress that the zipper wouldn't budge on last month slides like butter (or should I say trans-free canola margarine). It's now in the new pile of clothes I call the TBA (to be altered) pile.

It's now possible for me to enjoy the beautiful colors and fabrics that aren't always available in clothing for a woman my size. In fact, there is a red dress I have my eye on. I *will* wear this dress soon. When I do, you can be sure there will be a big party and a choir belting out the "Hallelujah Chorus" before my grand entrance!

LOST
24
POUNDS!

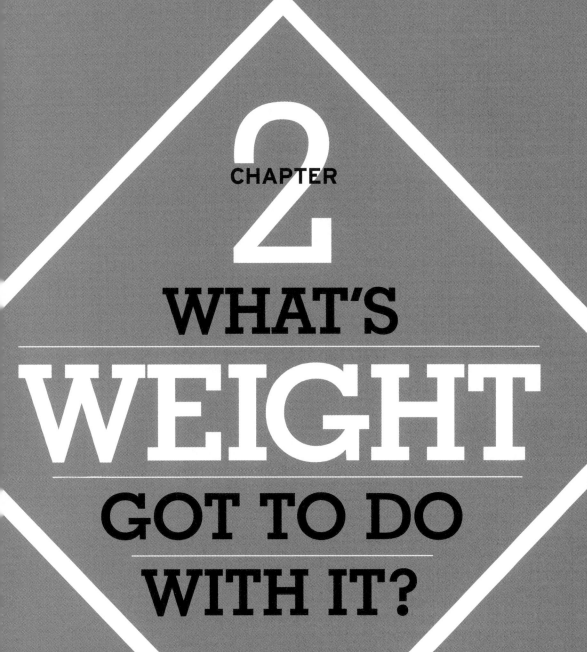

CHAPTER

2

WHAT'S WEIGHT GOT TO DO WITH IT?

At its core, diabetes is about blood sugar—or, more precisely, badly behaved blood sugar. The kind that likes to soar high and then plunge low, like an amusement-park roller coaster. Except the ride is no fun, because it leaves you tired and mentally fuzzy and maybe just a little cranky. It's also playing games with your weight.

You see, high blood sugar is a hallmark of insulin resistance, in which insulin can't do its job of escorting blood sugar into cells. Insulin resistance is a common precursor to diabetes. As you'll see, it also can make weight loss that much harder.

The beauty of the Diabetes DTOUR Diet is its one-two punch of weight loss and blood sugar control. We'll introduce you to a way of eating that will shave off any unwanted pounds *and* stabilize your blood sugar in a healthy range. What this means, if you already have diabetes, is that you could avoid or delay the use of medication (or reduce your current dosage). And if you have prediabetes, you could steer clear of full-blown diabetes for good.

Pretty amazing benefits, don't you think? And they're all yours, just for eating the DTOUR way. That's five—yes, five!—meals and snacks every day, featuring our fabulous Fat-Fighting 4!

As you follow DTOUR, you *will* lose weight—as much as 12 pounds and 4 inches in the first 2 weeks. That's a change you can see in your mirror. What you can't see is all the good stuff that's going on inside your body. In particular, getting rid of those extra pounds helps your body's cells respond to insulin more effectively. Insulin, you'll remember, is the hormone that escorts glucose—blood sugar—out of your bloodstream and into cells, where it's turned into energy. When insulin does its job, it keeps a tight rein on blood sugar, which means fewer peaks and valleys. Instead, your blood sugar stays on an even keel—and pounds melt away faster and easier.

DIABETES: A FOOD-CENTERED PROBLEM

If you picture the relationship between weight, insulin, and blood sugar as a triangle of sorts, with each "side" connecting to and influencing the other two, then standing smack at the center of the triangle is, you guessed it, *food!* Food matters in determining how much you weigh, how much insulin you produce, and how much your blood sugar rises and falls. But not all food has the same effect.

Now, you might be expecting yet another run-through of the "high this," "low that" diet debate. We're not going there, because we don't need to. The fact is, the science that explains how food influences blood sugar levels—and therefore insulin release and weight gain or loss—is solid, and has been for quite some time. That science, for the most part, focuses on carbs.

Dietary carbohydrates—the slices of rye in your turkey sandwich, the veggies in your salad, the chewy pizza crust—are broken down by your body into glucose, or sugar. The process itself is pretty straightforward: Food goes down, glucose goes up, and sensors in the pancreas—detecting the presence of glucose in the bloodstream—trigger the release of insulin, which then escorts the glucose into cells. Once the cells accept the glucose "package," blood glucose levels fall and the pancreas stops releasing insulin.

At least that's how it's *supposed* to work. And it can work that way when you're eating the right kind of carbs, in balance with lean proteins and healthy fats. What are the "right" kind of carbs? Glad you asked! We're talking about fiber-dense complex carbohydrates, which your body digests and absorbs relatively slowly. Simple carbs, on the other hand—white bread, potato chips, and almost all sweets—break down comparatively quickly. In response, insulin production kicks into overdrive in an effort to sweep all that glucose out of the bloodstream and into cells.

Sometimes, though, the cells decide not to answer when insulin comes a-knockin'. But the pancreas is persistent. It just churns out more insulin, which continues to pound on the cells' doors, determined to gain entry. This is insulin resistance, which we briefly talked about in Chapter 1.

The pancreas can keep pace for a while, but not forever. At some point, it tires out. That's when blood sugar levels skyrocket—generally, an indicator of type 2 diabetes.

Even before the onset of type 2, all that excess

Stop Here

TO CURB SODA cravings, try a seltzer-juice combo with no added sugar. Or keep a pitcher of water in the fridge. Add slices of orange, lemon, lime, or cucumber to give it kick.

insulin can cause trouble by undermining your weight-loss efforts. First, it helps liberate fatty acids from food, which means that more fatty acids are available for storage in fat cells. Second, insulin discourages fat cells from releasing stored fat. So if you're insulin resistant, you're more likely to store fat and gain weight.

FAT IS NOT YOUR FATE!

Research suggests that, by and large, our genes determine our weight range. But lifestyle—what we eat, how much we move—determines where we fall within that range.

Translation: You're not destined to be overweight, even if every relative on your mother's (or father's) side of the family happens to be. In general, lifestyle trumps genetics. For proof, we need look no further than the Pima Indians of Arizona and Mexico.

Extensive studies of the Pima population provide a great example of the interplay between genetics and lifestyle. Both Arizonan and Mexican Pimas are genetically predisposed to type 2 diabetes. Researchers have learned, for example, that Pimas carry a gene called FABP2 that may play a role in insulin resistance. Other studies have shown that another gene linked to type 2 diabetes and insulin resistance is more common in Pimas than in whites.

But, oh, what a difference a Western lifestyle makes.

Arizonan Pimas have the highest prevalence of type 2 diabetes on earth. Fully half of those between ages 30 and 64 are diabetic, and 95 percent of those with diabetes are overweight.

However, in a landmark 2006 study, researchers at the University of Wisconsin-Milwaukee discovered that Mexican Pimas have dramatically lower rates of diabetes and obesity. These two groups share a common genetic background, but their eating habits and physical activity levels are strikingly different.

As a result, the obesity rate among Arizonan Pima men is 10 times higher than that of their Mexican male counterparts. In fact, the obesity and diabetes rates among Mexican Pimas are comparable to the rates among other Mexicans with similar lifestyles, even though Pimas are genetically vulnerable to type 2. That's because Mexican Pimas eat about the same number of calories and grams of fiber as other Mexicans, and they tend to lead very active lifestyles. American Pimas, on the other hand, have adopted the lifestyle habits of most Americans—heavy on calorie-laden foods, light on exercise.

So don't blame your genes for putting you at risk of overweight and diabetes. Outsmart them with a healthy lifestyle—the kind you'll find with DTOUR!

THE HEAVY-HITTER HORMONES

In fairness, insulin isn't the only hormone that toys with your weight and your waistline. Some can even work to your weight-loss advantage. Just like insulin, though, these regulatory hormones sometimes run amok.

Scientists don't yet understand every mechanism that links overweight to high blood sugar and diabetes. But they're pretty confident that hormones and other chemicals released by fat cells will turn out to be key players. Here are a few of the biggies.

Resistin. As its name implies, this hormone—made only by fat cells—promotes insulin resistance. In fact, some experts have theorized that resistin is a direct link between obesity and type 2 diabetes. In studies of mice with elevated blood sugar, scientist Mitchell Lazar, MD, and his colleagues at the University of Pennsylvania School of Medicine in Philadelphia intentionally hindered resistin production in the animals. Their cells responded better to insulin, which made their blood sugar levels fall.

Leptin. As your body's energy requirements are met, insulin triggers cells to produce this "fullness hormone." In people of normal weight, leptin (from the Greek *leptos,* which means *thin*) tells the brain that it's time to stop eating. For some reason, this communication doesn't happen in people who are overweight, and researchers are trying to figure out why. It may be that these people are genetically predisposed to produce less leptin than usual. Without enough of the hormone, the brain may not get the "stop eating" message, causing a person to keep eating past the point of fullness. Result: weight gain.

Adiponectin. As fat cells expand, their chemical

FYI

CALORIES COUNT, BUT so does the quality of what you put in your mouth. Researchers from the ongoing Framingham Nutrition Studies found that women who ate almost 400 fewer calories per day but chose the least nutritious foods were 2½ times more likely to develop abdominal obesity—that is, belly fat—than women who ate fewer calories but made healthier choices. The first group also was at dramatically higher risk of type 2 diabetes and heart attack.

FYI

YOUR LIVER HOLDS extra glucose in reserve. It releases this stored glucose, called glycogen, when you need more than your bloodstream contains at that moment. Your body uses glycogen between meals, during sleep, and when you're in need of an extra burst of energy to fight or flee danger.

output changes in ways that actually increase the accumulation of body fat. One of these changes involves the hormone adiponectin.

Secreted by fat cells, adiponectin helps muscle cells burn glucose. It also makes cells more sensitive to insulin, which lowers the risk of diabetes—and discourages weight gain, to boot.

In fact, researchers at the University of Pennsylvania found that adiponectin can boost the rate at which the body burns calories without increasing appetite, a terrific advantage for weight loss. In a cruel twist of nature, however, levels of the hormone decline just when you need it most—as you gain weight. Researchers want to understand why this happens, because it could lead to a solution to overweight and obesity.

A FOOD-CENTERED SOLUTION

As you can see, science still has much to learn about why we gain and lose weight, and about how the body's various hormones and chemicals contribute to the process. But we can say with certainty that stabilizing your insulin levels improves your chances of weight-loss success—and dropping those extra pounds, in turn, can help steady your insulin production.

The best way to achieve both is with food.

Not just any kind of food, mind you. Remember those simple carbs we talked about earlier? They hit your bloodstream hard and fast, causing your blood sugar to soar. In response to this surge, your pancreas churns out insulin—so much, in fact, that your blood sugar slumps lower than it was before you ate. When it goes that low, you end up feeling fatigued and famished, and you're

FROM THE DTOUR DIETITIAN

You may have read that high-fructose corn syrup (HFCS) raises the risk of obesity and type 2 diabetes. But in 2008, both the American Medical Association (AMA) and the Center for Science in the Public Interest (CSPI) stated that HFCS has no more detrimental effect on health than regular sugar, according to current scientific evidence. How can this be? Let's consider the facts.

HFCS is a natural sweetener made from corn. Corn kernels contain corn starch, glucose (sugar) molecules connected together in long chains. Enzymes—like the ones in our bodies that digest food—break these long chains into individual glucose molecules to make corn syrup. Other enzymes convert about half the glucose in corn syrup to fructose, another sugar. That's how we get HFCS.

HFCS is as sweet as table sugar. But compared to sugar from cane or beets, HFCS is more stable and less expensive to produce, which is why it is added to everything from soda to spaghetti sauce.

HFCS is chemically similar to table sugar. Refined from sugar cane or beets, table sugar is a 50/50 mixture of fructose and glucose. HFCS is 55 percent fructose and 45 percent glucose. Not much of a difference.

Sugar, honey, and HFCS are digested the same. All are broken down to fructose and glucose in the digestive tract.

It's the fructose part of sugar and HFCS that has scientists worried. Large doses of fructose may interfere with the body's ability to metabolize fats and may be related to our growing obesity problem.

Fructose has redeeming qualities, too. It is the main sugar in fruit. What's more, fructose does not raise blood sugar or stimulate insulin as much as table sugar.

Here's the bottom line: Too much of any sugar—not just HFCS—isn't good for you. If you avoid products that contain HFCS and choose those loaded with sugar instead, you miss a very important point. The real issue, says the AMA and CSPI, is that excessive consumption of any sugars may lead to health problems. Amen.

—Barbara

desperate for an energy boost. You can see how this scenario—coupled with unhealthy food choices in such critical moments (can you say cappuccino and a chocolate-chip scone?)—could sabotage your efforts to lose weight *and* control your blood sugar.

Incidentally, another surefire way to crank up hunger and cravings—not to mention

FYI

the likelihood of making questionable food choices—is to cut calories to fewer than 1,000 a day. Restricting or eliminating an entire food group, such as carbohydrates, can have the same effect.

It's been found, for example, that just 3 days of strict dieting reduces levels of leptin (the stop-eating hormone) by 22 percent. And according to a study published in the journal *Appetite,* women who were asked to cut carbs for 3 days reported stronger food cravings— and ate 44 percent more calories from carb-rich foods on Day 4.

DTOUR FOR WEIGHT LOSS THAT LASTS

On the Diabetes DTOUR Diet, you will cut your calorie intake. Rest assured, though, that you'll get more than enough calories to fuel your body and brain throughout the day. And you'll *never* feel hungry. How is that possible? Because we've loaded DTOUR with high-fiber whole foods that your body will digest at a slow and steady pace. You won't experience the blood sugar spurts and sputters that can make you eat more than you should.

Now, if the phrase "high-fiber whole foods" has you thinking bland and boring, think again! The DTOUR menus and recipes are all about flavor and satisfaction. Yes, we *are* talking quesadillas, pancakes, garlic toast, and oven-fried chicken! Not what you'd expect to find on a weight-loss plan, right? They're all part of DTOUR, along with dozens of other meal and snack options that will surprise and tantalize your taste buds. *No willpower required!*

We'll lay out all of the details of eating DTOUR-style a bit later in the book. Here's a sneak peek to whet your appetite.

◆ On DTOUR, you're going to focus on foods and ingredients that deliver a healthy daily dose of our fabulous Fat-Fighting 4: fiber, calcium, vitamin D, and omega-3 fatty acids. As you'll learn in Part 2, these vital nutrients help melt away body fat, balance blood sugar, and improve cells' insulin response. That's an anti-diabetes trifecta!

◆ You'll be eating a DTOUR meal or snack every 3 to 4 hours throughout the day. That may be more often than you're accustomed to now, but it's going to help prevent the blood sugar roller coaster ride that's more likely to occur with the standard three square meals a day.

◆ You'll swap foods high in fast-burning simple carbohydrates—namely, refined sugar and white flour—for slow burners like fruits, vegetables, and whole grains. Here again, the idea is to avoid the rush of blood sugar and the subsequent surge in insulin that ultimately send your appetite into overdrive.

◆ You'll team these slow-burn carbs with lean proteins and healthy fats. Your body needs all three macronutrients in adequate amounts to function optimally. Shortchange it on even one, and you could unwittingly set yourself up for an assortment of health problems—not just diabetes.

What's great about DTOUR is that it works with your body to bring it back into balance. You'll feel so good eating this way—you'll have less fatigue, more energy, better concentration, a brighter mood—that you won't want to go back to your "old" diet. You'll be living DTOUR for life!

CHAPTER 3

IT'S ALL ABOUT THE ABOUT THE BELLY

While the Diabetes DTOUR Diet is great for losing inches all over, it's especially effective at whittling the waistline. Our eight DTOUR panelists lost a total of 40 inches around their middles over the course of 6 weeks. Wow! That's pretty impressive, especially when you consider that belly fat can be more stubborn than other body fat.

So what's the big deal about belly fat? Sure, it can keep you from zipping up your favorite pair of jeans. And yes, it creates an annoying paunch at your midsection. But its effects aren't just cosmetic. According to a raft of recent studies, a widening waistline is a strong predictor of insulin resistance and type 2 diabetes.

To understand why, we need to look beneath the skin surface, where excess fat packs in and around the abdomen. Because it lies so close to vital organs, it's long been suspected of causing trouble beyond keeping button-flies from buttoning. Now science is bearing this out: People who carry their weight around their middles—the so-called apple shape—are more likely to have type 2 diabetes, heart disease, Alzheimer's, and a host of other health problems. The real kicker? Even someone who doesn't look overweight from the outside can have too much of this fatty padding on the inside.

DTOUR targets the belly fat you can see, as well as the "invisible" fat under-

IS BELLY FAT MAKING YOU FAT?

Belly fat may have one more sneaky health effect: Too much of it could actually cause you to gain weight. Really!

How is this possible? The latest research suggests that a hunger-promoting hormone called neuropeptide Y, or NPY—previously thought to be produced only in the brain—is made in belly fat tissues, too. So in effect, any extra weight around your midsection could rev up your appetite, leading to overeating, weight gain—and more belly fat.

If these new studies are correct, as levels of NPY rise, you eat more, and you store more fat around your midsection. Then this belly fat pumps out more NPY, which triggers the production of even more fat cells. Talk about a vicious circle!

neath. Our Fat-Fighting 4 will trim your midsection directly by melting away pounds and indirectly by controlling your blood sugar and insulin response. These four supernutrients—fiber, calcium, vitamin D, and omega-3 fatty acids—get a boost from the fitness routine that starts in Phase 2 of DTOUR. It'll rev up your metabolism, burn more fat, and build more muscle across your middle. With benefits like these, belly fat doesn't stand a chance!

THE SNEAKY RISK FACTOR FOR DIABETES

Don't get us wrong: We're not opposed to body fat. In fact, you need a certain amount of the stuff to survive. Even the leanest among us have some 40 billion (that's right, 40 *billion!*) fat cells that pad and protect our internal organs and insulate us from the cold.

But trouble arises when we have too much of the wrong kind of body fat. You see, there are two kinds, each with its own characteristics and purpose.

One, known as subcutaneous fat, lies just beneath the skin. It's responsible for cellulite, back fat, the muffin top over the waistband—essentially, the bane of people in department-store dressing rooms everywhere! Most women carry subcutaneous fat in the breasts, hips, buttocks, and thighs; men, in the chest, abdomen, and lower back.

The other kind of fat, called visceral fat (or intra-abdominal fat or simply belly fat), lies deep within the abdomen, around the internal organs. In an average person, about 10 percent of total body fat is visceral, while 90 percent is subcutaneous. The ratio shifts to about 25:75 in someone who's very overweight.

Visceral fat is hidden under muscle, so it doesn't wiggle when you walk. But don't let that fool you! Visceral fat is a major health problem for anyone with blood sugar concerns. Why?

FYI

A 2008 STUDY of more than 44,000 women, published in the medical journal *Circulation*, found that—compared with women whose waist-lines measured 28 inches or less—those whose midsections measured 35 inches or more were 79 percent more likely to die early of heart disease or cancer. All the more reason to whittle your middle!

◆ Visceral fat is highly metabolic, which means that it breaks down quickly and enters the bloodstream directly. Once in the bloodstream, visceral fat cells travel around the body and park themselves in various tissues, including those of the pancreas. And the pancreas, you'll remember, is responsible for producing the insulin that helps regulate your blood sugar.

◆ Visceral fat also hampers the ability of the body's cells to communicate with one another via chemical signals. Though researchers don't fully understand why this interference occurs, it may help explain why people with too much visceral fat tend to be less sensitive to insulin: The hormone can't "talk" to the cells.

WHAT ABOUT BMI?

Years ago, when you wanted to know if you were overweight, you stepped on a scale—either your own or your doctor's. If the number was higher than you or your doctor liked, the answer was yes. Period.

Then came the introduction of body mass index (BMI)—a rough calculation of body size and bone mass—as a tool for assessing risk of weight-related health problems like diabetes and heart disease. Researchers continue to use BMI because the evidence is clear: At a BMI of 25, which indicates overweight, the risk of serious illness rises. A BMI of 30 or higher indicates obesity and an even greater risk.

While calculating BMI is rather easy, it does have limitations. For example, BMI doesn't account for muscle mass. This means it can overestimate body fat in those who are ultrafit, such as athletes and bodybuilders, and underestimate it in those who have lost muscle mass, which the elderly often do.

Today, it's generally agreed that if you store fat mainly around your middle, you're more likely to develop health problems than if your fat sits on your hips and thighs. This is true even if your BMI falls within the normal range. In fact, a 2008 analysis published in the *Journal of Clinical Epidemiology* concluded not only that BMI is a poor indicator of cardiovascular health, but also that waist size is the most accurate predictor of risk for diabetes, high blood pressure, and elevated cholesterol.

So if you just want a sense of whether you're gaining or losing weight, your bathroom scale (or your doctor's scale) will do the job. To get a handle on how your weight may be affecting your health, BMI is a better tool, and a tape measure may be the best. In terms of health risk, it's not how much you weigh, but where you carry your body fat that matters the most.

◆ While an excess of all-over body fat is a known health risk, visceral fat is especially suspect because it secretes chemicals that increase inflammation. Under normal circumstances, inflammation is a natural, healthy immune response. But when it becomes chronic, it can set the stage for a number of health problems, including type 2 diabetes.

Need more proof of the connection between visceral fat, insulin resistance, and diabetes? Consider the 2007 report from the International Day for the Evaluation of Abdominal Obesity (IDEA), a massive study involving 168,000 people from across the globe. According to the study data, women with the widest waists had a diabetes risk nearly *six times greater* than that of women with the slimmest waists. For men with the widest waists, diabetes risk was three times higher.

BAD NEWS FOR THE HEART, TOO

Both belly fat and insulin resistance are part of a cluster of conditions collectively known as metabolic syndrome. Though it has taken a while to gain acceptance as a diagnosis, metabolic syndrome is now recognized as a precursor to type 2 diabetes, as well as to heart disease.

In fact, excess belly fat is a risk factor for heart-related health problems in its own right. Here's why: Because visceral fat resides in the same anatomical "zip code" as your liver, it boosts production of LDL cholesterol, the bad kind that collects in your arteries and forms a waxy substance called plaque. Over time, plaque becomes inflamed, which causes the arteries to swell and restricts the flow of blood. It's a recipe for heart trouble, including an increased risk of high blood pressure and blood clots.

In one study, researchers from Queen's University in Kingston, Ontario, analyzed both body mass index and waist circumference in about 15,000 men and women who took part in the third National Health

Stop Here

HIDDEN BELLY FAT is most common among people who get little or no exercise, researchers say. If you're at a normal body weight but sedentary, you should ask your doctor about a simple, noninvasive test that detects hidden belly fat, according to a report in the journal Clinical Endocrinology. Called the brachial-ankle pulse wave velocity test, it predicts the presence of visceral fat by measuring how efficiently blood moves throughout the body. (Visceral fat can impede bloodflow.)

FYI

and Nutrition Examination Survey. The researchers found that for every 1-inch increase in the men's waist circumference, blood pressure rose by 10 percent, total cholesterol by 8 percent, and triglycerides—a type of blood fat—by 18 percent. HDL cholesterol, meanwhile, declined by 15 percent. That's not good, because HDL helps usher cholesterol out of the bloodstream and back to the liver, and from there out of the body. Women, by the way, showed similar changes.

ROLL THE (MEASURING) TAPE!

No matter which way you look at it, belly fat is bad news. Sure, the subcutaneous fat that pads the hips and thighs into a pear shape may be frustrating when you're trying on new pants. In terms of your health, though, it's not nearly as troublesome as visceral fat, the hallmark of an apple shape.

How can you tell if belly fat might be a problem for you? Researchers who want to measure a person's visceral fat use expensive, highly sophisticated technologies. But you can size up your midsection just as well with an item you can pick up at the dollar store: a tape measure.

To check your waist circumference, place the tape measure around your bare abdomen just above your hip bones. The tape should be snug, but it shouldn't compress your skin. Make sure it's parallel to the floor. Breathe normally, and don't suck in your stomach.

According to government guidelines, a woman whose waist circumference exceeds 35 inches is at higher risk of health problems, including insulin resistance and type 2 diabetes. For a man, the magic number is 40 inches.

Now, if your number is higher than it should be, let's give it some perspective:

Between 1960 and 2000, the average waist measurement among American women grew from 30 to 37 inches; for men, it went from 35 to 39 inches. According to a 2004 study with almost 27,000 participants, 60 percent of women were carrying too much belly fat, as were 39 percent of men.

Here's your advantage over these folks: You're about to embark on DTOUR! Over the next 6 weeks, the Diabetes DTOUR Diet will blast away belly fat with a combination of sensational food (featuring our Fat-Fighting 4!) and sensible exercise. Your waistbands will get a little looser—and you just might drop a size or two (or more!).

We do encourage you to measure your waist at the start of the program and again at the end, so you can see how much progress you've made. You can measure in between these end points, too, though how often you do is up to you. In

COMING SOON: A BLOOD TEST FOR BELLY FAT

To measure belly fat, researchers still depend on expensive, highly sophisticated equipment, such as CT and MRI scans. But a simple blood test may detect the presence of deep belly fat just as effectively, according to a 2007 study.

The blood test screens for RBP4, which is shorthand for *retinol-binding protein 4*. Secreted by fat cells and the liver, RBP4 may contribute to insulin resistance. And as levels of the protein increase, so does the amount of visceral fat.

A team of researchers from Beth Israel Deaconess Medical Center in Boston and the University of Leipzig in Germany analyzed abdominal fat samples from 196 people. Belly fat made more RBP4 than the subcutaneous fat that lies just beneath the skin, the researchers concluded. Further, compared with people of normal weight, those who were overweight had double or triple the levels of RBP4 in their blood.

Tests for RBP4 may identify people at high risk of diabetes and heart disease in time for them to adopt preventive measures, the researchers say. The test might also reveal how well such measures work.

There is one simple, tried-and-true method of lowering RBP4, and that's physical activity. A 2006 study by the same research team found that people with high RBP4 successfully lowered it with exercise. And as RBP4 levels went down, so did insulin resistance.

Stop Here

TO HELP PREVENT
mindless eating, keep your dirty dishes where you can see them. When researchers at Cornell University treated graduate students to a free chicken wing buffet, those whose dishes piled up ate 28 percent less than those whose plates were continually whisked away.

our opinion, "waistband watching" can work just as well. You'll know you're on track if your clothes are fitting better!

Remember, too, that as you're losing inches from your waist, you're improving your cells' insulin response, which means better blood sugar control and—if you're prediabetic—lower type 2 risk. Actually, your waist measurement can be a better predictor of your general health status than the bathroom scale; after all, DTOUR doesn't just melt away pounds, it also replaces body fat with calorie-incinerating muscle, which the number on the scale won't show.

So are you ready to start your DTOUR? Good! First, you'll want to get to know our fabulous Fat-Fighting 4, which are vital to your weight-loss success. They're the stars of Part 2, which is coming up next.

THE BELLY-BRAIN CONNECTION

Besides improving insulin response and balancing your blood sugar, getting rid of that belly fat may have another important benefit—for your brain.

Researchers at Kaiser Permanente, an Oakland, California-based health care organization, decided to analyze the medical exam records of 6,583 members whose belly fat measurements had been tracked over a 36-year period. The records didn't note waist circumferences, but they did document a specific measure of abdominal obesity called the *sagittal abdominal diameter* (SAD). A SAD of 25 centimeters is considered an indicator of excess visceral fat.

Using these data, the researchers determined that the more belly fat members had in middle age, the more likely they were to develop dementia later in life. Overall, 21 percent of those with large amounts of visceral fat developed dementia, compared with 15 percent of the rest of the study group. Also note-worthy: People of normal weight but with excess visceral fat had almost double the risk (1.89 times) of dementia of people of normal weight and no excess belly fat.

Checkpoint

If you're already on medication to help you manage your diabetes, you may be wondering if DTOUR can help you. Absolutely! In fact, Randy and Tom—two of our DTOURists—not only lost 44 pounds between them, but also were able to cut back significantly on their meds.

Before you embark on our program, though, we do want to pass on a couple of important caveats about losing weight on DTOUR.

1. Be sure to talk to your doctor first. On DTOUR, you're going to see results quickly—in as little as 2 weeks. As you slim down and your blood sugar stabilizes, you may find yourself needing less medication. Your doctor can help you monitor your progress and make adjustments in your daily doses as necessary. Also—and this is critical—never, ever cut back on your meds, or stop taking them altogether, without consulting your doctor.

2. Find out whether your medication can cause weight gain. It isn't true of all diabetes meds, but some can be quite fickle. They're very effective at controlling your blood sugar, but they also can make those extra pounds hang on for dear life. This happens for several reasons. Certain medications can cause you to retain fluid, which shows up on the scale, while others can ramp up your appetite. Also, because your body is using blood sugar much more efficiently, gaining weight is that much easier.

Of the major classes of diabetes meds currently available in the United States, these three are most likely to cause weight gain.

◆ Sulfonylureas (SULL-fuh-nil-u-ree-uhz), which include glipizide (Glucotrol and Glucotrol XL), glyburide (Micronase, Glynase, and Diabeta), and glimepiride (Amaryl)
◆ Meglitinides (meh-GLIT-in-ides), such as repaglinide (Prandin) and nateglinide (Starlix)
◆ Thiazolidinediones (THIGH-ah-ZO-li-deen-DYE-owns), which include rosiglitazone (Avandia) and pioglitazone (Actos)

The typical weight gain with any of these medications is no more than 10 pounds. Still, when you already have pounds to lose, you probably would rather not see the scale going in the opposite direction. (By the way, insulin can have the same effect; there's an average weight gain of 9 pounds for those just starting treatment.)

You may want to ask your doctor about switching to a weight-neutral medication. Though it won't take off pounds, it won't add any, either. But here's the thing: Even if your doctor changes your prescription or adjusts your dosage, that alone won't be enough to help you lose weight. Slimming down and controlling your blood sugar always begins with changing your lifestyle. That's why DTOUR can be so effective at getting you to the weight you want.

DTOUR WINNER!

Randy Sumey, 40
POUNDS LOST: 23
INCHES LOST: 4
BLOOD SUGAR: DROPPED
182 POINTS!

BEFORE **AFTER**

I was recently diagnosed with type 2 diabetes. When my doctor told me, I wasn't surprised. My father had it, and my 16-year-old son, Justin, was diagnosed with it 3 years ago. Justin was at 260 pounds then. Not anymore, though. He lost all the weight with help from a nutritionist who taught him how to make proper food choices. When he was diagnosed, my wife, Kris, and I were committed to helping him get healthy, but he did most of the hard work himself. He took control of his health. I knew I had to do that, too.

My doctor told me I'd have to take medication, but if I lost weight, I might be able to stop one day. That motivated me. I don't want to take pills for the rest of my life. So when Kris heard about the DTOUR program and suggested that we try following it together, I thought I'd give it a shot. (See Kris's story on page 12.)

I didn't expect to lose much weight; in fact, we were told not to expect to lose more than 8 pounds in a month. But the scale just kept going down, down, down.

Not that it was easy. It was tough to adapt to the smaller portions. When you work hard all day like I do, you want to come home to a nice meal. What I've learned is that you have to redefine "a nice meal." I think we are.

We hardly eat out now, too. We had stopped ordering from the local pizza place for a month, and a delivery guy showed up out of nowhere with a free pizza. They were worried about us!

Justin is our primary motivator. If Kris and I eat something we shouldn't, he says, "Put that away." I was impressed with the way he helped us stick with this program.

I've tried some new foods that I like; hummus is my favorite. We've learned to be conscious of portions. I can't believe the amount of food we used to eat at one sitting! My migraines have also improved. I used to get them if I waited too long between meals. Now that I eat every 2½ to 3 hours, I haven't had one.

I feel really good. My clothes fit better. I'll definitely continue the program. My main goal is to get off my medication and get down to between 200 and 220 pounds. When I started DTOUR, my fasting blood sugar was 281; at our final check-in, it was 99. So I'm hopeful that one day, I won't have to take medications at all.

I look forward to being healthier and having even more energy than I do now. I want to be around for my kids, too; I want to play football with my son without having to sit down so often. I want to be an example for him as much as he's been an example for me.

BLOOD SUGAR:
DOWN
182
POINTS!

PART 2

THE DTOUR FAT-FIGHTING 4

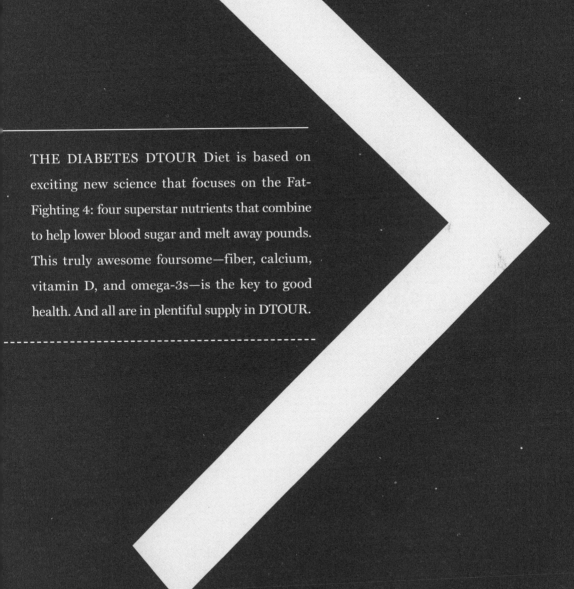

THE DIABETES DTOUR Diet is based on exciting new science that focuses on the Fat-Fighting 4: four superstar nutrients that combine to help lower blood sugar and melt away pounds. This truly awesome foursome—fiber, calcium, vitamin D, and omega-3s—is the key to good health. And all are in plentiful supply in DTOUR.

FAT-FIGHTER #1

FIBER

FILL UP TO SLIM DOWN

Whole foods tempt us with their come-hither hues—the jewel-toned berries and lush, leafy greens; the luminous beans; the rich, earthy grains. Like bees to flowers, we're drawn to them. That's a good thing, because underneath those beautiful exteriors, whole foods pack some serious nutrition, including a mother lode of fiber.

A half century of research has proven fiber to be the Swiss Army knife of nutrients. Name just about any health problem—high blood sugar or type 2 diabetes, for example—and a high-fiber diet probably can help treat it, if not prevent it in the first place.

Trying to lose weight? Then fiber-rich foods definitely are the way to go. Case in point: Researchers at the University of Minnesota found that people who ate the most vegetables, fruits, and other fiber-rich foods lost 2 to 3 pounds more per month than those on lower-fiber diets.

With all the good things it has going for it, fiber ought to be a dietary mainstay. Yet a full two-thirds of us are getting 15 grams a day, at most. That's about half of the recommended 25 to 30 grams a day!

Why are so many of us coming up so short? The answer, at least in part, is that fiber-rich whole foods must compete with processed foods for our dietary favor. The latter's very name suggests their inherent weakness: Processed foods are pretty much devoid of fiber.

DTOUR is all about whole foods—fruits, veggies, beans, and whole grains. They're the staple ingredients of our menus and recipes, which are as easy to make as they are fabulous to eat! You'll enjoy stir-fries, bean tostadas, pasta primavera, and pancakes—yes, pancakes!—on this diet. And no worries about fiber: You'll be getting between 26 and 29 grams every day, depending on your calorie level. You'll eat great, lose weight, and rein in your blood sugar. That's the DTOUR promise!

THE 411 ON FIBER

So just what is fiber? Simply put, it's the component of a plant food that passes through the digestive system pretty much intact. The term *fiber* actually describes a group of plant compounds, each with different functions and health benefits and each generally categorized as soluble or insoluble.

Soluble fiber is the kind that dissolves in water and turns into a thick gel during digestion. The humble apple, which contains a modest 80 calories but an impressive 5 grams of fiber, is an excellent source of a particular soluble fiber called pectin. If the name rings a bell, it's because pectin is used as a thickener in foods like jams and jellies. The same properties allow pectin to "thicken" in your digestive tract. The result: You feel fuller after eating.

Soluble fiber's gummy texture also may interfere with carbohydrate and glucose absorption in the intestines, leading to lower blood sugar and insulin. With your blood sugar on an even keel, you're better able to manage hunger and cravings.

FIBER BY ANY OTHER NAME

What is fiber, anyway? Food scientists, nutritionists, and medical experts have debated this question since nutritionist E. H. Hipsley introduced the term *dietary fiber* in 1953.

Even the FDA, which regulates food labeling, has no formal, written definition of dietary fiber. It uses the definition created by AOAC International, a professional association of analytical chemists that sets standard methods for laboratory analysis.

Experts do agree on one thing: Fiber is derived from the edible parts of plants that are not broken down by the human digestive system. But some believe a clearer, universally accepted definition of dietary fiber would ensure that the total fiber counts on food labels are accurate and consistent.

In recent years, several organizations have attempted to narrow the definition of dietary fiber. For example, the National Academy of Sciences—the organization that issues Recommended Dietary Allowances—has suggested phasing out use of the terms *insoluble fiber* and *soluble fiber* in favor of *dietary fiber* and *added fiber*. According to the proposed definitions, dietary fiber is derived from plants, while added fiber is incorporated into foods during processing. *Total fiber*, then, would be the sum of dietary fiber and added fiber.

The definitions may be tricky, but the most important facts remain: A fiber-rich diet helps prevent type 2 diabetes and obesity, and the best source of fiber is whole foods.

Another benefit of soluble fiber is its ability to lower cholesterol. One study found that for every gram of soluble fiber consumed in a diet of primarily fruits, veggies, and whole grains, blood cholesterol could decline by as much as 2 percent.

Unlike soluble fiber, insoluble fiber—your grandmother called it roughage—doesn't dissolve in water. Because it stays solid, it adds bulk to bowel movements. It also speeds the passage of food through the digestive tract, which means the intestines have less time to absorb carbohydrates. The result: Your blood sugar stays on an even keel.

This is one reason for insoluble fiber's impressive ability to reduce diabetes risk. When Finnish researchers tracked 4,316 men and women ages 40 to 69 over 10 years, they found that the people who ate the most fiber from cereal grains were 61 percent less likely to develop type 2 diabetes than those who ate the least.

Among the best sources of insoluble fiber are whole wheat flour, wheat bran, and many vegetables; for soluble fiber, top-notch sources include oats, peas, beans, apples, and citrus fruits. That said, plant foods vary greatly in the types and amounts of fiber they contain. Your best bet is to vary your food choices—which is exactly what you'll be doing on DTOUR!

FEEL FULL ON FEWER CALORIES (NO KIDDING!)

As we mentioned earlier, fiber is a must-have for any weight-loss plan—or at least the ones that produce results. Large-scale studies have shown that people who follow high-fiber diets tend to have lower body weights and less body fat than those who don't. For example, when Tufts University researchers reviewed the findings of several weight-loss studies, they concluded that increasing fiber intake by 14 grams per day could lower a person's calorie intake by 10 percent.

Why fiber promotes weight loss isn't rocket science.

Stop Here

WHILE HIGH-FIBER FOODS are good for your health, bad things—gas, bloating, and cramping—can happen when you add too much fiber to your diet too quickly. It's best to increase your fiber intake gradually, over a period of a few weeks, to allow the natural bacteria in your digestive system to adjust to the change. Also be sure to drink plenty of water; otherwise, all that fiber will make for hard (and hard-to-pass) stool.

First, fiber-rich foods tend to require more chewing. More chewing means it takes longer to eat a meal, which allows time for your brain to get the message that your body has gotten its fill. So, you're less likely to overeat.

Further, high-fiber foods tend to have more volume. In other words, they take up more room in your belly, so that I'm-full feeling lingers long after you've taken your last bite. Studies have shown that a fiber-packed breakfast—say, a slice of whole grain toast spread with peanut butter or a bowl of oatmeal with berries—

PEANUT BUTTER: FIBER-FULL INDULGENCE

On the Diabetes DTOUR Diet, a "weakness" for peanut butter works to your advantage. That's because when it comes to weight loss and blood sugar control, PB is A-OK. Here's why.

It helps you lose weight. Yes, PB packs 180 to 210 calories per serving. But its winning combo of fiber and protein—2 grams and 8 grams per serving, respectively—fills you up and keeps you feeling full longer, so you eat less overall. Plus, there's nothing more indulgent than licking peanut butter off a spoon—and indulgence (in moderation) helps dieters master cravings and stay on track.

It's a diabetes foe. Peanuts can reduce your risk of diabetes and heart disease. A 2002 study published in the *Journal of the American Medical Association* found that consuming 1 ounce of nuts or peanut butter (about 2 tablespoons) at least 5 days a week can lower the risk of diabetes by almost 30 percent.

It's packed with belly-flattening fat. Peanut butter is rich in heart-healthy monounsaturated fat. In one study, people with insulin resistance who ate a diet high in monos had less belly fat than people who ate more carbohydrates or saturated fat.

The fat and calorie counts of most brands of peanut butter are similar, but there are other indicators of a healthy pick. Here's what to look for.

◆ **Sodium:** Counts can range from 40 to 250 milligrams per 2-tablespoon serving. Organic versions tend to have less.
◆ **Sugar:** Natural brands have 1 to 2 grams, about half as much as commercial brands.

PS: No need to select reduced-fat PB. It contains about the same number of calories as full-fat brands, if not more—thanks to ingredients intended to make up for the missing fat, such as added sugar.

reduces food intake not only for the rest of the morning, but also at lunch.

Finally, high-fiber foods deliver more food for fewer calories. A fiber-rich pear, for example, delivers 5.5 grams of fiber for a calorie price tag of just 150 calories. Nutritionists refer to this as low energy density.

Of all the fiber-rich food choices, whole grains seem to have an especially strong connection to both weight loss *and* heart health. A team of researchers at the University of Pennsylvania was the first to confirm this link, in a study involving 50 overweight men and women with metabolic syndrome. All of the study participants cut their calorie intakes for 12 weeks. The key difference: Half were instructed to strive for more whole grains in their diets, while the rest were told to choose refined grains.

By the end of the study, the members of both groups had dropped between 8 and 11 pounds and showed about the same change in waistline measurements. Those eating the whole grains, however, lost a higher percentage of body fat. As a bonus, their blood levels of C-reactive protein (CRP) declined by 38 percent. CRP is a marker for the chronic low-level inflammation that's a predictor of heart disease. By comparison, CRP levels remained unchanged among those eating refined grains.

Among the food sources of insoluble fiber, whole grains are the superstars. In a 2007 meta-analysis of several studies involving more than 700,000 people, researchers at the Harvard School of Public Health concluded that two extra servings of whole grains a day could reduce a person's risk of diabetes by a full 21 percent.

Across the Atlantic, German researchers made a similar finding when they tracked the eating habits of more than 25,000 men and women. Those who consumed the most fiber from whole grain cereals—about 17 grams per day—were 27 percent less likely to develop diabetes than those who ate the least (less than 7 grams per day).

FYI

AS YOU'RE CHECKING out food labels, keep your eye on two numbers for the biggest weight-loss payoff: the percentage of calories from fat and the number of grams of fiber.

In a Tufts University study that tracked the daily fat and fiber consumption of 824 women, those who got less than 13 grams of fiber and consumed more than 35 percent of their calories from fat were up to 13 times more likely to be overweight than those who ate more fiber and less fat.

AN ANSWER TO BLOOD SUGAR MEDS?

When you lose weight, you automatically improve insulin's ability to sweep blood sugar out of the bloodstream and into cells. But that isn't the only way fiber helps to rein in blood sugar. Soluble fiber appears to play an especially important role. Its secret: a quality called viscosity, which causes the stomach to empty at a more leisurely pace. This, in turn, slows the digestion of starches and sugars and reduces spikes in blood sugar.

Among the food sources of soluble fiber are beans and legumes, which appear to work their own magic on diabetes. One noteworthy study, which appeared in the *American Journal of Clinical Nutrition*, tracked the dietary habits of 64,227 healthy middle-aged Chinese women for close to 5 years. The research team that conducted the study, from Vanderbilt University Medical Center and the Shanghai Cancer Institute in China, found that the women who consumed the most legumes were 38 percent less likely to develop type 2 diabetes. Those with high intakes of soybeans, in particular, saw their risk plummet even further—by 47 percent.

What about the fiber in fruits and veggies? Its effect on blood sugar isn't quite so clear. The German study mentioned above, for example, found no particular asso-

C YOU LATER, DIABETES!

Many fruits and veggies are rich in vitamin C, an antioxidant that offers potent protection against disease. At least one study has shown that a high vitamin C intake may lower diabetes risk.

For the study, which appeared in the *Archives of Internal Medicine*, British researchers collected data on 21,831 men and women who didn't have diabetes at the outset. The study lasted for 12 years; during that time, 735 people developed type 2.

When the researchers compared the participants' blood levels of vitamin C, they noticed that the group with the most C in their blood was 62 percent less likely to have been diagnosed with diabetes. According to the researchers, the chances of these folks getting type 2 in the future were 22 percent lower.

FROM THE DTOUR DIETITIAN

A whole grain food retains the three main components of a grain seed: bran, germ, and endosperm. Whole grains may be cracked, flaked, ground, or popped. Follow these steps into a whole new world of whole grains.

◆ Look for the phrase "100 percent whole grain" on product labels. Don't be fooled by the word "multigrain"; these products may or may not be made with whole grains. And "made with whole grains" does not mean "100 percent whole grains."

◆ Aim for at least 3 servings of whole grains spread throughout the day. One serving equals one ounce of bread, cereal, crackers, or other whole grains.

◆ Watch those portion sizes. Whole grains still contain carbohydrates. One cup of whole grain rice or pasta can affect blood sugar the same as three slices of bread.

◆ Get adventurous. Besides whole wheat bread, oatmeal, and brown rice, try barley, whole wheat pasta, popcorn, whole rye bread and crackers, corn tortillas, and wild rice.

—Barbara

ciation between fruit and vegetable consumption and diabetes risk. On the other hand, based on data collected from more than 2,000 people over the course of 10 years, Australian researchers were able to conclude that a person could lower his or her diabetes risk by 24 percent just by eating 5 grams of fiber from vegetable sources every day.

So eat your fruits and veggies—and your beans and whole grains. No matter where you're getting your fiber, it's going to do your blood sugar a whole lot of good. Actually, fiber works so well that if you take insulin or diabetes medication, you may need to lower your dosage (with your doctor's okay, of course). That was the case for Tom and Randy, two of our DTOUR test panelists; our fiber-rich menus and recipes helped them lower their blood sugar by 78 and 182 points, respectively.

FYI

SOME RESEARCHERS HAVE calculated that if Americans doubled their fiber intake, they could shave 100 calories from their diets each day. This one change could trim off 10 pounds per year.

Stop Here

PREVENTION OFFERS a handy Fiber Up food finder to help you plan fiber-rich meals. To use it, log on to www.prevention. com/fiberup.

FIBER'S PARTNERS IN PREVENTION

Coincidentally, the same whole foods that provide your daily fiber fix also contain an abundance of phytochemicals. You've probably heard of them; they're natural substances in plant foods that have the power to heal and prevent disease, including type 2 diabetes and heart disease. In fact, one study that recently appeared in the *British Journal of Nutrition* reported that phytochemicals may lower the risk of metabolic syndrome as well as diabetes complications.

In this study, polyphenols were found to be particularly beneficial. They, along with carotenoids, are among the most avidly studied classes of phytochemicals. The carotenoids include the beta-carotene in broccoli, sweet potatoes, pumpkins, and carrots; the lutein in leafy greens, such as kale and spinach; and the lycopene in tomatoes and pink grapefruit. Polyphe-

FROM THE DTOUR DIETITIAN

It's normal for your weight to go up and down over the course of a day. The scale takes in everything, including the meal you haven't yet digested, that cup of coffee or water you drank, and solid waste. Just 2 cups of water weighs 1 pound, so if you're retaining fluid because you consumed more sodium or carbohydrates than usual (or if you're constipated), your weight will rise—but only temporarily.

By contrast, body fat changes slowly over time. This may help keep things in perspective: To gain 1 pound of body fat in a day, you'd have to consume 3,500 calories more than you burn. That's roughly the equivalent of 50 chocolate chip cookies. We doubt you've eaten that much in one sitting!

To rein in your scale anxiety, weigh yourself just once a week, ideally first thing in the morning. Pay attention, too, to other changes—like how your clothes are fitting and how much energy you have. These can be even better measures of success!

—Barbara

nols are abundant in apples, red grapes, berries, onions, teas, and wines.

Though researchers still have much to learn about these and other phytochemicals, here's a snapshot of their key findings so far.

◆ Broccoli contains a slew of phytochemicals besides beta-carotene—among them the carotenoids lutein and quercetin, as well as sulforaphane and indoles. Collectively, they may protect against diabetes complications as well as certain cancers.

◆ The beta-carotene in cantaloupes, mangoes, carrots, sweet potatoes, and spinach also may delay or prevent the onset of diabetes complications.

◆ Another carotenoid, lycopene, may reduce heart disease risk. It's found in abundance in tomatoes and tomato products.

◆ Blueberries and raspberries are rich in ellagic acid, which may lower blood cholesterol.

Think about it: All this fabulous protective power—and fiber, too! Now you can see why plant foods of all kinds are such an important part of DTOUR.

EASY WAYS TO GET YOUR FIBER FILL

You're going to be getting a lot of fiber on DTOUR, perhaps more than you're accustomed to eating. So we've put together a list of tips for you to follow now, before you start the plan. Don't try them all at once; your digestive tract may not forgive you. Instead, choose one or two that seem doable to you. By the way, these same strategies guided us in developing the DTOUR menus and recipes. So think of them as a head start!

HOW FIBER WORKS*

We tend to think of fiber as a digestive aid of sorts, and that certainly is one of its most important functions. But it is just one of many, as this chart shows.

IN THE . . .	FIBER ACTS TO . . .	AND BENEFITS YOUR HEALTH BY . . .
Stomach and small intestine	• create a sense of fullness • trap cholesterol and fats • slow absorption of sugars	• regulating weight • lowering cholesterol • improving blood sugar levels
Large intestine (colon)	• cause fermentation and promote growth of healthy bacteria • absorb water, adding "bulk" to stool	• enhancing the immune system to fight infection and chronic disease • promoting regularity and elimination, minimizing constipation

*Reprinted with permission from the National Fiber Council

◆ Select a breakfast cereal that provides 5 or more grams of fiber per serving. Another option: Add 2 tablespoons of unprocessed wheat bran to your favorite nonsugary cereal.

◆ Switch to a whole grain bread that contains at least 2 grams of fiber per serving. Read labels to make sure you're getting the real thing. You should see whole wheat, whole wheat flour, or another whole grain in the top spot on the ingredient list.

◆ Eat whole fruit instead of drinking fruit juice. Berries, along with pears, apples, and oranges, are good sources of fiber.

◆ Swap meat for legumes two or three times per week. Black beans, chickpeas, and edamame (whole soybeans) are high in fiber, low in fat, and packed with lean protein. Toss them in salads, or add them to chili or soups.

◆ Visit your local natural-foods store and experiment with some of the more exotic whole grains, such as buckwheat, millet, barley, and quinoa.

◆ Take advantage of ready-to-use vegetables. Mix chopped frozen broccoli into prepared spaghetti sauce or nibble on baby carrots.

SOURCES OF SOLUBLE AND INSOLUBLE FIBER

On DTOUR, you'll be getting a healthy mix of both types of fiber from top-notch sources like these.

Soluble Fiber
◆ Apples
◆ Beans and legumes
◆ Berries (blueberries, strawberries)
◆ Nuts and seeds
◆ Oatmeal and oat bran
◆ Pears

Insoluble Fiber
◆ Barley
◆ Brown rice
◆ Bulgur
◆ Carrots
◆ Celery
◆ Tomatoes
◆ Wheat bran
◆ Whole grain breads and breakfast cereals
◆ Zucchini

◆ Add some roughage to your snacks. Fresh fruits, raw vegetables with fat-free dip, and low-fat popcorn are all good choices.

◆ Experiment with Indian and Middle Eastern cuisines, which feature whole grains and legumes as part of the main meal. You might whip up Indian dal or Middle Eastern tabbouleh—a cracked-wheat salad flavored with lemon, fresh parsley, mint, chopped tomatoes, and spices.

◆ Add ½ cup of chickpeas, either cooked or canned, to a pot of your favorite soup. You'll boost its total fiber count by 6 grams. Be sure to rinse canned chickpeas to reduce their sodium content.

◆ Steam your broccoli, cauliflower, and carrots before eating them, and you'll get 3 to 5 grams of fiber per serving—up to twice the amount in the raw veggies. Heat makes fiber more available.

◆ Use uncooked oatmeal instead of bread crumbs in meat loaf. Add ¾ cup of oats per pound of lean ground beef, and you'll boost the total fiber count to more than 8 grams.

◆ Top your fat-free ice cream with sliced fresh berries. One-half cup of raspberries provides 4 grams of fiber; the same amount of strawberries or blueberries packs 2 grams.

DTOUR WINNER!

Jean Nick, 48
POUNDS LOST: 20
INCHES LOST: 6½
BLOOD SUGAR: STABLE

BEFORE

AFTER

My self-image was fine. My general health was good. But at 48, I was concerned that my extra pounds could threaten my future health. When I met my birth mother several years ago (I was adopted at birth), I learned that she had type 2 diabetes with many complications and she was taking insulin multiple times a day. I didn't want her present to be my future. I wanted to stay healthy and active.

I also worried about my partner Tom's diabetes. (See Tom's story on page 84.) He kept it under good control, but his extra weight put him at risk of complications. The time was right, and the program, which stressed whole, natural foods, was a good fit for us.

As Tom said, portion sizes were our problem: too much healthy food. The first few days, it was a challenge to measure out portions—and to think about eating smaller portions. My brain said, *A table-spoon of this, an ounce of that—I'm going to starve*. But it wasn't so bad. When I ate the measured portions, they were perfectly fine and filled me up. After 3 or 4 days, I thought, *Two tablespoons—that's an awful lot!* There were days I could not finish all my meals and snacks.

I also liked that we could make the plan flexible. We grow a lot of our own food and buy from local farmers, so we modified the menus to match the local produce in season. But we stuck very strictly to portion sizes.

We didn't do the exercise component of the program because neither of us felt we needed more activity than we already get. We run a farm, which means I do 2 to 3 hours of physical labor before I go to my day job, and then usually a couple more hours after I get home.

The main change for me is that I need to spend a little more time cooking, but that's something I really want to have as a priority in my life anyway. Unfortunately, with two full-time jobs—writer and farmer—it's been easy to fall into the habit of grabbing food that's quick but not so healthy. Now Tom and I sit at the table and talk and eat tasty, healthy food. My daughter ate dinner with us recently. She said, "This isn't diet food. It's *good*."

I've lost 20 pounds so far. It was a kick to jump on the scale at our check-in, especially after the first 2 weeks—I lost a pound a day. Now it's a couple of pounds a week, which is still great. I've dropped from a size 20 to a size 16, and even some of those 16s are too big now.

We'll continue to eat this way, no question. This isn't a weight-loss diet. It's a sensible way to eat, and it will keep us both healthy and active. It took me a long time to find the right guy, so I want to keep him around as long as possible and keep us both able to do the activities we love.

LOST
20
POUNDS!

5

FAT-FIGHTERS #2 AND #3: CALCIUM & VITAMIN D

THE DYNAMIC DUO OF DIABETES CONTROL

Surprised to see calcium and vitamin D among our Fat-Fighting 4? We admit, they probably are not the first nutrients that come to mind for weight loss or diabetes management. Strong bones and teeth? Definitely. Healthy blood pressure and cholesterol? Perhaps.

But the latest evidence from the research front is impossible to ignore: The combination of calcium and vitamin D appears to enhance fat burning as well as cellular insulin response. That's a surefire formula for better blood sugar control!

Despite their impressive and growing résumés of health benefits, both calcium and vitamin D tend to come up short in the typical American diet. When you think about it, this could help explain—to some degree—why obesity and diabetes have become so prevalent here.

We're doing our part to help correct this dietary deficit by loading our DTOUR menus and recipes with calcium- and vitamin D–rich ingredients. Eating the DTOUR way, you'll get a generous 1,200 milligrams of calcium plus 155 IU of vitamin D per day, on average. And that's just from foods—delectable dishes like stuffed bell peppers, French onion soup, and rice pudding with raspberries.

Because getting enough vitamin D from diet alone can be a challenge, we do recommend a D supplement for everyone on DTOUR. You might benefit from supplemental calcium, too, depending on your age and health status. (We'll say more about this a bit later in the chapter.) As much as possible, though, we want you to get your calcium and vitamin D from foods. The reason: There may be nutritional "supporting players" in foods that allow the superstars to work their magic. Oh yes, and foods are so much more satisfying and delicious than supplements!

CALCIUM PUTS FAT CELLS ON A DIET

Around the time you were learning about the basic four food groups in elementary school, you probably got a lesson or two about how milk—and, more precisely, the calcium in milk—helps build your bones. In fact, about 99 percent of the calcium in your body resides in your bones and teeth. The remaining 1 percent has a lot going on, too—helping your heart to beat, your blood to clot, and your nerves to communicate with each other. As you can see, your body needs calcium to thrive.

It's only fairly recently that researchers began to suspect a connection between calcium and weight loss. In 2002, a research team at the University of Tennessee put 32 people—all overweight—on calorie-restricted diets that included varying amounts of dietary calcium. Over the 6 months of the study, the people who ate three servings of dairy (including low-fat milk, cheese, and yogurt) lost 70 percent more weight—an average of 24 pounds—and 64 percent more body fat than those who ate just one serving a day.

Understandably, this study made national headlines. Ever since, experts have been debating the role of calcium—mainly from dairy foods—in weight loss. Now, common sense will tell you that you can't expect to slim down by eating a pint of Ben & Jerry's every day. (We know—we're disappointed, too!) On the other hand, if you make a point of stocking your daily diet with low-fat, calcium-rich choices—as you'll be doing on DTOUR—you will stack the weight-loss odds in your favor. (PS: The DTOUR Diet leaves room for ice cream, too!)

So how might calcium help burn body fat? Researchers are still looking for the answer. One theory, from Michael Zemel, PhD, who led the University of Tennessee study, focuses on the role of the hormone calcitriol in fat cells.

Here's how it may work: Low blood levels of calcium cause levels of calcitriol to rise. In response, the body hoards calcium by sending more into fat cells, prompting the cells to store more fat and burn less. The reverse also appears to be true: In a calcium-rich diet, calcitriol production falls, and less calcium is shuttled into fat cells. So less fat is stored and more is burned. In essence, a lack of calcium somehow makes fat cells hang on to fat—perhaps an evolutionary vestige of our caveman ancestors, whose bodies adapted to endure times of famine.

The University of Tennessee study relied on dairy foods to cover the participants' calcium needs. At least for weight loss, foods seem a better choice than calcium

FYI

STRANGE BUT TRUE: People who live farthest from the equator have higher rates of heart disease and high blood pressure. Experts think it's because they get less exposure to the sun's ultraviolet rays, which makes them more likely to be deficient in vitamin D.

supplements. It's the total mix of nutrients in foods that provides the benefit, rather than calcium in isolation.

Considering all the fabulous foods that double as outstanding calcium sources, it's hard to fathom that we're not getting enough of the mineral in our daily diets. Yet many of us are missing the mark. According to a 2008 study, only 40 percent of American women between ages 20 and 49 are at or above the recommended intake of 1,000 milligrams of calcium a day; among women over 50, just 27 percent are getting the recommended 1,500 milligrams a day. (Calcium levels are of particular concern for women, because they're much more likely than men to develop osteoporosis.)

Your body has two ways of meeting its calcium needs. One is by metabolizing the mineral from calcium-rich foods and supplements, which is by far the healthiest option. The other is by absorbing it from bones, which is what happens when your blood level of calcium falls too low.

Remember the hormone calcitriol that we mentioned earlier? Well, here's where it really comes into play. When you don't have enough calcium in your bloodstream, small glands called the parathyroids (so named because they sit on the surface of the thyroid) trigger the release of calcitriol. Calcitriol, in turn, encourages the release of calcium by breaking down bone. It also increases the kidneys' ability to reabsorb calcium, so you lose less in urine.

The fact is, you're losing calcium constantly—at every bathroom break; to your skin, hair, and nails; even in your perspiration. In a study at Purdue University, women who exercised for an hour a day sweated away about 92 milligrams of calcium. Incidentally, that's about one-third the amount in a glass of milk.

Another by-product of calcitriol is that as blood levels of the hormone rise, more calcium gets pushed into the smooth muscle cells that line the arteries. The arteries narrow, and boom—up goes blood pressure. As we've discussed

FYI

IN THE LANDMARK DASH (Dietary Approaches to Stop Hypertension) study, people who followed a diet packed with low-fat dairy products and other healthy food choices were able to lower their blood pressure in just 8 weeks. Calcium can't take all the credit for the improvement, but it definitely made a difference, experts say.

elsewhere, insulin resistance and diabetes seem to go hand in hand with heart disease; high blood pressure can drive heart disease risk even higher.

The solution, of course, is to keep blood calcium at a healthy level. Then calcitriol won't rise, fat cells won't hoard fat, and blood pressure will remain normal. The best way to meet your body's calcium needs is with food—and the Diabetes DTOUR Diet is chock-full of yummy, calcium-rich choices!

FROM D-FICIENCY TO D-FENSE

We can't really talk about calcium without bringing vitamin D into the conversation, since D's most important function is to help the intestines absorb calcium.

TURN TOWARD THE SUN

On a sunny (or even cloudy) day, as you take your dog for a stroll or just walk to the mailbox and back, the sun's ultraviolet B rays strike your skin, literally creating vitamin D. How much D your skin makes depends on several factors, including where you live, what season and time of day it is, whether there's cloud cover or smog, and whether you're wearing sunscreen.

Age and skin color play roles, too. People over 50 don't synthesize vitamin D as well as younger folks. In fact, an average 70-year-old makes only 25 percent as much vitamin D as a 20-year-old. Melanin, the pigment that gives skin its color, also affects its ability to produce vitamin D; generally, the higher the concentration of melanin, the lower the level of D. That's why black Americans have half as much vitamin D in their blood, on average, as whites.

Given all the warnings about excessive sun exposure causing wrinkles and skin cancer, you may be concerned about soaking up the sun's rays. No worries! All you need is 10 to 15 minutes of sun time to safely synthesize a healthy dose of vitamin D.

Simply head outside on a sunny day, leaving your arms and legs uncovered. (But do protect your face, which has thinner, more sensitive skin.) Forgo the sunscreen for this brief period of time, because it hinders your body's ability to make vitamin D. After 15 minutes, you should apply sunscreen if you're planning to stay outdoors. Use a product with an SPF of at least 15, even on hazy or cloudy days.

At the risk of stating the obvious, if your gut can't absorb calcium, your body can't use it.

As you'll see a bit later in the chapter, calcium and vitamin D appear to work together to help fight type 2 diabetes. But vitamin D has benefits in its own right: It has shown promise in helping to protect against heart disease, as well as certain cancers and autoimmune diseases. Since the risk of heart disease rises in the presence of diabetes, we'll spend just a few moments on vitamin D's cardiovascular benefits.

To start, vitamin D plays a fundamental role in the heart's ability to pump blood and in the structure of heart cells. It also may turn down chronic inflammation, which a growing body of research is implicating as a key risk factor for heart disease.

For a recent study, Harvard researchers tracked more than 1,700 men and women for 5 years to determine if low blood levels of vitamin D led to heart disease. None of the participants had heart disease at the start of the study, but 28 percent were running low on vitamin D. Those in the D-deficient group were 60 percent more likely to develop heart disease than those who had enough D.

Since this was just an observational study, the researchers can't say for sure why vitamin D appeared to have heart-protective effects. Whatever the mechanism, though, the findings advance the case for satisfying your body's vitamin D requirements.

Just as with calcium, many of us—an estimated 60 percent of Americans—aren't getting enough vitamin D, according to a survey by the Centers for Disease Control and Prevention. If we're low on vitamin D, then our shortfall of calcium makes sense. As we said earlier, our bodies can't use calcium without D. People who are deficient in vitamin D typically absorb just 10 to 15 percent of their dietary calcium, compared with 30 to 40 percent for people who are meeting their D needs.

If you're over age 50 or African American, or if you're vegan or lactose intolerant, you're more likely to experience a D deficiency than the general population. Overweight may be a risk factor, too. Though the body stores vitamin D in fat and releases it into the bloodstream on an as-needed basis, this process doesn't go quite so smoothly in the presence of extra pounds. Instead, excess body fat seems to act as a sort of trap, preventing vitamin D from entering the bloodstream.

One other possible explanation for our national D deficit: sunscreen. You see, the human body synthesizes its own vitamin D when exposed to the sun's ultraviolet rays. Though it's highly controversial, a growing number of experts believe that since we've become so indoctrinated in the use of sunscreen, we don't give sunlight a chance to penetrate our well-protected hides. In effect, we're setting ourselves up for deficiency.

Our bodies need all the vitamin D they can get, whether it comes from sunlight (about 10 minutes a day of unprotected exposure), from food, or from supplements— or, ideally, a combination of the three. To learn more about how safe sun exposure can boost your body's supply of D, see "Turn Toward the Sun" on page 62.

THE ANTIDIABETES "A TEAM"

If calcium and vitamin D can do so much good individually, just imagine their potential when they work together! This powerhouse pair may turn out to be the most potent diabetes defense around.

When researchers at the Tufts–New England Medical Center and other Boston-area institutions launched their exploration of the relationship between calcium, vitamin D, and type 2 diabetes, they already knew that other research findings had linked low blood levels of D to insulin resistance and type 2. Their landmark study, published in 2006, provided compelling evidence that adequate amounts of vitamin D, in tandem with calcium, reduce diabetes risk.

For their analysis, the research team collected data from 83,779 women who already had enrolled in the long-running Nurses' Health Study. Every 2 to 4 years over the course of 2 decades, the researchers assessed the women's intakes of calcium and vitamin D from both foods and supplements.

At the outset, none of the women was diabetic. That changed by the study's end, when more than 4,800 women had been diagnosed with the disease. But the researchers also noticed this: The women who had been

FYI

THE AVERAGE FEMALE body contains about 2 pounds of calcium; the typical male body, just over 2½ pounds.

taking in more than 1,200 milligrams of calcium and more than 800 IU of vitamin D a day were 33 percent less likely to have developed diabetes than women who had been getting lesser amounts of both nutrients.

A more recent study, also from Tufts, determined that chronically low levels of vitamin D could raise a person's risk of type 2 diabetes by as much as 46 percent. In this meta-analysis, people who were consuming between three and five servings of dairy foods a day—including milk, which typically is fortified with vitamin D—were 14 percent less likely to develop diabetes than those who were taking in less than 1½ servings a day.

Stop Here

AVOID CALCIUM SUPPLEMENTS made with unrefined oyster shell, bone meal, or dolomite. They may contain lead or other hazardous substances. Leave chelated calcium supplements on the shelf, too. They're pricier, but no better than other forms of calcium.

Interestingly, this research team did not believe that getting more D by itself would be enough to stop diabetes. Drawing on other published evidence, they concluded that the combination of calcium and vitamin D—in daily doses of 1,200 milligrams and 1,000 IU, respectively—would be the most effective preventive.

Because the Tufts studies were population-based, they don't reveal precisely how calcium and vitamin D might help to derail diabetes. One explanation is that the two nutrients may enhance cellular insulin response and reduce chronic inflammation, which is a known diabetes risk factor.

The calcium–vitamin D combination is a boon to weight loss, too—though in at

DAILY INTAKES OF CALCIUM AND VITAMIN D

Below are the National Academy of Sciences' current daily recommendations for calcium and vitamin D, along with the safe daily upper limit for each.

AGE	CALCIUM	VITAMIN D
19 to 50 years	1,000 mg	200 IU
51 to 70 years	1,200 mg	400 IU
71 years and over	1,200 mg	600 IU
Safe upper limit	2,500 mg	2,000 IU

FYI

least one way that you might not expect. According to a 2008 study published in the *Journal of Nutrition*, this talented team helps protect against the weakening of bones that sometimes occurs in dieters. For this study, researchers at the University of Illinois assigned 130 middle-aged, overweight men and women to one of two groups. One group followed a diet that provided three servings of dairy products a day and derived 30 percent of total calories from protein, 40 percent from carbs, and 30 percent from fat. The diet for the other group had a slightly different mix of macronutrients—15 percent of calories from protein, 55 percent from carbs, and 30 percent from fat—and just two servings of dairy a day.

Over the course of 12 months, the researchers tracked the weight, bone mineral content, and bone density of all the participants. The results: Bone density remained stable in the first group but declined in the second group. The researchers concluded that the combination and/or interaction of calcium and vitamin D with dietary protein helped to protect the participants' bones while they slimmed down.

There's one more bonus benefit of this nutritional dynamic duo that we should mention: It appears to lower LDL cholesterol, the bad kind that builds artery-clogging plaques and sets the stage for heart disease. According to a study that appeared in the *American Journal of Clinical Nutrition*, dieters who took 600 milligrams of supplemental calcium and 200 IU of supplemental vitamin D a day—which are not even the recommended minimums—cut their LDL cholesterol by 14 percent. Total cholesterol declined by 9 percent. Researchers speculate that calcium may prevent the absorption of dietary fat, which reduces the liver's production of LDL.

GETTING THE CALCIUM AND D YOU NEED

When you consider all that calcium and vitamin D can do for your body, you have plenty of good reasons to make sure you're getting enough of both nutrients. Never fear: The Diabetes DTOUR Diet covers your nutritional bases, and then some! Our menus and recipes deliver 1,200 milligrams of calcium and 155 IU of vitamin D, on average, every day. These levels, in combination with a vitamin D supplement, meet or beat the government guidelines for most people. (They are lower than the amounts some experts are recommending for therapeutic purposes, but the jury is still out on just how much calcium and vitamin D is necessary and safe.)

Our diet does feature a variety of dairy foods and dairy-based dishes, since dairy is just about the best dietary source of calcium around. Just three glasses of fortified fat-free milk offers more than 1,000 milligrams of calcium, plus 400 IU of vitamin D. But what if you can't do dairy because you're lactose intolerant? One option is to use lactose-free or soy-based products; the fortified varieties are just as nutritious as the "real thing," and they taste great, too! You also might try using Lactaid or another supplement

Stop Here

AVOID COD LIVER OIL. While it's super rich in vitamin D (1 tablespoon contains about 1,400 IU), it may cause an overdose when taken on top of the D made by your body and the amount you get from food.

FOOD SOURCES OF CALCIUM

From fish to beans to greens, calcium crops up in a wide variety of tasty foods.

FOOD	AMOUNT	CALCIUM (MG) PER SERVING
Yogurts, nonfat	8 oz	400
Soy milk, fortified	1 c	368
Sardines, oil-packed, drained	3 oz	325
Milk, fat-free	1 c	300–350
Tofu, firm, prepared with nigari (a natural solidifier)	½ c	253
Salmon, canned, with bone	3 oz	181
Collards, cooked	½ c	178
Spinach, cooked	½ c	146
Oatmeal, fortified, instant	1 packet	99–110
White beans, canned	½ c	96

that contains lactase, an enzyme that helps your body digest lactose. You can get significant amounts of calcium from nondairy sources like fortified tofu; canned salmon and sardines (with their bones); and dark green, leafy vegetables. See the chart for your best choices.

As for vitamin D, if the latest research is any indication, even current government guidelines—which range from 200 IU to 600 IU, based on age—may be falling short. How much higher they ought to be is the subject of considerable debate. Based on what we know so far, we think it makes good sense for everyone to take supplemental vitamin D.

How much do you need in supplement form? If you're age 70 or younger, 400 IU a day—in combination with the DTOUR menus and recipes—will cover your body's needs and then some. If you're 71 or older, your goal is a bit higher—600 IU a day. That's because your body may not be synthesizing its own D as efficiently.

You also might consider taking extra calcium and vitamin D as nutritional insurance—if, for example, you spend a lot of your time indoors (which means your skin may not be synthesizing vitamin D) or you're at risk of osteoporosis. Your doctor can help you decide whether you require more than the recommended amounts of these nutrients, and which of the following choices would best suit your needs.

A multivitamin. Many multis contain both calcium and vitamin D, but in varying amounts. For example, One-A-Day Women's provides 450 milligrams of calcium

FOOD SOURCES OF VITAMIN D

Fish and fortified foods are excellent sources of vitamin D.

FOOD	AMOUNT	VITAMIN D (IU) PER SERVING
Salmon, cooked	3½ oz	360
Mackerel, cooked	3½ oz	345
Sardines, oil-packed, drained	1¾ oz	250
Tuna, oil-packed, drained	3 oz	200
Quaker Nutrition for Women Instant Oatmeal	1 packet	154
Soy milk, fortified	1 c	100
Milk, fortified, fat-free, low-fat, or whole	1 c	98
Cereal, fortified	¾–1 c	40-50

and 800 IU of vitamin D, while Centrum supplies 200 milligrams of calcium and 400 IU of vitamin D. Be sure to read product labels when deciding what to buy.

Individual supplements. You can get your calcium from chewable supplements such as Tums (a calcium-based antacid) or Viactiv soft chews. Traditional supplements take one of two forms: calcium carbonate or calcium citrate. Though calcium citrate can be taken anytime, calcium carbonate should be paired with a meal to improve absorption.

A calcium–vitamin D combo. What's nice about a combination supplement is that you get both nutrients in the proper ratio, and you cut down on the number of pills that you need to swallow. Look for a supplement that contains vitamin D_3 (also known as cholecalciferol); it's more potent and more easily absorbed by the body than D_2.

We do urge you to talk with your doctor before you add any of these supplements to your self-care regimen. Since DTOUR delivers generous amounts of calcium and vitamin D, you need to be careful not to go overboard on your daily intake. Rather than too much or too little of either nutrient, you should aim for "just right"!

CHAPTER 6

FAT-FIGHTER #4:

OMEGA-3s

GOOD FOR YOUR HEART—AND YOUR WAISTLINE

If fat were a celebrity, all of Hollywood would be lining up to hire its publicist. Talk about an image transformation! A mere decade or so ago, America had become a no-fat zone, with dietary fat being blamed for health concerns from weight gain to heart disease. But something odd happened: Even though we were cutting our fat intake, we weren't getting any healthier, and our waistlines weren't getting any narrower.

It seems that in our zeal to slash fat, we were depriving our bodies of an important macronutrient. That's right: Our bodies depend on fat to function as they should. Maybe we *had* been consuming too much of it, but then we drifted to the other extreme, consuming way too little. As it turns out, we have to eat fat to lose weight!

Most experts agree that the right fats, in the right amounts, can be—make that *should* be—part of a healthy diet. By the right fats we mean omega-3 fatty acids, the kind that help melt away pounds and lower heart disease risk (which tends to be higher in those with blood sugar issues). These fats also may improve cells' insulin response!

Virtually every meal and snack in DTOUR delivers a delicious dose of omega-3s. Depending on which calorie level of our diet is best for you, you'll be getting between 2.5 and 2.7 grams over the course of a day. That's well above the recommended 1.1 grams for women and 1.6 grams for men.

DTOUR derives its omega-3s from a variety of foods, including fish, walnuts, and flaxseed. Of these, cold-water fish, such as salmon, albacore tuna, and sardines, are by far the most abundant sources of the two types of omega-3s: eicosapentaenoic acid (EPA) and docosahexaenoic acid (DHA). (Don't worry; you're only eating them—not pronouncing them!) We've also included foods that supply alpha-linolenic acid (ALA), another kind of fatty acid that your body cleverly converts into omega-3s.

We know that not everyone is a fan of fish. Though you have many other meal options on DTOUR, we urge you to give one or two of our fish dishes a try. One of our test panelists professed a profound aversion to "fin food" until she tried our fish tacos on Day 3. Now she's hooked—pardon the pun!

GOOD FATS MAKE A COMEBACK

Fish—and therefore omega-3s—have been a staple of the human diet since, well, our caveman ancestors mastered the skill of catching them. From an evolutionary perspective, our bodies are hardwired to require these beneficial fats to carry out their most basic biochemical tasks.

Still, omega-3s are relative newcomers to the nutritional scene. In fact, they were on the verge of extinction from our modern diet, with agricultural practices and cooking methods nearly eliminating them from our food supply.

Today, omega-3s seem to be just about everywhere. Just push your cart through the aisles of any supermarket and you'll find omega-3s added to all manner of foods and beverages, including breakfast cereals, eggs, orange juice, and margarine. Even some pet foods have them! It shows how far these beneficial fats have come, capturing the attention of nutrition scientists and food manufacturers alike.

GO FISH, BUT HOLD THE MERCURY

Fish may be our biggest nutritional catch-22. On the one hand, they're rich in health-boosting omega-3 fatty acids; on the other, they contain mercury. Too-high blood levels of mercury have been linked to an increased risk of heart disease. Our advice: Eat up to 12 ounces a week of low-mercury fish choices while going easy on others (and avoiding some altogether). Here's what to pick and what to skip:

Eat often*	Eat in moderation**	Avoid
Salmon	Albacore tuna (water-packed)	King mackerel
Shrimp	Lobster	Shark
Tilapia	Mahimahi	Swordfish
Tuna (water-packed)	Monkfish	Tilefish

*Up to three 4-ounce servings per week

**One 4-ounce serving per week

The potential health benefits of omega-3s first came to light in the mid-1970s, when a Danish research team conducted observational studies of Greenland Inuits. This population showed a very low rate of heart disease, which the researchers attributed to their traditional diet rich in fish. Since then, other observational studies have drawn a similar conclusion: Populations that eat fish on a regular basis, such as native Alaskans and Japanese, have low rates of death from heart disease. Omega-3s appear to protect the heart by reducing inflammation, preventing the blood clots that can cause heart attacks, slowing a rapid heartbeat, and relaxing the blood vessels so blood can flow freely. (We'll explore the heart-healthy effects of omega-3s later in the chapter.)

Omega-3s are fats of the unsaturated variety—a category that also includes nut oils and vegetable oils. Omega-6s, found in vegetable oils as well as breakfast cereals and whole grain breads, come under the "unsaturated" umbrella as well. Though our bodies need both kinds of omegas, we tend to eat them in disproportionate amounts— roughly 15 to 17 times more 6s than 3s. The ratio of the two should be just about equal. When it isn't, and it stays out of sync for a prolonged period, it can pave the way to an assortment of health problems, including heart arrhythmias, depression, and certain autoimmune and inflammatory diseases.

Stop Here

EATING FISH A FEW TIMES A WEEK is fine; in fact, it's recommended! Fish oil supplements are another story. Please don't take them without consulting your doctor first, because they can interact with other medications. For example, if you use aspirin or another med to reduce blood clotting, adding a fish oil supplement to the mix may increase the risk of bleeding.

BANISHER OF BODY FAT, SLAYER OF FAT CELLS

When you're getting enough omega-3s in your diet— and that's a guarantee on DTOUR—they can do some pretty amazing things for you. Some of the most exciting research currently under way is exploring the potential for omega-3s to help shrink your waistline.

Like all other fats—whether good or bad—omega-3s promote satiety, the feeling of contentment at the end of a meal that signals you've eaten your fill. (That's why most of us would scale a 10-foot fence if we knew a full-fat chocolate-chip cookie was waiting on the other side.)

Omega-3s may go one better, however. The results of a 2007 study published in the *American Journal of Clinical Nutrition* suggest that omega-3s may help burn body fat, shrink abdominal fat cells, and thwart certain genes that trigger inflammation in belly fat.

For this study, a team of French researchers assigned 27 women with type 2 diabetes to one of two groups. All of the women consumed a diet that provided 55 percent of calories as carbohydrates, 15 percent as protein, and 30 percent as fat. In addition, one group took 3 grams of omega-3s in supplement form every day, while the other group got a placebo.

FROM THE DTOUR DIETITIAN

You might have read that the omega-3 fats in fish oil are better for your heart than those from other food sources. What are the facts?

The omega-3 fats found in fish and marine mammals (EPA and DHA, mostly) consist of long molecular chains. They are more efficiently absorbed and used in the body than the short-chain omega-3s found in walnuts, hemp seed, and wild greens. Although the exact mechanism is unknown, the long-chain omega-3s have been shown to reduce arterial plaque, promote blood vessel dilation, lower triglyceride levels, and protect against heart disease. The FDA has even approved a prescription-only fish oil, called Lovaza, to lower triglycerides.

What about flax and flaxseed oil? Both provide beneficial alpha-linolenic acid (ALA), a short-chain omega-3 fatty acid. You can get your recommended daily amount of omega-3 fats from 1 tablespoon of ground flaxseed (1.8 grams).

Note that whole flaxseeds aren't particularly digestible; your best bet is to run them through a home coffee grinder, if you have one. Or buy flax meal instead; it's a good source of soluble fiber that can help lower blood cholesterol. Sprinkle it on oatmeal or in your morning smoothie for an added nutty taste and extra fiber.

Although some experts says flax is just fine at a cool room temperature, I prefer to store mine in the refrigerator or freezer. It can turn rancid when exposed to heat.

—Barbara

Over the next 2 months, the researchers tracked the women's blood sugar and insulin sensitivity, as well as their body weight, body mass index, and body fat percentage. The researchers also measured blood levels of certain substances that cause inflammation. (It's known that carrying excess body fat raises blood levels of these substances, while losing weight reduces their numbers and also improves insulin sensitivity.)

By the end of the study, women who took the omega-3 supplement had lost significantly more trunk fat—3 pounds of it, compared with less than ½ pound for those taking the placebo—yet their body weights remained the same. Moreover, their fat cells shrank by 6.2 percent, while the fat cells in the placebo group actually got bigger (by only 1.2 percent, but still!). Other markers, such as blood sugar and insulin sensitivity, remained about the same for both groups.

Another study, this one conducted by researchers at the University of Georgia in Athens, investigated the effect of DHA—which, you'll remember, is a specific type of omega-3—on immature fat cells. The researchers harvested these cells, called preadipocytes, from laboratory mice. They discovered that DHA—in amounts that we humans can get from foods and supplements—may prevent the formation of new fat cells and encourage existing fat cells to kill themselves (a process known as programmed cell death, or apoptosis).

In this study, DHA appeared to encourage fat cells to release their stores of fatty acids, which is what we mean when we talk about burning fat. The researchers concluded that if people consume more omega-3s, their reward might well be flatter bellies and a lower risk of overweight and metabolic syndrome.

OMEGA-3s ♥ DIABETIC HEARTS

Though few clinical studies have examined the direct impact of omega-3s on diabetes risk, other research offers convincing evidence of the potential benefits of these good fats for people with blood sugar issues. In particular, omega-3s may reduce insulin resistance and inflammation, raise good HDL cholesterol, lower triglycerides, and improve the function of the tissue that lines arteries. These cardiovascular effects are important, since heart disease is a common complication of diabetes.

For one study, researchers at the University of Western Australia and the West Australian Heart Research Institute in Perth randomly divided 63 people—all overweight and with high blood pressure—into four groups. The first group ate fish once a day, the second followed a calorie-restricted diet, the third combined the fish meal with the calorie-restricted diet, and the fourth continued their usual eating habits. Over the course of 4 months, the people in group 3—those following a calorie-restricted diet with fish—were best able to manage their blood sugar and blood cholesterol levels.

Later on, a research team from Kyoto, Japan, decided to investigate whether EPA—one of the two types of omega-3s—could lower levels of a particularly nasty

A BETTER OMEGA BALANCE

You need both kinds of essential fatty acids—omega-3s and omega-6s—to stay healthy. The problem is that most of us eat not nearly enough of the former and way too much of the latter.

Scientists believe that humans evolved on a diet of roughly equal proportions of omega-3s and omega-6s. Today, we get 10 to 20 times more omega-6s than our Stone Age ancestors. Those excess omega-6s come from vegetable oils, from the prepared and packaged foods made with those oils, and from animals and poultry raised on grains instead of grass.

These large amounts of omega-6s hinder the good work of omega-3s. The solution: Try to limit your omega-6 intake to no more than four times your omega-3 intake, or about 6 grams a day. On DTOUR,

the proper omega balance is built right in to the menus and recipes, so you needn't worry about counting grams. If you want to start working on your ratio now, here are four easy ways to get more omega-3s and fewer omega-6s:

◆ Avoid snacks and baked goods made with omega-6-rich vegetable oils, such as corn, cottonseed, safflower, and sunflower.
◆ Make or buy salad dressing with olive oil. Bottled dressings are made with soybean or canola oil.
◆ Use olive or canola oil for cooking and baking instead of corn, safflower, or sunflower oil.
◆ Look for margarine and mayonnaise made with canola oil. Many brands are made with oils that are high in omega-6s.

blood fat called small, dense low-density lipoprotein (sdLDL). For their study, the researchers recruited 44 men, all overweight and with type 2 diabetes. The men were divided into two groups, both of which followed a heart-healthy diet, but one group also took 1.8 grams of EPA daily.

In just 3 months, the men who were taking the EPA significantly reduced their levels of sdLDL. As a bonus, their levels of C-reactive protein (CRP) declined as

FROM THE DTOUR DIETITIAN

Trans fats appeared in our food supply more than 50 years ago when we thought it was a good idea to eat more plant sources of fats (like margarines made with partially hydrogenated vegetable oils) and fewer saturated fats (like butter). All was well until researchers discovered that trans fats produced from partially hydrogenated oils were linked to heart disease. Oops. Now food manufacturers are scrambling to remove trans fats from our food supply.

What's so hard about that? It's difficult, say some foodies, to find more healthful fats with favorable stability and cooking properties. Pure liquid vegetable oils, for example, are more likely to become rancid than those that are partially hydrogenated.

So why not just stick with butter, which is free of trans fats? We could. But butter is high in saturated fat, which is bad for our arteries, too.

Fortunately, food manufacturers have been tinkering with their product standards so that many of today's soft tub and liquid margarines are low in saturated fat and free of trans fats. What's more, it's easy to find this information on product labels, since both types of fats must be listed.

As trans fats make their exit, watch for other types of fats to start cropping up. Interesterified fats, for example, are free of trans fats yet have desirable cooking properties and stability. Be cautious, however: Some research has shown that interesterified fats may raise blood sugar.

And believe it or not, certain natural trans fats actually may be beneficial for our health. The conjugated linoleic acid (CLA) in meat and dairy, for example, is a naturally occurring trans fat that's being studied for its ability to reduce body fat and improve immune function.

For now, read labels and choose products with zero trans fats. Enjoy butter and other highly saturated fats in modest amounts. And fill your shopping basket with naturally low-fat staples—fresh fruits, vegetables, whole grains, beans, fish, poultry, lean meat, and low-fat dairy.

–Barbara

well. CRP, you'll remember, is considered a marker for chronic inflammation, which can damage the arterial lining and encourage clot formation. A growing body of research points to elevated CRP as a risk factor for metabolic syndrome and type 2 diabetes, in addition to heart disease.

For further evidence of the heart-healthy effects of omega-3s, we can turn to a 2008 University of Pittsburgh study involving more than 800 Japanese, Japanese American, and white American men. Now, Japanese men tend to smoke like chimneys, which is a major risk factor for heart disease. Still, they showed less severe atherosclerosis (narrowing of the arteries) than did their American-born counterparts. They also had double the blood levels of omega-3s. Their better heart health, the researchers concluded, probably stems from their lifelong consumption of fish, about 3½ ounces almost every day.

Not all studies have produced such glowing assessments of the omega-3s. One meta-analysis, which compiled and evaluated data from more than 20 studies, concluded that fish oil supplements could lower triglycerides. Unfortunately, they also appeared to raise LDL cholesterol, the bad kind that contributes to artery-clogging plaques. The increase wasn't significant, and the studies did use supplements rather than foods. Still, it shows that we have much to learn about what the omega-3s can do and—just as important—how they do it.

9 WAYS TO SNEAK IN MORE 3s

FYI

IN 2005, Americans ate 16.2 pounds of fish and shellfish per person.

The Diabetes DTOUR Diet is designed to satisfy your body's omega-3 needs—as well as your taste buds! Your daily dose is spread across each day's menu, so you'll get a little bit at every meal and snack.

To help ease you into the omega-3 habit, we've compiled a list of our favorite tips and techniques for taking advantage of these beneficial fats. Take them for a test-drive now, before you embark on DTOUR. They'll also serve as helpful guideposts while you're on the plan, helping you to stay the course while you're slimming down.

◆ Rebalance your dietary ratio of omega-3s to omega-6s. It's simple: As you increase your intake of omega-3-rich foods, cut way back on processed foods, refined grains, and supermarket cooking oils—the chief sources of omega-6s in the average diet.

◆ Munch a DTOUR salad every day—a potent combo of leafy greens and veggies dressed with walnut, canola, or flaxseed oil and a sprinkling of sesame seeds.

◆ Eat salmon or another type of cold-water fish two or three times a week. You'll get those beneficial omega-3s—and if the fish is replacing red meat in your diet, you'll probably be consuming less saturated fat.

◆ For lunch, help yourself to a tuna sandwich. Make your tuna with canola-oil mayo.

◆ Try tofu—really! Tofu and other products made with soybeans are good sources of omega-3s. You can always add tofu to stir-fries, but for variety, try pureeing it with peanut butter for a fluffy sandwich spread or blending soft tofu with a banana for a breakfast smoothie.

◆ Add 1½ tablespoons of ground flaxseed or 1 teaspoon of flaxseed oil to your diet every day. You can mix the seeds into low-fat cottage cheese or the oil into a smoothie.

◆ Use canola oil to cook and flaxseed oil for salad dressings. (Flaxseed oil breaks down when it's heated, so it's not good for cooking.)

RECOMMENDED DAILY INTAKES OF OMEGA-3 FATS

Currently, there are no formal government guidelines regarding daily intake of the omega-3 fats. The following recommendations come from the American Heart Association, so bear in mind that they're geared toward heart disease prevention and treatment. Incidentally, the DTOUR menus and recipes meet or exceed the dosage at every level.

IF YOU HAVE . . .	TAKE THIS
Diabetes without known coronary heart disease (CHD)	At least 0.5 g per day each of EPA and DHA, plus 1 g per day of ALA. To meet these goals, eat fish (preferably fatty fish) at least twice a week and consume oils and foods rich in ALA, such as flaxseed, canola, and soybean oils; ground flaxseed; and walnuts.
Known CHD	1 g of EPA and DHA daily, preferably as fatty fish
High triglycerides	2–4 g of EPA and DHA daily in capsule form (with your doctor's consent)

◆ Eat walnuts. As nuts go, they're the only kind rich in omega-3s. They may be good for the heart, too. When researchers in Spain asked a group of volunteers to eat 8 to 13 walnuts a day in tandem with a heart-healthy diet, this group showed 64 percent stronger artery-pumping action and 20 percent fewer of the gunky molecules that lead to atherosclerotic plaque than did a control group who followed the heart-healthy diet but skipped the nuts.

◆ Consider switching to eggs enriched with omega-3s. Many producers now add sources of omega-3 fats such as flaxseed and canola oil to the hens' feed to increase the healthy fats in their eggs. Look for cartons that carry the USDA-certified label; these eggs have been inspected, so you can feel confident that their claims (such as "omega-3 enhanced") are legit.

FOOD SOURCES OF ALA

You can boost your daily intake of omega-3s by consuming more ALA, which your body converts to omega-3s. Among the best sources:

FOOD	ALA
Flaxseed oil, 1 Tbsp	6.6 g
Ground flaxseed, 2 Tbsp	3.2 g
Canola oil, 1 Tbsp	1.6 g
Walnut oil, 1 Tbsp	1.4 g
Soybeans, cooked, 1 c	1.1 g
Soybean oil, 1 Tbsp	1.0 g
Walnuts, 2 Tbsp	1.0 g
Firm tofu, ½ c	0.7 g

Checkpoint

Before you embark on DTOUR, you'll need to decide on your goal weight. The wrong way to arrive at that magic number? Just pluck it out of the sky. For example, you want to weigh what Kelly Ripa weighs. Or what you weighed in high school. Or what you weighed for about 36 hours at the height of a nasty bout of the flu.

The right way to arrive at your goal weight: Use body mass index (BMI) and waist size.

While not perfect, BMI is the tool of choice among weight-loss experts. To calculate your BMI, divide your weight by your height in inches squared. Then multiply that number by 703. (Or go to the BMI calculator under the Weight Loss tab at www.prevention.com; we'll do the math for you.) Here's how to interpret your result.

IF YOUR BMI IS . . . 30 OR ABOVE
Sane solution: Aim to lose 10 percent of your body weight.
◆ If you currently weigh 190 pounds, that means a 19-pound weight loss. You'll drop a few sizes and lower your disease risk in the process. For safe and healthy weight loss, try not to exceed 2 pounds per week.
◆ If you can maintain that for at least a month, then set another 10 percent goal. Continue this step-by-step approach until you're satisfied with your weight or your BMI drops below 30.

IF YOUR BMI IS . . . 25 TO 29.9
Sane solution: Measure your middle.
◆ Evidence suggests that where you carry that extra weight is more important than how much you lug around. Belly fat is the most dangerous. A waist measurement that exceeds 35 inches for women or 40 inches for men means too much belly fat—a risk factor for metabolic syndrome, diabetes, and heart disease. If you're in the danger zone, try to lose 5 to 10 percent of your body weight and also shrink your waistline. (The DTOUR Workout can help.)
◆ If your waist is less than 35 inches, your biggest health benefit will come from exercising and maintaining your current weight.

IF YOUR BMI IS . . . BELOW 25
Sane solution: Check your waistline.
◆ Slim folks can have too much belly fat, too. If you do, your goal should be regular exercise, not weight loss.

DTOUR WINNER!

Thomas Colbaugh, 54
POUNDS LOST: 21
INCHES LOST: 3
BLOOD SUGAR:
DROPPED 78 POINTS

BEFORE

AFTER

I've always been active. I played baseball and football in high school and football in college. I've been a ski instructor for 17 years. I also run a sustainable poultry farm with my partner, Jean. (See Jean's story on page 54.)

I'm in my midfifties now, and I'm not as active as I was in my youth. But until DTOUR, I still ate like a football player. Not surprisingly, I gained weight. I'd been diagnosed with diabetes almost 20 years before I met Jean, and I started taking oral medication to manage it at about the same time I met her.

My father had diabetes, and it cost him his life. Before that, it also cost him one of his limbs and his ability to enjoy an activity he loved, golf. I also love golf, but my extra weight had affected my game. I had to use a golf cart, but I wanted to walk because that's the way the game should be played.

When Jean asked me if I wanted to do the DTOUR plan together, I agreed. We were both overweight. For us, it wasn't so much that we ate unhealthy foods. Mostly, we just ate too much healthy stuff. Portions were a problem, and I ate way too many sweets.

The plan wasn't hard. In fact, it was pretty easy, because the menu is laid out for you. I did substitute plain yogurt for the milk; I tend to overdo it on milk, which puts weight on me, so I stick to yogurt.

I lost 5 pounds the 1st week. By the end of the 2nd week, I'd lost 14. My blood sugar was falling after the 3rd day. The day before we started DTOUR, my fasting blood sugar was 135. Today, at our final check-in, it was 57.

I'm working to cut back on my meds, and another adjustment is obviously due. I take two oral diabetes medications, metformin and gliperide, that increase my appetite. But losing weight helped me reduce my dosage. Before DTOUR, I was taking eight pills a day. Now I take two, and according to this morning's test, even that's too much. Fewer meds means I'm less hungry now. I look forward to getting off medication completely.

I sleep well and wake up revved and ready to go. It definitely helped that I was following the plan with Jean. We have a great relationship and want to stay together for a good long time.

My golf game's improved, too. I recently played at Bethpage Black, a course on Long Island, New York, that hosted the US Open in 2002. I wouldn't have been able to play had I still been carrying that extra 21 pounds on me, since you have to walk the course and it's up and down hills. I'd like to lose 20 or 30 more pounds. It will take longer than it did when we first started, but that's because I've lost so much weight already.

BLOOD SUGAR: DOWN 78 POINTS!

PART 3

HIT THE ROAD: START LOSING

YOU'RE EAGER to start DTOUR, aren't you? Then let's get to it! First, we'll go over some basics of the plan. Then we'll move on to the 2-Week Fast Start, when you can expect to lose up to 13 pounds and start whittling away at your blood sugar, too—just by eating tasty, satisfying food. How fabulous is that?

CHAPTER

7

(HOW TO)
GET ON
DTOUR!

We've talked about why losing weight is your number one strategy for reining in wayward blood sugar, and how the nutritional muscle of our Fat-Fighting 4 can wrestle into submission even the most stubborn pounds. That brings us to the *what* of DTOUR—the 6-week plan that will get you on the road to a trim and fit physique while leaving high blood sugar far behind.

Actually, DTOUR is two plans in one. On the 2-Week Fast Start, you'll get in the swing of eating DTOUR-style with detailed daily menus that make the most of the Fat-Fighting 4. With five meals and snacks a day, you'll never feel like you're dieting! But the scale will tell a different story: Depending on your starting weight, you can lose up to 13 pounds in these first 2 weeks. (Our test panelists Kris, Randy, and Tom are living proof!)

After the 2-Week Fast Start, you'll shift into cruise control with our 4-Week Total Transformation. You'll continue eating five times a day, only now you'll be going freestyle—choosing from among a tempting array of meal and snack options to build your own daily menus. You'll add an easy walking routine, plus strength-training moves that will combine to ramp up your body's fat-burning power. And you'll take steps to improve your sleep habits and manage stress—both of which are vital to weight loss and blood sugar control. But this phase of DTOUR—like the 2-Week Fast Start—is all about the food!

So, what changes will you see at the end of 6 weeks? Again, it depends on where you're starting. In the 6 weeks that our eight test panelists followed DTOUR, they lost a grand total of just under 130 pounds and 40 inches. For almost all of our panelists, blood sugar remained stable or dropped measurably—in Randy's case, by an incredible 182 points!

You have a lot to look forward to over the next 6 weeks. (Did we mention the *food*?) Before you jump in, though, we want to acquaint you with the DTOUR How-Tos. These four simple, sensible rules form the foundation of our diet. In fact, once you finish the 6 weeks of DTOUR, the How-Tos can help ensure that your weight and blood sugar level remain healthy and stable. Stick with them, and they can keep you fit and vital for years to come.

DTOUR HOW-TO #1:
TRACK YOUR CALORIES

Notice we didn't say *count*. If you're a numbers type and counting calories helps you stay on track, by all means carry on. On the other hand, if—like many dieters—you consider this task only slightly more tolerable than having a root canal, then DTOUR is your diet dream come true. We've already done the calculations for you; all you need to do is eat!

Just remember this: Even if you don't count calories, calories still count. And if your objective is to lose weight, you need to burn more calories than you consume. It's that simple, and we all know it instinctively. Still, we need an occasional reminder that, at the end of the day, it's how any effective diet works.

Back in 1971, the average woman consumed 1,542 calories a day. Now it's more like 1,877 calories—an increase of 22 percent. This may seem reasonable, until we consider that only 19 percent of adults today are highly active. Translation: Very few of us are burning enough calories on a daily basis to compensate for the number going in. That's a surefire formula for gaining weight rather than losing.

So, you do want to keep an eye on your calorie intake. But guessing at a number can be a gamble. If you're off by even 100 calories a day, you can end up gaining between 6 and 10 pounds in a year. Experts say this is one reason why women in their forties today are about 25 pounds heavier than women of the same age back in 1960.

We're all different, and so are our calorie needs, which are based on age, gender, and activity level, among other factors. In general, though, both women and men can lose as much as 2 pounds a week by limiting their calories to no more than 1,600 calories a day.

On DTOUR, you have two calorie levels to choose

Stop Here

IF YOUR DINNER PLATES are extralarge, your hips may be, too. Downsize your plates to 8 or 9 inches in diameter. Research has shown that when people use smaller dinnerware and silverware, they automatically rein in their portions.

from: 1,400 and 1,600. If you're a relatively sedentary woman who's short in stature, the 1,400-calorie plan is about right for you. For women who are tall or physically active and for men, the 1,600-calorie plan is the better option. Just bear in mind that at the higher calorie level, you may occasionally need to dip a little lower if you want to speed up weight loss or break through a plateau.

Now, here's the best part: Once you've chosen your calorie level, DTOUR takes care of the rest! The 2-Week Fast Start is carefully structured to provide approximately the same number of calories per day, give or take a few. Once you graduate to the 4-Week Total Transformation, you get to choose your meals and snacks—but even as you mix and match, your daily calories will stay on track. How's that for easy?

USE YOUR BEAN, BEAT DIABETES

The government's latest dietary guidelines recommend eating 3 cups of beans each week. Follow these tips to pick the best beans of the bunch.

Buy canned—they're just as healthy. Dried beans need to be soaked and then boiled for hours before they're ready to eat. Who has time for that? Canned varieties, which are ready to eat, can be just as nutritious.

Don't eat beans (or any other food) from cans that are dented or bulging. Small dents and dings are okay, but if you find a badly dented or swollen can in your cupboard, or if a can spurts liquid when it's opened, don disposable gloves and toss out the contents and can (don't recycle it) right away. Unsure? Err on the side of caution and get rid of it anyway.

Go for low sodium. Low-sodium canned beans are exactly the same price as regular beans, but they have more than two-thirds less sodium. That's a decrease from about 720 milligrams per cup—almost a third of the daily max of 2,300 milligrams—to 220. Rinse beans in a colander under cold water for 1 minute to wash away another quarter of the sodium.

Beat the bloat, silence the toots. Before you dig in to a mess of beans, pop Beano tablets, or sip peppermint tea after.

DTOUR HOW-TO #2: PRACTICE PORTION CONTROL, SERIOUSLY!

Though you don't need to count calories on DTOUR, you will need to pay attention to your portion sizes. Different portion sizes of the same foods determine your calorie intake—and, frankly, they're often responsible for thwarting the best-laid weight-loss plans.

Before you begin DTOUR, you'll want to make sure that you have the following equipment on hand: measuring cups, a food scale, and a set of measuring spoons. In practice, it takes mere moments to weigh and measure your food. Those few seconds can determine whether you'll be slipping into your skinny jeans or squeezing into a bigger size.

Studies show just how easily portion distortion can lead to calorie overload. In one study conducted on 2 consecutive days over each of 3 weeks, Pennsylvania State University researchers asked 32 volunteers to choose as many food portions as they wanted. But the portion sizes changed: What were normal-size portions in week 1 became 50 percent larger by week 2 and doubled in size by week 3.

Compared with the 1st week of the study, women ate 335 more calories per day in the 2nd week and 530 more per day in the 3rd week. For men, the news wasn't any better: Compared with week 1, their calorie intakes increased by 504 and 812 calories per day in weeks 2 and 3, respectively.

At home, it's easy to practice portion control. Keep your measuring tools right on your kitchen counter and use them to measure the ingredients in your meals and snacks, as well as the actual serving sizes. Place the correct portion on your plate and leave the serving dishes on the counter. That way, you'll think twice before helping yourself to seconds!

Monitoring portions is a bit more challenging when

Stop Here

MANY PEOPLE MISTAKE THIRST for hunger, so stay hydrated to keep your metabolism in high gear. Options include water, sparkling water, herbal or black teas, coffee, and low-calorie beverages such as diet lemonade. Limit caffeinated drinks (coffee and diet colas) to no more than two a day. Since caffeine acts as a diuretic, it actually can leave you thirstier.

you eat out, but you can do it. (You have to! Who wants to cook every night?) You probably realize that, at many restaurants, one "serving" of anything—from appetizer to dessert—is more like two (or three, or four!). So, ask your server to bring you a to-go box along with your meal and wrap up half of your food to take home before you even dig in to the rest. In addition, the visual guide on page 99 can help you visualize proper portion sizes when your measuring tools aren't handy. Just make a photocopy and tuck it in your purse or wallet, then refer to it as you need to until you've perfected your eyeballing technique.

Once you've reached your goal weight, you might switch to measuring just grains (such as pasta and breakfast cereal) and fats (such as nuts, oils, and salad dressings). Few people gain weight by eating lots of low-calorie, nutrient-dense fruits and vegetables. Grains and fats, though, can blow your calorie budget quickly. Get lax about their portions and you could add hundreds of calories to your daily intake. An extra ⅓ cup of berries or broccoli is far less risky—and besides, their high fiber content makes eating too much of them far less likely.

DTOUR HOW-TO #3: FEAST ON THE FAT-FIGHTING 4

On DTOUR, the majority of foods that you'll weigh and measure are *whole foods*. In other words, they're in or close to their natural state, with nothing added—no sugars, fats, or artificial anything. Oatmeal and strawberries are whole foods; cream-filled oatmeal pies and strawberry toaster pastries are not.

Whole foods also happen to be the best sources of our Fat-Fighting 4. Stick with the DTOUR menus and recipes and you're sure to get at least—if not more than—the recommended daily intake of each of these supernutrients. Here's a snapshot of how they'll help you achieve your weight-loss and blood sugar goals; for more detailed descriptions, turn back to Part 2.

Fiber. All whole foods are high in fiber, which satisfies your hunger, helps reduce the number of calories absorbed by your body, and keeps your blood sugar from skyrocketing after a meal. Along with fruits, veggies, and whole grains, don't overlook another outstanding fiber source: beans. Red or black, pink or speckled, dry or canned, beans are nutritional gems. One cup of cooked beans provides a whopping 13 grams of fiber and 15 grams of protein, with zero saturated fat. They also offer respectable doses of calcium and another diabetes fighter, magnesium.

According to the 2006 National Health and Nutrition Examination Survey, adults who regularly ate beans weighed 6.6 pounds less than those who didn't, even though they ate 199 calories *more* daily. They also had smaller waistlines, consumed less total and saturated fat, and were 22 percent less likely to become obese.

Calcium and vitamin D. Whether you choose fat-free milk or a soy beverage, low-fat yogurt or reduced-fat cheese, the calcium and vitamin D you'll be getting are sure to put you on the fast track to weight loss. In a study that appeared in the *Journal of the American Dietetic Association,* nutritionists at Northern Illinois University put 14 women on a reduced-calorie diet that included 3 cups of either fat-free milk or soy milk daily. All of the women got the same number of calories and the same amounts of protein, fat, calcium, and vitamin D. After 8 weeks, both groups had lost about the same number of pounds and the same percentage of body fat. They had also shrunk their bellies by the same number of inches.

On DTOUR, you'll easily take in about 1,200 milligrams of calcium and about 155 IU of vitamin D every day from a variety of sources—not just dairy. If you choose soy milk, make sure it's fortified with at least 30 percent of the Daily Value of calcium per serving. Since the Daily Value of calcium is 1,000 milligrams, a serving of soy milk should supply roughly 300 milligrams.

Omega-3 fatty acids. Put fish on your dish—along with walnuts, flaxseed, and tofu. Research from Spain suggests that it's easier to stay slim when you're consuming omega-3s and monounsaturated fats. In contrast, the omega-6 fats (prevalent in corn oil and baked goods) cause the ab fat to pile on.

Incidentally, when you follow DTOUR, you'll automatically limit your intake of trans fats. These bad-for-you fats, which are found mostly in processed foods and bakery products, have no redeeming nutritional value.

FYI

SEVENTY-EIGHT PERCENT of successful losers sit down to breakfast every day. That's according to the National Weight Control Registry, a database of more than 5,000 people who've lost more than 30 pounds and kept it off for at least a year.

DTOUR HOW-TO #4: EAT EVERY 3 HOURS

If you're accustomed to the standard three square meals a day, DTOUR will ask you to up the ante. Our menus provide for three meals and two snacks every day, each containing a mix of complex carbs, lean protein, and beneficial fats, plus a healthy dose of each of the Fat-Fighting 4.

When you eat smaller meals more often, your blood sugar stays on an even keel, which in turn helps tame hunger and control weight. Studies have shown that even among people with essentially the same caloric intakes, those who eat fewer times per day are likely to weigh more.

We don't need to tell you what happens when you wait too long to eat. Your blood sugar plummets, and so does your ability to make healthful choices. When researchers in the United Kingdom asked workers to choose a snack just after lunch, 70 percent picked foods like candy bars and potato chips. That percentage shot up to 92 percent when workers chose snacks in the late afternoon. It's no surprise, really. At that hour, their blood sugar probably was plummeting, prompting cravings and an urge for quick energy.

Small, frequent meals also keep your metabolism humming. You can think of your metabolism as a wood-burning fire: If you don't stoke the flames and add wood at regular intervals, it eventually goes out. The same is true for your body. Stoke it with nutritious fuel every few hours and you'll keep your metabolism elevated, your blood sugar stable, and your body operating at its peak.

There is one corollary to DTOUR's five-meals-and-snacks-a-day rule, and it's this: *You must eat breakfast.* It really is the most important meal of the day, especially if you want to lose weight. When you skip your morning meal, you may crave more high-calorie foods later in the day. As a result, you may eat more throughout the day than you would otherwise.

Research supports the breakfast-and-weight-loss connection. One recent study published in the *British Journal of Nutrition* tracked the diets of nearly 900 adults. It concluded that when people ate more carbohydrates, protein, and fat in the morning, they stayed satisfied and ate less over the course of the day than those who ate their bigger meals later on. Can't stomach an early breakfast? Then wait until 9:00, 10:00, or even 11:00 a.m. It still will keep you from overeating.

A final note: While it's important for everyone to eat approximately every 3 hours throughout the day, it's especially so if you're on diabetes medication. Waiting more than 5 hours between meals, or skipping a meal entirely, can cause your blood sugar to plunge.

DEAR (FOOD) DIARY

Though DTOUR spells out your daily menus and meal and snack options, we've also included space for you to write down what you eat every day. That's because research shows that keeping a food diary can increase—even double—weight loss.

For one study, researchers at Kaiser Permanente's Center for Health Research asked 1,685 volunteers to attend 20 weekly group sessions led by nutritionists and behavioral counselors. At the sessions, the participants were encouraged to consume about 500 fewer calories a day, eat plenty of fruits and vegetables, and engage in moderate-intensity exercise for 180 minutes (3 hours) a week. They also were asked to keep records of their daily food intake and physical activity. Those who kept a food diary on 6 or more days a week lost an average of 18 pounds in 6 months, compared with an average of 9 pounds for those who chose not to track their eating and exercise habits.

You may prefer to write in a separate notebook or journal or to type your notes on the computer (which you can do at www.dtour.com). Feel free to use whatever method works best for you. If you're creating your own format, you might want to include the following information along with what you eat and drink and how much (in either calories or number and sizes of portions):

◆ **When:** the time of day you ate
◆ **Where:** at the refrigerator, in your car, in bed, etc.
◆ **What you were doing:** driving, watching TV, etc.
◆ **How you felt:** your mood before, during, and after eating

If you've never kept a food diary before, these tips can help.

◆ Record your food intake when you eat, rather than saving the task for the end of the day. It's hard to recall what you had for breakfast, and how much, at 9 o'clock at night.
◆ Write down everything—even the five jellybeans from your co-worker's candy dish, the cheese sample at the super- market, and the handful of french fries from your spouse's burger basket.
◆ Tailor your diary to your unique food challenges. For example, if you tend to eat mindlessly, focus on weighing and measuring portions. If you're an emotional eater, record your moods and try to connect them to your eating patterns.

PERFECT PORTIONS: YOUR CHEAT SHEET

Knowing what to eat is half the battle. But to lose weight and manage your blood sugar, you need to know how much to eat, too. The list below provides the correct serving sizes for the top food sources of the Fat-Fighting 4.

CALCIUM AND VITAMIN D

Cheese, light or nonfat, 1 ounce	Low-fat cottage cheese, $\frac{1}{2}$ cup	calcium and Vitamin D, 8 ounces	Yogurt, flavored light fat-free or low-fat, 6 ounces ($\frac{2}{3}$ cup)
Fat-free milk, 8 ounces	Low-fat milk (skim or 1%), 8 ounces	Yogurt, fat-free plain, 8 ounces (1 cup)	
Fat-free ricotta cheese, $\frac{1}{3}$ cup	Low-fat soy or rice milk fortified with		

FIBER

Beans and Legumes (Serving size = $\frac{1}{2}$ cup cooked)

Black beans	Garbanzo beans (chickpeas)	Lentils	Navy beans
Dried peas	Kidney beans	Lima beans	Pinto beans

Fruits

Apple, pear (1 whole small or medium fruit)	Banana ($\frac{1}{2}$)	Canned, cooked, chopped fruit ($\frac{1}{2}$ cup)	Citrus fruits (1 whole small or medium fruit)
	Berries ($\frac{1}{2}$ cup)		

Soy products (Serving size = $\frac{1}{2}$ cup cooked)

Miso	Soybeans	Tempeh	Tofu

Starchy vegetables (Serving size = $\frac{1}{2}$ cup unless otherwise noted)

Corn	Peas	Sweet potato or yam, baked, plain, 1 small or $\frac{1}{2}$ large	Sweet potato or yam, plain, mashed
Lima beans	Potato, baked, 1 small or $\frac{1}{2}$ large		

Vegetables (Serving size = 1 cup raw, $\frac{1}{2}$ cup cooked

Artichoke	Carrots	Green peppers	Spinach
Asparagus	Cauliflower	Lettuce	Squash
Broccoli	Celery	Mushrooms	Tomato
Brussels sprouts	Cucumber	Onions	Zucchini
Cabbage	Green beans	Pumpkin	

Whole grains (Serving size = ¹/₂ cup cooked)

Barley	Oatmeal	Rice, brown or wild (¹/₃ cup)	Spelt
Buckwheat	Quinoa	Rye	Whole wheat
Millet			Whole wheat pasta

Whole grain products

Bread, 1 slice	Cereal, cooked, ¹/₂ cup	English muffin, ¹/₂	Rice cakes, 2
Bread, reduced-calorie, 2 slices	Cereal, ready to eat, 1 ounce	Pita or wrap, ¹/₂ of 8-inch diameter	Tortilla, 6-inch diameter

OMEGA-3 FATTY ACIDS

Fish Serving size = 3 ounces cooked

Catfish	Haddock	Shellfish (shrimp, crab, lobster)	Tuna
	Salmon		

Plants

Canola oil, 1 tablespoon	Nuts: almonds, peanuts, walnut halves, 1 ounce	Olive oil, 1 tablespoon	Seeds: pumpkin, sesame, sunflower, ¹/₂ ounce
Flaxseed, 1 tablespoon		Safflower oil, 1 tablespoon	

HANDY PORTION CONTROL

Feel sheepish about carrying your measuring cups and spoons into your favorite restaurant? Well, we do, too. So here's the next best thing: a (literally) handy guide to estimating portion sizes.

HAND	EQUIVALENT	FOODS	CALORIES
Fist	1 c	Rice	200
		Pasta	75
		Fruit	40
Palm	3 oz	Meat	160
		Fish	160
		Poultry	1601
Handful	1 oz	Nuts	170
		Raisins	85
2 handfuls	1 oz	Chips	150
		Popcorn	120
		Pretzels	100
Thumb	1 oz	Peanut butter	170
		Hard cheese	100
Thumb tip	1 tsp	Cooking oil	40
		Mayonnaise	35
		Butter	35
		Sugar	15

DTOUR WINNER!

Scott Newhard, 38
POUNDS LOST: 16
INCHES LOST: 5½
BLOOD SUGAR:
DROPPED 14 POINTS

BEFORE

AFTER

I don't have a family history of diabetes. What I do have is a history of traditional Pennsylvania Dutch cooking. Both sides of my family were raised on farms and ate lots of red meat, butter, and lard, in big portions.

I don't work on a farm; I work in an office. So does my wife. Although she wasn't overweight, I certainly was. I was eating way too much, and I had no idea what a sensible portion looked like. If I didn't eat every 5 to 6 hours, I got shaky. My wife suggested that I give DTOUR a try, and I agreed.

I bought a food scale, shopped for the foods on the menus, and prepared my own lunches (my wife cooked dinner). The menus were tasty, and I liked the variety. I also discovered that I like cottage cheese, which I'd never had before. The 1st day was rough; I was very hungry toward the end of the day. I also craved sugar for the 1st week. I love sweets!

But by the 2nd day, the hunger was gone. So were the cravings for sweets by the end of the 1st week. My office has a communal candy jar, and I hit it just once in the entire 6 weeks of the test plan. My colleagues were very supportive. They put the candy jar in someone's cubicle so I didn't see it.

I got serious about exercise, too. I'd worked out before DTOUR, but off and on, maybe a couple of times a week. This time, I walked on my treadmill and lifted weights 6 days a week.

When I started the program, my fasting blood sugar was 91. This morning, at our final check-in, it was 77. I eat every few hours, instead of one big meal at the end of the day like I used to, and I think that's really helped a lot. I've always had a lot of energy, but I feel lighter and healthier, and the shakiness is gone. I used to have highs and lows, peaks and valleys. Now I feel phenomenal.

I plan to have a few beers this weekend, a few wings, and then go back to following the plan and watching my portions. My goal weight is 170 pounds. I can't stress the importance of portion sizes enough. My wife and my two young sons are eating healthier food and smaller portion sizes, and they're getting outside to play more often. It's my goal to stay healthy a long time so I can keep up with my boys—and DTOUR has really shown me how I can do that.

LOST
16
POUNDS!

8

THE 2-WEEK FAST START

At last—the moment you've been waiting for! You're about to take your first steps on the road to a healthy weight, balanced blood sugar, and your best health ever. We're confident that DTOUR will help you succeed beyond your wildest expectations. You're going to love the changes you see and feel. And they start right here, right now!

For the next 2 weeks, we've made eating healthfully as effortless as possible. Every day of the Fast Start features a complete menu of our Awesome 4some meals and snacks. Preparation is a breeze; every recipe equals one serving, so you just need to measure or count the ingredients.

There's a reason we've done all the legwork for you. We know how challenging changing habits can be. And chances are that DTOUR is a whole new way of eating for you. So, we want you to use the next 2 weeks to acclimate to the components of the DTOUR diet. Not obsess over them, but rather just pay attention to them—the food choices, the portion sizes, the meal frequency. Over time, they will become second nature to you. That's important, because eating DTOUR-style isn't just for the next 6 weeks, it's for life.

But the Fast Start is much more than a dress rehearsal for what's to come. It produces results on its own. Based on our DTOUR test panel, you can expect to lose up to 13 pounds over the next 2 weeks. *Thirteen pounds!* Our panelists also lost up to 4 inches off their waists, while their blood sugar remained stable or began a steady decline. And these are just the measurable changes. Down to the person, our test panel told us how much better they felt—with more energy, less mental fog, and fewer mood shifts than they'd experienced pre-DTOUR. That's what balancing your blood sugar can do for you!

Your own results will depend on where you're starting from and how closely you follow the Fast Start. But, given our panelists' incredible outcomes, aren't you ready to give our plan a try?

A QUICK TOUR OF THE FAST START

In addition to the menus, each day of the Fast Start consists of three sections: "How Did You Do?", "Balance Your Blood Sugar," and "Succeed All Day." We've also provided space for you to note your weight and your waist measurement on certain days. Here's how you can use the pages ahead as your road map for the next 2 weeks. (Remember, too, that you can do your tracking electronically at www.dtour.com.)

"How Did You Do?" We encourage you to take these each day to reflect on how the Fast Start is working for you. You might write about how you mastered a craving, why you fell prey to a jelly doughnut at work, or what helped you keep the lid on the cookie jar after an unpleasant phone call. It's important to celebrate every victory—even the small ones!—and to acknowledge any lessons learned.

Measure Yourself. You'll see this section just twice during the Fast Start—on Day 1 and again on Day 8. It's intended to help you track your progress by noting changes in your weight and your waist measurement. In general, we recommend weighing yourself once a week and measuring your waist once a month. Make sure you do your weigh-ins at about the same time on the appointed days, because the number you see on the scale goes up and down over the course of the day. (For a refresher on how to get the most accurate waist measurement, see page 30.)

Balance Your Blood Sugar. If you have diabetes, you can use this section to record up to five blood sugar readings a day. (Your doctor can tell you how often you should be checking your blood sugar.) As you progress on DTOUR, you're bound to see these numbers improve.

Succeed All Day. In this section, you'll find a selection of tips and techniques that can help you stay on course toward your weight-loss goal. You needn't try every one; read through them and choose one or two that appeal to you. Each is proof that even the smallest steps can make a big difference in your weight-loss efforts.

A WORD ABOUT THE MENUS

For ease of use, we've broken out the 1,400- and 1,600-calorie plans into separate menus for each day. Really, though, they aren't all that different. On either plan, you'll be getting approximately 40 percent of your calories from carbohydrates, 25 percent from protein, and 35 percent from fat. Saturated fat—the bad-for-you kind—accounts for no more than 7 percent of your total caloric intake.

Whichever calorie level you choose, you're sure to get your daily fix of the Fat-Fighting 4. On the 1,400-calorie plan, our Awesome 4some meals and snacks deliver about 26 grams of fiber, 1,200 milligrams of calcium, 144 IU of vitamin D, and 2.5 grams of omega-3s per day. These numbers change slightly for the 1,600-calorie plan, which averages 29 grams of fiber, 1,200 milligrams of calcium, 165 IU of vitamin D, and 2.7 grams of omega-3s per day.

To get the best results from the Fast Start, you'll want to follow these few simple rules.

Pick the right plan. Women who are short in stature or who have been fairly sedentary should go with the 1,400-calorie plan. The 1,600-calorie plan is best for women who are tall or very active and for men of all builds and fitness levels. Another option is to try the 1,600-calorie plan for 1 week. If you lose weight, stick with it; if not, switch plans.

Follow the menus exactly. We've designed all of the DTOUR menus to ensure that you're eating about every 3 hours—which will keep your tummy happy and your blood sugar steady—and that you're getting the maximum benefit from the Fat-Fighting 4. Portion sizes are critical. Use your measuring tools throughout the Fast Start; before you know it, you'll be able to eyeball proper portions.

Choose the best ingredients for your Awesome 4some meals and snacks.

◆ Each day, you'll fill up on fiber-rich whole foods. Fresh fruits and veggies are preferable, but frozen fruits (without added sugar) and veggies (without butter or sauces) contain as much fiber and nutrients as fresh. For salads, we recommend dark, leafy greens (romaine, spinach leaves), which contain more nutrients than iceberg lettuce, but use whatever type you prefer.

◆ For these 2 weeks, use a scale to weigh fruit to get an idea of what a serving looks like.

◆ Select no-sugar-added, fat-free or low-fat yogurts that contain no more than 100 calories and no more than 15 grams of total carbohydrates per serving. Look for brands enriched with vitamin D (not all are).

◆ Opt for fat-free milk or low-fat soy or rice beverage fortified with calcium and vitamin D.

◆ Opt for soft tub or liquid margarines with zero grams of trans fats and no more than 1 gram of saturated fat per serving.

◆ If you use canned beans, rinse them thoroughly to remove as much sodium as possible.

◆ It's fine to enjoy your cup of coffee or tea at breakfast. Black is best, but you can add a sprinkle of sugar-free sweetener and a splash of fat-free milk or low-fat soy or rice beverage if you like.

◆ You may have sparkling water or reduced-calorie beverages (diet lemonade, for example), as long as they contain no more than 20 calories per serving.

◆ For light ice cream, look for products that provide no more than 2 grams of saturated fat and no more than 20 grams of total carbohydrate per serving.

Now, let's get started!

DAY 1

1,400 CALORIES

BREAKFAST

☐ Veggie omelet: Heat 1 teaspoon canola, peanut, or olive oil in a skillet. Add ¼ cup egg substitute (or 1 egg white); ½ cup spinach leaves; ½ cup chopped mushrooms; and as much onion, garlic, and herbs as desired. Cook over low heat until set. Top with ¼ cup reduced-fat cheese.

☐ ½ cup fat-free milk or low-fat, calcium-enriched soy or rice beverage

☐ 1 slice reduced-calorie whole grain toast spread with 1 teaspoon trans-free canola margarine

LUNCH

☐ Tuna sandwich: Mix 2 ounces water-packed tuna with 2 tablespoons reduced-fat mayonnaise (or 2 teaspoons regular mayonnaise). Spread on 1 slice whole grain bread *or* 2 slices reduced-calorie whole grain bread. Top with green or red leaf lettuce; 1 small tomato (½ cup), sliced; and 4 large black olives, chopped.

SNACK

☐ 8 ounces (1 cup) fat-free plain yogurt *or* 6 ounces (⅔ cup) no-sugar-added, fat-free or low-fat flavored yogurt, topped with ¾ cup fresh blueberries or blackberries

DINNER

☐ 3 ounces grilled chicken breast with garlic herb seasoning (such as Mrs. Dash)

☐ ⅔ cup cooked brown or wild rice

☐ 2 cups grilled or roasted vegetables (mushrooms, onions, zucchini, yellow squash, bell peppers) tossed with 2 teaspoons olive oil and salt-free herb seasoning to taste

SNACK

☐ 1 small apple (4 ounces), sliced, spread with 2 teaspoons peanut butter

1,600 CALORIES

BREAKFAST

☐ Veggie omelet: Heat 2 teaspoons canola, peanut, or olive oil in a skillet. Add ½ cup egg substitute (or 2 egg whites), ½ cup spinach leaves, ½ cup chopped mushrooms, 2 tablespoons chopped onion, 1 teaspoon chopped or minced garlic, and herbs as desired. Cook over low heat until set. Top with 2 tablespoons shredded reduced-fat cheese.

☐ 1 slice whole grain toast or 2 slices reduced-calorie whole grain toast spread with 1 teaspoon trans-free canola margarine

☐ 1 cup fat-free milk or low-fat, calcium-enriched soy or rice beverage

LUNCH

☐ Tuna sandwich: Mix 3 ounces water-packed tuna with 2 tablespoons reduced-fat mayonnaise (or 1 tablespoon regular mayonnaise). Spread on 1 slice whole grain bread *or* 2 slices reduced-calorie whole grain bread. Top with green or red leaf lettuce; 1 small tomato (½ cup), sliced; and 4 large black olives, chopped.

SNACK

☐ 8 ounces (1 cup) fat-free plain *or* 6 ounces (⅔ cup) no-sugar-added, fat-free or low-fat flavored yogurt, topped with ¾ cup fresh blueberries or blackberries and 1 tablespoon chopped walnuts

DINNER

☐ 3 ounces grilled chicken breast with garlic herb seasoning (such as Mrs. Dash)

☐ ⅔ cup cooked brown or wild rice

☐ 2 cups grilled or roasted vegetables (mushrooms, onions, zucchini, yellow squash, bell peppers) prepared in 1 tablespoon olive oil, sprinkled with Mrs. Dash or other salt-free herb seasoning

SNACK

☐ 1 small apple (4 ounces), sliced, spread with 2 teaspoons peanut butter

HOW DID YOU DO?

BALANCE YOUR BLOOD SUGAR

	TIME	READING
CHECK 1		
CHECK 2		
CHECK 3		
CHECK 4		
CHECK 5		

MEASURE YOURSELF

Starting weight: _____ pounds

Starting waistline: _____ inches

> Success is the sum of small efforts, repeated day in and day out.
> —ROBERT J. COLLIER

SUCCEED ALL DAY

To think before you binge, use the HALT technique. Before you scarf down that box of mini-doughnuts or plow through a bag of chips, ask yourself, "Do I want to eat this because I'm *h*ungry, *a*ngry, *l*onely, or *t*ired?" Often, simply knowing what's driving your urge to overeat can short-circuit it.

Take a "gratitude break." Tick off one thing or person you're grateful to have in your life. Are you grateful that the sun is shining after days of rain? Duck out of the office to soak up the sunshine. Do you appreciate your supportive spouse? Send an e-mail to say so—and don't forget to say why.

1,400 CALORIES

BREAKFAST

☐ 1 cup cooked oatmeal topped with 2 tablespoons walnut halves (about 8) and ½ teaspoon ground cinnamon and/or 1 teaspoon sugar substitute

☐ ½ cup fat-free milk or low-fat, calcium-enriched soy or rice beverage

LUNCH

☐ Chicken salad: Mix 2 cups mixed greens, ½ cup chopped tomato, ½ cup sliced cucumber, and ¼ cup chopped carrot. Top with 2 ounces chicken breast. Drizzle with avocado yogurt dressing (¼ cup mashed avocado, ½ cup fat-free plain yogurt, and vinegar and/or herbs to taste).

☐ 1 ounce (2 slices) whole grain crispbread crackers

SNACK

☐ 1 ounce string cheese

☐ 1 small pear or other fruit (4 ounces)

DINNER

☐ 1 cup Progresso Healthy Classics or Campbell's Healthy Request canned beef barley soup

☐ Spinach salad: Toss 3 cups fresh spinach with 1 tablespoon each olive oil and balsamic vinegar dressing. Top with 2 tablespoons shredded reduced-fat mozzarella cheese.

☐ 1 slice whole grain bread or 2 slices reduced-calorie, high-fiber whole grain bread

SNACK

☐ 1 medium orange

☐ 3 tablespoons unsalted raw cashews (about 18)

1,600 CALORIES

BREAKFAST

☐ 1 cup cooked oatmeal topped with 3 tablespoons walnut halves (about 12) and cinnamon and/or sugar substitute to taste

☐ 1 cup fat-free milk or low-fat, calcium-enriched soy or rice beverage

LUNCH

☐ Chicken salad: Mix 2 cups mixed greens, ½ cup chopped tomato, ½ cup sliced cucumber, and ¼ cup chopped carrot. Top with 3 ounces chicken breast. Drizzle with avocado yogurt dressing (¼ cup mashed avocado, ½ cup fat-free plain yogurt, and vinegar and/or herbs to taste).

☐ 1 ounce (2 slices) whole grain crispbread crackers

☐ 2 tablespoons hummus

SNACK

☐ 1 ounce mozzarella string cheese

☐ 1 small pear or other fruit (4 ounces)

DINNER

☐ 1½ cups Progresso Healthy Classics or Campbell's Healthy Request canned beef barley soup

☐ Spinach salad: Toss 2 cups fresh spinach with 1 tablespoon each olive oil and balsamic vinegar dressing. Top with 2 tablespoons shredded reduced-fat mozzarella cheese.

☐ 1 slice whole grain bread or 2 slices reduced-calorie, high-fiber whole grain bread

SNACK

☐ 1 medium orange

☐ 2 tablespoons unsalted raw cashews (about 12)

HOW DID YOU DO?

BALANCE YOUR BLOOD SUGAR

	TIME	READING
CHECK 1		
CHECK 2		
CHECK 3		
CHECK 4		
CHECK 5		

The only way to discover the limits of the possible is to go beyond them into the impossible.
—ARTHUR C. CLARKE

SUCCEED ALL DAY

Go cold turkey on trigger foods. Can't have just one cheese curl or chocolate-chip cookie? Indulging a craving affects your brain the same way that thinking about cocaine affects an addict's brain. That surprising comparison comes from studies conducted by researchers at Brookhaven National Laboratory in Upton, New York, who scanned the brains of 12 people as they sampled their favorite foods. **Develop a bedtime routine.** Do the same thing every night before going to sleep. For example, take a warm bath and then read for 10 minutes before going to bed. Soon you'll connect these activities with sleeping, and doing them will help make you sleepy.

1,400 CALORIES

BREAKFAST

❒ Peanut butter banana toast: Spread 1 slice reduced-calorie whole grain toast with 2 tablespoons all-natural peanut butter and $\frac{1}{2}$ medium banana, sliced.

❒ $\frac{1}{2}$ cup fat-free milk or low-fat, calcium-enriched soy or rice beverage

LUNCH

❒ Mixed-Up Salad: Mix 2 cups vegetable greens, $\frac{3}{4}$ cup 1% cottage cheese, and $\frac{1}{2}$ cup mandarin orange slices with 2 tablespoons light Italian salad dressing. Top with 2 tablespoons chopped unsalted raw almonds (about 12) or walnut halves (about 8).

❒ 5 whole grain crackers (such as Triscuits)

SNACK

❒ 6 ounces no-sugar-added, fat-free or low-fat yogurt

❒ 2 tablespoons chopped walnuts

DINNER

❒ Grilled fish tacos: Tuck 1 ounce grilled salmon or other fish and $\frac{1}{2}$ cup shredded cabbage seasoned with rice vinegar into each of 2 corn tortillas. Top each with 1 tablespoon reduced-fat sour cream.

❒ Grilled or roasted vegetables: Marinate 2 cups eggplant, mushrooms, green beans, and onion in 2 tablespoons light Italian dressing. Grill or roast.

SNACK

❒ 2 tablespoons hummus

❒ 2 rye crisp crackers

1,600 CALORIES

BREAKFAST

❒ Peanut butter banana toast: Spread 1 slice reduced-calorie whole grain toast with 2 tablespoons all-natural peanut butter and $\frac{1}{2}$ medium banana, sliced.

❒ 1 cup fat-free milk or low-fat, calcium-enriched soy or rice beverage

LUNCH

❒ Mixed-Up Salad: Mix 2 cups vegetable greens, 1 cup 1% cottage cheese, and $\frac{1}{2}$ cup mandarin orange slices with 2 tablespoons light Italian dressing. Top with 2 tablespoons chopped unsalted raw almonds (about 12) or walnut halves (about 8).

❒ 5 whole-grain crackers (such as Triscuits)

SNACK

❒ 6 ounces no-sugar-added, fat-free or low-fat flavored yogurt

❒ 2 tablespoons raw walnut halves

DINNER

❒ Grilled fish tacos: Tuck $1\frac{1}{2}$ ounces grilled salmon or other fish and $\frac{1}{2}$ cup shredded cabbage seasoned with rice vinegar into each of 2 corn tortillas. Top each with 1 tablespoon reduced-fat sour cream.

❒ Grilled or roasted vegetables: Marinate 2 cups eggplant, mushrooms, green beans, and onion in 2 tablespoons light Italian dressing and 1 teaspoon olive oil. Grill or roast.

SNACK

❒ 2 tablespoons hummus

❒ 2 rye crisp crackers

HOW DID YOU DO?

BALANCE YOUR BLOOD SUGAR

	TIME	READING
CHECK 1		
CHECK 2		
CHECK 3		
CHECK 4		
CHECK 5		

The future belongs
to those who
believe in the beauty
of their dreams.
—ELEANOR ROOSEVELT

SUCCEED ALL DAY

Let loose with laughter—or tears. Both are stress melters. When you laugh, your muscles go limp and the knots unkink. Tears help cleanse the body of substances that accumulate in times of stress.

Turn in only when you're sleepy. If you can't fall asleep within 15 to 20 minutes, get up and leave your bedroom. Go into the living room and read until you're tired again. Or sit in a chair and think pleasant thoughts: a dream vacation or standing by a waterfall. This should help calm you so you can return to bed and sleep.

1,400 CALORIES

BREAKFAST

- ❐ 1 ounce (about 1 cup) flaxseed-enriched whole grain cereal

- ❐ 1 cup fat-free milk or low-fat, calcium-enriched soy or rice beverage

- ❐ 2 tablespoons unsalted raw almonds (about 17)

LUNCH

- ❐ Cheese quesadilla: Place 2 ounces reduced-fat cheese on 1 whole wheat tortilla. Fold tortilla in half and cook in small skillet over medium heat until cheese melts and tortilla is browned on both sides. (You can also microwave on medium power for 30 to 45 seconds.) Garnish with 1½ cups chopped lettuce and tomato, ¼ cup salsa, 2 tablespoons avocado, and 1 tablespoon reduced-fat sour cream.

SNACK

- ❐ 1 medium banana spread with 1 tablespoon all-natural peanut butter

DINNER

- ❐ 3 ounces oven-roasted beef or pork tenderloin

- ❐ 2 cups roasted vegetables (½ cup potato plus 1½ cups nonstarchy vegetables, such as green beans, bell peppers, eggplant, zucchini or yellow squash, onion, and garlic) tossed in 1 tablespoon olive oil and baked at 400°F for 30 to 40 minutes.

SNACK

- ❐ 2 whole grain fig cookies

- ❐ 1 cup fat-free milk or low-fat, calcium-enriched soy or rice beverage

1,600 CALORIES

BREAKFAST

- ❐ 1 ounce (about 1 cup) flaxseed-enriched whole grain cereal

- ❐ 1 cup fat-free milk or low-fat, calcium-enriched soy or rice beverage

- ❐ 3 tablespoons chopped almonds

LUNCH

- ❐ Cheese quesadilla: Place 1 ounce shredded chicken and 2 ounces reduced-fat cheese on two 6-inch or one 12-inch whole wheat tortilla. Fold tortilla in half and cook in small skillet over medium heat until cheese melts and tortilla is browned on both sides. (You can also microwave on medium power for 30 to 45 seconds.) Garnish with 2 cups chopped lettuce and tomato, ¼ cup salsa, 2 tablespoons avocado, and 1 tablespoon reduced-fat sour cream.

SNACK

- ❐ 1 medium banana spread with 1 tablespoon all-natural peanut butter

DINNER

- ❐ 3 ounces oven-roasted beef or pork tenderloin

- ❐ 2 cups roasted vegetables (½ cup potato plus 1½ cups nonstarchy vegetables, such as green beans, bell peppers, eggplant, zucchini or yellow squash, onion, and garlic) tossed in 1 tablespoon olive oil and baked at 400°F for 30 to 40 minutes.

SNACK

- ❐ 2 whole grain fig cookies

- ❐ 1 cup fat-free milk or low-fat, calcium-enriched soy or rice beverage

HOW DID YOU DO?

BALANCE YOUR BLOOD SUGAR

	TIME	READING
CHECK 1		
CHECK 2		
CHECK 3		
CHECK 4		
CHECK 5		

Our greatest glory
is not in never
falling, but in rising
every time we fall.
—CONFUCIUS

SUCCEED ALL DAY

Choose the right craving "cure." To defang a craving, identify your current emotion (e.g., bored, anxious, angry) and complete this sentence: "I feel _____ because of _____." Now, find an activity that releases that emotion. If you're stressed, for example, channel your nervous energy into cleaning out a closet or tackling yard work.

Try moving meditation. Qigong (chee-gung), an active Chinese meditation routine incorporating fluid, dancelike movements and controlled breathing, elicits the body's relaxation response, studies have found. Classes often are held at YMCAs, gyms, and community centers. Find a local instructor at the National Qigong Association's Web site, www.nqa.org.

1,400 CALORIES

BREAKFAST

❐ ½ whole grain bagel spread with
1 tablespoon low-fat cream cheese and
1 teaspoon 100 percent fruit spread

❐ 1 cup fat-free milk or low-fat, calcium-
enriched soy or rice beverage

LUNCH

❐ Taco No Taco Salad: Mix 2 ounces grilled
fish, chicken, or lean beef with ⅓ cup brown
rice and ½ cup cooked red, black, or pinto
beans. Top with 1 tablespoon shredded
reduced-fat cheese. Microwave on medium
power for 45 seconds. Top with ½ cup salsa
and 1 tablespoon reduced-fat sour cream.
Serve over 2 cups mixed lettuce greens.

SNACK

❐ ¼ cup walnuts or pecans mixed with
6 ounces low-fat plain yogurt or light yogurt
sweetened with noncalorie sweetener.
Sprinkle with ground cinnamon to taste.

DINNER

❐ 3 ounces grilled salmon

❐ ½ cup fruit salsa (chopped melon and
mango)

❐ 2 cups spinach leaves with 2 tablespoons
chopped unsalted raw pecans and ¾ cup
sliced red onion

❐ 1 tablespoon oil-and-vinegar dressing

❐ 1 cup fat-free milk or low-fat, calcium-
enriched soy or rice beverage

SNACK

❐ 1 ounce spreadable reduced-fat cheese

❐ 1 medium pear, sliced

1,600 CALORIES

BREAKFAST

❐ ½ whole grain bagel spread with
2 tablespoons natural peanut butter

❐ 1 cup fat-free milk or low-fat, calcium-
enriched soy or rice beverage

LUNCH

❐ Taco No Taco Salad: Mix 3 ounces grilled
fish, chicken, or lean beef with ⅓ cup brown
rice and ½ cup cooked red, black, or pinto
beans. Top with 2 tablespoons shredded
reduced-fat cheese. Microwave on medium
power for 45 seconds. Top with ½ cup salsa
and 2 tablespoons reduced-fat sour cream.
Serve over 2 cups mixed lettuce greens.

SNACK

❐ ¼ cup walnuts or pecans mixed with
6 ounces low-fat plain yogurt or light yogurt
sweetened with noncalorie sweetener.
Sprinkle with ground cinnamon to taste.

DINNER

❐ 3 ounces grilled salmon

❐ ½ cup fruit salsa (chopped melon and
mango)

❐ 2 cups spinach leaves with 2 tablespoons
chopped unsalted raw pecans and ¼ cup
sliced red onions

❐ 1 tablespoon oil-and-vinegar dressing or
2 tablespoons light Italian dressing

❐ 1 slice reduced-calorie, high-fiber bread

❐ 1 cup fat-free milk or low-fat, calcium-
enriched soy or rice beverage

SNACK

❐ 1 ounce spreadable reduced-fat cheese

❐ 1 medium pear, sliced

HOW DID YOU DO?

BALANCE YOUR BLOOD SUGAR

	TIME	READING
CHECK 1		
CHECK 2		
CHECK 3		
CHECK 4		
CHECK 5		

> Nothing great was ever achieved without enthusiasm.
> —RALPH WALDO EMERSON

SUCCEED ALL DAY

Practice safe cravings. Plan ways to enjoy craved foods in controlled portions. Order a slice of pizza instead of a whole pie, or share a piece of restaurant cheesecake with two friends.

Stub out the butts. Nicotine stimulates the nervous system and disturbs sleep. But if you're a habitual smoker who can't fall or stay asleep, insomnia is the least of your worries. Quit. Today. You'll help protect your health and sleep better, too. At the very least, avoid nicotine within 1 hour of bedtime.

DAY 6

1,400 CALORIES

BREAKFAST

❒ Super White Egg: Heat 1 teaspoon canola oil in a small skillet. Add 1 whole egg and then 1 egg white or ¼ cup egg substitute around the outside of the whole egg. Cook over low heat until set. Top with 2 tablespoons chopped tomato or salsa.

❒ 1 slice reduced-calorie, high-fiber whole grain toast spread with 1 teaspoon trans-free canola margarine

❒ 1 cup fat-free milk or low-fat, calcium-enriched soy or rice beverage

SNACK

❒ 6 ounces no-sugar-added, fat-free or low-fat flavored yogurt

❒ 4 dried apricot halves

LUNCH

❒ Pile 'Er High Turkey and Ham Sandwich: Pile 1 ounce *each* sliced ham, turkey, and low-fat cheese on 1 slice reduced-calorie, high-fiber whole wheat bread. Spread 1 additional slice bread with 1 tablespoon reduced-fat mayonnaise (or 1 teaspoon regular mayonnaise) and 1 tablespoon mustard, if desired. Top with ½ cup shredded romaine lettuce and ½ tomato, sliced.

❒ 8 baby carrots dipped in 1 tablespoon low-fat ranch dressing

DINNER

❒ Beef- or Chicken-Broccoli Stir-Fry: Stir-fry 4 ounces lean beef or chicken breast and 1 cup broccoli, 1 cup carrots, and ½ cup onion in 1 tablespoon olive oil and 2 tablespoons low-sodium teriyaki sauce. Serve over ⅓ cup cooked brown or wild rice.

SNACK

❒ 3 cups light microwave popcorn

❒ 16 ounces sugar-free seltzer water

1,600 CALORIES

BREAKFAST

❒ Super White Egg: Heat 1 tablespoon canola oil in a small skillet. Add 1 whole egg and then 1 egg white or ¼ cup egg substitute around the outside of the whole egg. Cook over low heat until set. Top with 2 tablespoons chopped tomato or salsa.

❒ 2 slices reduced-calorie, high-fiber whole grain toast spread with 1 teaspoon trans-free canola margarine

❒ 1 cup fat-free milk or low-fat, calcium-enriched soy or rice beverage

SNACK

❒ 6 ounces no-sugar-added, fat-free or low-fat flavored yogurt

❒ 4 dried apricot halves

LUNCH

❒ Pile 'Er High Turkey and Ham Sandwich: Pile 1 ounce sliced ham, 2 ounces sliced turkey, and 1 ounce sliced reduced-fat cheese on 1 slice reduced-calorie, high-fiber whole wheat bread. Spread 1 additional slice bread with 1 tablespoon reduced-fat mayonnaise (or 1 teaspoon regular mayonnaise) and 1 tablespoon mustard, if desired. Top with ½ cup shredded romaine lettuce and ½ tomato, sliced.

❒ 16 baby carrots dipped in 1 tablespoon low-fat ranch dressing

DINNER

❒ Beef- or Chicken-Broccoli Stir-Fry: Stir-fry 4 ounces lean beef or chicken breast and 2 cups broccoli, carrots, and onion in 1 tablespoon olive oil and 2 tablespoons low-sodium teriyaki sauce. Serve over ⅔ cup cooked brown or wild rice

SNACK

❒ 3 cups light microwave popcorn

❒ 16 ounces lemon-lime seltzer water

HOW DID YOU DO?

BALANCE YOUR BLOOD SUGAR

	TIME	READING
CHECK 1		
CHECK 2		
CHECK 3		
CHECK 4		
CHECK 5		

SUCCEED ALL DAY

Reach out a helping hand. Under stress, we tend to focus on ourselves. But helping someone else in distress—even if it's just running an elderly neighbor to the store—can help us put our own worries in perspective.

Move the TV out of your bedroom. Your spouse may grumble, but if you're a chronic late-night talk-show buff, go cold turkey. The bed and bedroom are for sleep and sex. That's it. No reading. No talking on the telephone. No worrying.

> First say to yourself
> what you would be;
> and then do what
> you have to do.
> —EPICTETUS

1,400 CALORIES

BREAKFAST

❒ 3 buckwheat or whole wheat pancakes (6" diameter) spread with 1 teaspoon trans-free canola margarine and 1 tablespoon 100 percent fruit spread *or* 2 tablespoons sugar-free syrup, if desired, and sprinkled with 1 tablespoon chopped walnuts

❒ 8 ounces fat-free milk or low-fat, calcium-enriched soy or rice beverage

LUNCH

❒ Chicken Caesar salad: Top 3 cups romaine lettuce with 2 ounces skinless cooked chicken and ½ cup mandarin oranges packed in juice or water, drained. Drizzle on 2 tablespoons light Caesar dressing and top with 1 tablespoon Parmesan cheese.

❒ 1 ounce whole grain crackers

SNACK

❒ 1 cup apple slices

❒ 2 tablespoons walnut halves

DINNER

❒ 4 ounces (3 ounces cooked) top sirloin, grilled or broiled

❒ ½ oven-baked potato (about 3 ounces): Preheat oven to 400°F. Slice potato lengthwise, drizzle cut side with 1 teaspoon olive oil, and bake with cut side down for 30 minutes or until brown.

❒ Garlic roasted asparagus: Toss 10 medium (5-7") asparagus spears or 1 cup cut asparagus in 1 teaspoon olive oil and chopped garlic to taste. Roast with the potato for 20 minutes.

SNACK

❒ 1 cup fat-free milk or low-fat, calcium-enriched soy or rice beverage

❒ 5 vanilla wafers or 3 graham cracker squares (1½ sheets)

1,600 CALORIES

BREAKFAST

❒ 4 buckwheat or whole wheat pancakes (6" diameter) spread with 1 teaspoon trans-free canola margarine and 1 tablespoon 100 percent fruit spread *or* 2 tablespoons sugar-free syrup, if desired, and sprinkled with 1 tablespoon chopped walnuts

❒ 8 ounces fat-free milk or low-fat, calcium-enriched soy or rice beverage

LUNCH

❒ Chicken Caesar salad: Top 3 cups romaine lettuce with 3 ounces skinless cooked chicken and ½ cup mandarin oranges packed in juice or water, drained. Drizzle on 2 tablespoons light Caesar dressing and top with 1 tablespoon Parmesan cheese.

❒ 1 ounce whole grain crackers

SNACK

❒ 1 cup apple slices

❒ ¼ cup walnut halves (about 16)

DINNER

❒ 4 ounces (3 ounces cooked) top sirloin, grilled or broiled

❒ 1 small oven-baked potato: Preheat oven to 400°F. Slice potato lengthwise, drizzle cut side with 1 teaspoon olive oil, and bake with cut side down for 30 minutes or until brown.

❒ Garlic roasted asparagus: Toss 10 medium (5-7") asparagus spears or 1 cup cut asparagus in 1 teaspoon olive oil and chopped garlic to taste. Roast with the potato for 20 minutes.

SNACK

❒ 1 cup fat-free milk or low-fat, calcium-enriched soy or rice beverage

❒ 5 vanilla wafers or 3 graham cracker squares

HOW DID YOU DO?

BALANCE YOUR BLOOD SUGAR

	TIME	READING
CHECK 1		
CHECK 2		
CHECK 3		
CHECK 4		
CHECK 5		

SUCCEED ALL DAY

Eliminate sensory cues. Smells, sights, and sounds are all powerful triggers. So whether you're, say, paying bills or reading the newspaper, be sure to station yourself far away from the kitchen and the cupboard full of snacks.

Recite the Serenity Prayer. This prayer is a time-tested way to get calm quick: "God, grant me the serenity to accept the things I cannot change, the courage to change the things I can, and the wisdom to know the difference."

If you let your fear of consequence prevent you from following your deepest instinct, your life will be safe, expedient and thin.
—KATHARINE BUTLER HATHAWAY

1,400 CALORIES

BREAKFAST

❏ Fruit smoothie: In a blender, combine 1 cup fat-free milk or low-fat, calcium-enriched soy or rice beverage; 6 ounces (¾ cup) fat-free plain yogurt; ½ cup sliced or chopped strawberries; 2 tablespoons chopped walnuts; and 4 tablespoons flaxseed meal. Add ground cinnamon and/or sugar substitute to taste. Blend for 15 seconds.

LUNCH

❏ Tuna melt: Preheat oven to 450°F. Toast ½ whole grain English muffin. Combine ¼ cup (1 ounce) water-packed tuna, drained; 1 tablespoon reduced-fat mayonnaise (or 1 teaspoon regular mayonnaise); 1 tablespoon minced dill pickle and/or chopped celery; and 1 ounce reduced-fat cheese. Spoon mixture onto toasted muffin. Place in oven for 5 to 10 minutes or microwave on high power for 30 seconds, or until cheese melts.

❏ 8 baby carrots dipped in 1 tablespoon reduced-fat ranch dressing

❏ 1 cup fat-free milk or low-fat, calcium-enriched soy or rice beverage

SNACK

❏ 1 medium orange or tangerine

❏ 2 tablespoons unsalted dry-roasted almonds (about 12)

DINNER

❏ 3 ounces chicken breast, grilled or roasted with 2 tablespoons barbecue sauce

❏ 1 slice sourdough bread spread with 1 teaspoon olive oil and minced garlic to taste and toasted

❏ Colorful Coleslaw: Mix 1 cup shredded red and green cabbage and carrots with 2 tablespoons reduced-fat coleslaw dressing (or 1 tablespoon regular coleslaw dressing)

SNACK

❏ 2 squares graham crackers (1 sheet)

❏ 1 tablespoon all-natural peanut butter

1,600 CALORIES

BREAKFAST

❏ Fruit smoothie: In a blender, combine 1 cup fat-free milk or low-fat, calcium-enriched soy or rice beverage; 6 ounces (¾ cup) fat-free plain yogurt; ½ cup sliced or chopped strawberries; 2 tablespoons chopped walnuts; and 2 tablespoons flaxseed meal. Add ground cinnamon and/or sugar substitute to taste. Blend for 15 seconds.

LUNCH

❏ Tuna melt: Preheat oven to 450°F. Toast 1 whole grain English muffin. Combine ½ cup (2 ounces) water-packed tuna, drained; 2 tablespoons reduced-fat mayonnaise (or 1 tablespoon regular mayonnaise); 1 tablespoon minced dill pickle and/or chopped celery; and 1 ounce reduced-fat cheese. Spoon mixture onto both halves of toasted muffin. Place in oven for 5 to 10 minutes or microwave on high power for 30 seconds, or until cheese melts.

❏ 16 baby carrots dipped in 1 tablespoon reduced-fat ranch dressing

❏ 1 cup fat-free milk or low-fat, calcium-enriched soy or rice beverage

SNACK

❏ 1 medium orange or tangerine

❏ 2 tablespoons unsalted dry-roasted almonds (about 12)

DINNER

❏ 3 ounces chicken breast grilled or roasted with 2 tablespoons barbecue sauce

❏ 2 slices sourdough bread each spread with 1 teaspoon olive oil and minced garlic to taste and toasted

❏ Colorful Coleslaw: Mix 1 cup shredded red and green cabbage and carrots with 2 tablespoons reduced-fat coleslaw dressing (or 1 tablespoon regular coleslaw dressing)

SNACK

❏ 3 squares graham crackers (1½ sheets)

❏ 1 tablespoon all-natural peanut butter

HOW DID YOU DO?

BALANCE YOUR BLOOD SUGAR

	TIME	READING
CHECK 1		
CHECK 2		
CHECK 3		
CHECK 4		
CHECK 5		

MEASURE YOURSELF

Week 2 weight: _____ pounds

Winning isn't everything, but wanting to win is.
—VINCE LOMBARDI

SUCCEED ALL DAY

Picture yourself fit. Every time a food you crave pops into your head, think, *Stop!* Then, focus on a healthy image—say, you, lean and fit, walking or running. After a while, your brain will dismiss the food image, and the craving will subside.

Ban work from the bedroom. If you pay bills, study, or work on your laptop in your bedroom, your brain associates this location with work rather than sleep. (Even crafts like scrapbooking are "work" to the brain.) Consider relocating your "office"—including your computer—to another room. Eventually, your brain will associate the bedroom only with sleep and sex if you use it only for those things.

1,400 CALORIES

BREAKFAST

❏ Fruit yogurt cup: Stir ¼ cup low-fat granola, 2 tablespoons flaxseed meal, and 1 tablespoon chopped unsalted raw nuts into 6 ounces no-sugar-added, fat-free flavored yogurt. Add ground cinnamon and/or sugar substitute to taste.

LUNCH

❏ Lean-Body Salad: Combine 2 cups mixed dark greens, ½ cup canned chickpeas, and 1 ounce shredded reduced-fat mozzarella cheese. Drizzle with 2 tablespoons light Italian dressing.

❏ 1 medium peach or ½ cup peaches canned in juice or water

SNACK

❏ 1 medium orange or 1 cup fresh strawberries

❏ 2 tablespoons unsalted raw nuts (almonds, peanuts, cashews, walnuts, pistachios)

DINNER

❏ 3 ounces lean roast beef

❏ 2 cups raw or 1 cup cooked spinach tossed with 1 teaspoon olive oil and 1 teaspoon balsamic vinegar

❏ ⅔ cup brown rice cooked with 1 teaspoon olive oil

SNACK

❏ 3 cups light microwave popcorn

❏ 1 ounce low-fat mozzarella string cheese

❏ 16 ounces light lemonade

1,600 CALORIES

BREAKFAST

❏ Fruit yogurt cup: Stir ¼ cup low-fat granola, 1 tablespoon flaxseed meal, and 2 tablespoons chopped unsalted raw nuts into 6 ounces no-sugar-added, fat-free flavored yogurt. Add ground cinnamon and/or sugar substitute to taste.

LUNCH

❏ Lean-Body Salad: Combine 1 ounce white-meat turkey or chicken with 2 cups mixed dark greens, ½ cup canned chickpeas, and 1 ounce shredded reduced-fat mozzarella cheese. Drizzle with 2 tablespoons light Italian dressing.

❏ 1 medium peach or ½ cup peaches canned in juice or water

SNACK

❏ 1 medium orange or 1 cup fresh strawberries

❏ ¼ cup unsalted raw nuts (almonds, peanuts, cashews, walnuts, pistachios)

DINNER

❏ 4 ounces lean roast beef

❏ 2 cups raw or 1 cup cooked spinach tossed with 1 teaspoon olive oil and 1 teaspoon balsamic vinegar

❏ ⅔ cup brown rice cooked with 1 teaspoon olive oil

SNACK

❏ 3 cups light microwave popcorn sprinkled with 2 tablespoons Romano cheese

❏ 16 ounces light lemonade

HOW DID YOU DO?

BALANCE YOUR BLOOD SUGAR

	TIME	READING
CHECK 1		
CHECK 2		
CHECK 3		
CHECK 4		
CHECK 5		

> The significance of a man is not in what he attains but in what he longs to attain.
>
> —KAHLIL GIBRAN

SUCCEED ALL DAY

See the glass as half full. Optimists live longer than pessimists, according to a study of more than 1,100 people tracked for 30 years by the Mayo Clinic. In a separate study of 999 men and women ages 65 to 85, Dutch researchers found that optimistic participants were 77 percent less likely than the pessimists to die of cardiovascular diseases.

Time your last caffeine break. Avoid coffee, tea, and other caffeinated foods and drinks such as chocolate and colas for 6 to 8 hours before you turn in. Even if you don't think caffeine affects you, it could be disrupting the quality of your sleep: While caffeinated products remain in the body for an average of 3 to 5 hours, they can affect some people for up to 12 hours.

1,400 CALORIES

BREAKFAST

❏ 1 egg scrambled in 1 teaspoon canola or olive oil and topped with $\frac{1}{2}$ cup salsa

❏ 1 whole grain English muffin, toasted and spread with 2 tablespoons 1% cottage cheese

❏ 1 cup fat-free milk or low-fat, calcium-enriched soy or rice beverage

LUNCH

❏ Chicken salad: Top 2 cups mixed dark greens with 2 ounces cooked chicken breast; 2 stalks celery, chopped; and $\frac{1}{4}$ cup sliced green or red grapes. Drizzle with 2 tablespoons light honey mustard dressing (such as Newman's Own).

❏ 1 slice reduced-calorie whole grain bread

❏ 1 teaspoon trans-free canola margarine

SNACK

❏ 1 cup watermelon (or other melon)

❏ 6 ounces no-sugar-added, fat-free or low-fat flavored yogurt

❏ 1 tablespoon dry-roasted mixed nuts

DINNER

❏ Preheat oven to 350°F. Place 4 ounces fresh halibut or other fish (4 ounces raw equals 3 ounces cooked) onto square piece of foil. Top with 1 cup chopped or thinly sliced bell peppers and onions. Season with salt-free seasoning (such as Mrs. Dash), garlic powder, lemon juice, and pepper. Wrap in foil and bake for 20 to 30 minutes or until the fish flakes easily.

❏ Toss $\frac{1}{2}$ cup sliced or diced red potatoes in 1 tablespoon olive oil. Place on cookie sheet and season with garlic, onion, or a salt-free seasoning (such as Mrs. Dash). Bake at 350°F for 30 to 45 minutes or until browned.

SNACK

❏ $\frac{1}{4}$ cup unsalted raw cashews, almonds, walnuts, or other nuts

1,600 CALORIES

BREAKFAST

❏ 1 egg scrambled in 1 teaspoon canola or olive oil and topped with $\frac{1}{4}$ cup salsa

❏ 1 whole grain English muffin, toasted and spread with 3 tablespoons 1% cottage cheese

❏ 1 cup fat-free milk or low-fat, calcium-enriched soy or rice beverage

LUNCH

❏ Chicken salad: Top 2 cups mixed dark greens with 2 ounces cooked chicken breast; 2 stalks celery, chopped; and $\frac{1}{4}$ cup sliced green or red grapes. Drizzle with 2 tablespoons light honey mustard dressing (such as Newman's Own).

❏ 2 slices reduced-calorie whole grain bread

❏ 2 teaspoons trans-free canola margarine

SNACK

❏ 1 cup watermelon (or other melon) chunks

❏ 6 ounces no-sugar-added, fat-free or low-fat flavored yogurt

❏ 2 tablespoons dry-roasted mixed nuts

DINNER

❏ Preheat oven to 350°F. Place 4 ounces fresh halibut or other fish (4 ounces raw equals 3 ounces cooked) onto square piece of foil. Top with 1 cup chopped or thinly sliced bell peppers and onions. Season with salt-free seasoning (such as Mrs. Dash), garlic powder, lemon juice, and pepper. Wrap in foil and bake for 20 to 30 minutes or until the fish flakes easily.

❏ Toss 1 cup sliced or diced red potatoes in 1 tablespoon olive oil. Place on cookie sheet and season with garlic, onion, or a salt-free seasoning (such as Mrs. Dash). Bake at 350°F for 30 to 45 minutes or until browned.

SNACK

❏ $\frac{1}{4}$ cup unsalted raw cashews, almonds, walnuts, or other nuts

HOW DID YOU DO?

BALANCE YOUR BLOOD SUGAR

	TIME	READING
CHECK 1		
CHECK 2		
CHECK 3		
CHECK 4		
CHECK 5		

> If you don't know
> where you are going,
> you might wind
> up someplace else.
> —YOGI BERRA

SUCCEED ALL DAY

Lead yourself not into temptation. If you're feeling shaky about your willpower, avoid locations and anything else that might trigger cravings, from cooking or food programs on TV to the snack aisles of supermarkets or convenience stores.

Reflect on your values. Going through a rough patch? Taking time to reflect on and affirm your personal values can help you cope. Researchers had 85 people undertake either a values-affirming task or a neutral task before undergoing a stressful lab test. Those who had affirmed their values released less cortisol, a stress hormone, than members of the control group did.

DAY
11

1,400 CALORIES

BREAKFAST

❒ Good-Morning Blend: Stir 2 tablespoons mixed dried fruits, 2 tablespoons flaxseed meal, and 2 tablespoons chopped unsalted raw almonds, walnuts, or pecans into 6 ounces no-sugar-added, fat-free flavored yogurt.

LUNCH

❒ Roast beef sandwich: Spread 1 teaspoon regular mayonnaise and 1 teaspoon mustard on 2 slices reduced-calorie whole grain bread or toast. Add 2 ounces lean roast beef. Top with $\frac{1}{2}$ cup chopped romaine lettuce and $\frac{1}{2}$ tomato, sliced.

SNACK

❒ 4 dried apricot halves or 3 dried plums (prunes)

❒ 7 walnut halves

DINNER

❒ $\frac{2}{3}$ cup cooked whole grain pasta tossed in 1 teaspoon olive oil and minced garlic to taste

❒ 3 ounces (about 5) lean turkey, chicken, or soy meatballs (such as Tyson Fully Cooked Italian Meatballs)

❒ 1 teaspoon grated Parmesan cheese

❒ Cucumber salad: On a bed of 1 cup mixed greens, arrange 1 cup cucumber slices, 10 halved cherry tomatoes, and $\frac{1}{4}$ cup chopped red onion. Drizzle with 1 tablespoon light Italian dressing.

SNACK

❒ 1 cup fat-free milk or low-fat, calcium-enriched soy or rice beverage

❒ 5 vanilla wafers or 3 graham cracker squares

1,600 CALORIES

BREAKFAST

❒ Good-Morning Blend: Stir 2 tablespoons mixed dried fruits, 2 tablespoons flaxseed meal, and 3 tablespoons chopped unsalted raw almonds, walnuts, or pecans into 6 ounces no-sugar-added, fat-free flavored yogurt.

LUNCH

❒ Roast beef sandwich: Spread 1 teaspoon regular mayonnaise and 1 teaspoon mustard on 2 slices reduced-calorie whole grain bread or toast. Add 4 ounces lean roast beef. Top with $\frac{1}{2}$ cup chopped romaine lettuce and $\frac{1}{2}$ tomato, sliced.

SNACK

❒ 4 dried apricot halves or 3 dried plums (prunes)

❒ 7 walnut halves

DINNER

❒ $\frac{3}{4}$ cup cooked whole grain pasta tossed in 2 teaspoons olive oil and minced garlic to taste

❒ 4 ounces (about 6) lean turkey, chicken, or soy meatballs (such as Tyson Fully Cooked Italian Meatballs)

❒ 2 teaspoons grated Parmesan cheese

❒ Cucumber salad: On a bed of 1 cup mixed greens, arrange 1 cup cucumber slices, 10 halved cherry tomatoes, and $\frac{1}{4}$ cup chopped red onion. Drizzle with 1 tablespoon light Italian dressing.

SNACK

❒ 1 cup fat-free milk or low-fat, calcium-enriched soy or rice beverage

❒ 5 vanilla wafers or 3 graham cracker squares

HOW DID YOU DO?

BALANCE YOUR BLOOD SUGAR

	TIME	READING
CHECK 1		
CHECK 2		
CHECK 3		
CHECK 4		
CHECK 5		

SUCCEED ALL DAY

Portion out a serving. If you can't beat a food craving, try this trick: Before you dig in, dole out a small amount of the food on a small plate. Then put the rest away.

Log off and tune out an hour before bed. The light from a TV or computer monitor mimics the intensity of sunlight, which fools your brain and body into thinking it's *not* time to sleep.

> The thing always happens that you really believe in; and the belief in a thing makes it happen.
> —FRANK LLOYD WRIGHT

DAY 12

1,400 CALORIES

BREAKFAST

❑ ½ cup cooked oatmeal or 1 cup whole oat cereal (such as Cheerios) topped with ¼ cup unsalted raw walnuts or other nuts. Add ½ teaspoon ground cinnamon and/or 1 teaspoon sugar substitute.

❑ 1 cup fat-free milk or low-fat, calcium-enriched soy or rice beverage

LUNCH

❑ Pesto pizza: Split and toast a whole grain English muffin. Spread with 1 tablespoon basil pesto sauce or ½ teaspoon olive oil seasoned with fresh basil. Top each half with 1 slice reduced-fat cheese and 1 slice tomato or 1 tablespoon canned tomatoes, drained. Broil or bake at 450°F until cheese melts.

SNACK

❑ 2 fresh or dried figs

❑ 12 almonds or ½ ounce other nuts

DINNER

❑ Shrimp salad bowl: Mix together ⅓ cup cooked brown rice and 2 tablespoons crumbled feta cheese. Arrange on 2 cups mixed greens. Top with 3 ounces grilled or sautéed shrimp or other fish. Drizzle with 2 tablespoons light Italian dressing.

❑ 2 rye crisp crackers spread with 2 tablespoons low-fat ricotta or 1% cottage cheese

SNACK

❑ 6 ounces no-sugar-added, fat-free or low-fat flavored yogurt

❑ 1 medium orange or ¾ cup blueberries, raspberries, or blackberries

1,600 CALORIES

BREAKFAST

❑ 1 cup cooked oatmeal or 1 cup whole oat cereal (such as Cheerios) topped with ¼ cup unsalted raw walnuts or other nuts. Add ½ teaspoon ground cinnamon and/or 1 teaspoon sugar substitute.

❑ 1 cup fat-free milk or low-fat, calcium-enriched soy or rice beverage

LUNCH

❑ Pesto pizza: Split and toast a whole grain English muffin. Spread with 2 tablespoons basil pesto sauce or 1 teaspoon olive oil seasoned with fresh basil. Top each half with 1 slice reduced-fat cheese and 1 slice tomato or 1 tablespoon canned tomatoes, drained. Broil or bake at 450°F until cheese melts.

SNACK

❑ 2 fresh or dried figs

❑ 12 almonds or ½ ounce other nuts

DINNER

❑ Shrimp salad bowl: Mix together ½ cup cooked brown rice and 2 tablespoons crumbled feta cheese. Arrange on 2 cups mixed greens. Top with 4 ounces grilled or sautéed shrimp or other fish. Drizzle with 2 tablespoons light Italian dressing.

❑ 2 rye crisp crackers spread with 3 tablespoons low-fat ricotta or 1% cottage cheese

SNACK

❑ 6 ounces no-sugar-added, fat-free or low-fat flavored yogurt

❑ 1 medium orange or ¾ cup blueberries, raspberries, or blackberries

HOW DID YOU DO?

BALANCE YOUR BLOOD SUGAR

	TIME	READING
CHECK 1		
CHECK 2		
CHECK 3		
CHECK 4		
CHECK 5		

SUCCEED ALL DAY

Know thy stressors. When you perceive that you're not in control, levels of stress hormones rise. Devise solutions to "uncontrollable" sources of stress (a long commute, your partner's sloppiness) to help defuse them.

Prepare your bladder for bed. If middle-of-the-night bathroom visits routinely disrupt your slumber, be proactive. Make it a habit to empty your bladder before you turn in, and don't drink more than 4 ounces of fluids within an hour of bedtime.

> If you don't like something, change it. If you can't change it, change your attitude. Don't complain.
> —MAYA ANGELOU

1,400 CALORIES

BREAKFAST

❑ ½ whole grain bagel spread with
1 tablespoon low-fat cream cheese

❑ 1 cup fat-free milk or low-fat, calcium-enriched soy or rice beverage

LUNCH

❑ Bean tostada: Preheat oven to 400°F. Bake 1 corn tortilla (6-inch diameter) until crisp (about 5 to 10 minutes). Spread with ½ cup cooked pinto beans and 2 tablespoons shredded reduced-fat Mexican-blend cheese. Return tortilla to oven for 5 to 10 minutes until cheese melts, or microwave on medium power for 30 to 45 seconds. Top with ¼ cup salsa.

❑ Cabbage salad: Combine 1 cup shredded cabbage with 1 tomato, chopped, and drizzle with 2 tablespoons light ranch or creamy Italian dressing.

SNACK

❑ 1 kiwi or small orange

❑ 12 whole almonds

DINNER

❑ Oven-fried chicken: Preheat oven to 350°F. Toss 4 ounces raw chicken breast in 1 tablespoon light Italian dressing. Coat with 2 tablespoons seasoned bread crumbs and spray lightly with canola oil spray. Place chicken on a lightly oiled cookie sheet. Bake for 30 minutes, or until browned on the outside and no longer pink inside.

❑ 3-bean salad: Toss ½ cup cooked green beans, ¼ cup cooked chickpeas, ¼ cup cooked red beans, and 2 tablespoons chopped onion with 2 tablespoons light Italian dressing.

SNACK

❑ ½ cup light ice cream

❑ 1 tablespoon chopped walnuts

1,600 CALORIES

BREAKFAST

❑ ½ whole grain bagel spread with
2 tablespoons low-fat cream cheese and
2 ounces lox (smoked salmon)

❑ 1 cup fat-free milk or low-fat calcium-enriched soy or rice beverage

LUNCH

❑ Bean tostadas: Preheat oven to 400°F. Bake 2 corn tortillas (6-inch diameter) until crisp (about 5 to 10 minutes). Spread with ½ cup cooked pinto beans and 2 tablespoons shredded reduced-fat Mexican-blend cheese. Return tortillas to oven for 5 to 10 minutes until cheese melts, or microwave on medium power for 30 to 45 seconds. Top with ¼ cup salsa.

❑ Cabbage salad: Combine 1 cup shredded cabbage with 1 tomato, chopped, and drizzle with 2 tablespoons light ranch or creamy Italian dressing.

SNACK

❑ 1 kiwi or small orange

❑ 1 ounce whole almonds (about 23)

DINNER

❑ Oven-fried chicken: Preheat oven to 350°F. Toss 5 ounces raw chicken breast in 1 tablespoon light Italian dressing. Coat with 2 tablespoons seasoned bread crumbs and spray lightly with canola oil spray. Place chicken on lightly oiled cookie sheet. Bake for 30 minutes, or until browned on the outside and no longer pink inside.

❑ 3-bean salad: Toss ½ cup cooked green beans, ¼ cup cooked chickpeas, ¼ cup cooked red beans, and 2 tablespoons chopped onion with 2 tablespoons light Italian dressing.

SNACK

❑ ½ cup light ice cream

❑ 1 tablespoon chopped walnuts

HOW DID YOU DO?

BALANCE YOUR BLOOD SUGAR

	TIME	READING
CHECK 1		
CHECK 2		
CHECK 3		
CHECK 4		
CHECK 5		

To climb steep
hills requires slow
pace at first.
—SHAKESPEARE

SUCCEED ALL DAY

Keep a stash of Tootsie Rolls. They're sweet. They're chewy. They're chocolaty good. Best of all, these tiny treats will quash a chocolate craving for fewer calories and less fat. What's not to love?

Swap the bubbly for a bubble bath. If you tend to "relax" with alcohol, swap it for some of the tension tamers in this book. Abusing alcohol raises levels of triglycerides and can lead to high blood pressure and heart failure.

1,400 CALORIES

BREAKFAST

❒ Veggie omelet: Heat 1 teaspoon canola, peanut, or olive oil in a skillet. Add ½ cup egg substitute (or 1 egg white); 1 cup spinach leaves; ½ cup chopped mushrooms, onion, and garlic; and herbs as desired. Cook over low heat until set. Top with 2 tablespoons shredded reduced-fat cheese.

❒ 1 slice whole grain toast spread with 1 teaspoon trans-free canola margarine

❒ 1 cup fat-free milk or low-fat, calcium-enriched soy or rice beverage

LUNCH

❒ Tuna salad: Mix 3 ounces water-packed tuna, drained, with 2 stalks celery, chopped; 4 green olives, chopped; and 1 tablespoon reduced-fat mayonnaise (or 1 teaspoon regular mayonnaise). Add 1 tablespoon seasoned rice vinegar, if desired. Serve on a bed of 2 cups mixed dark greens. Top with 1 tablespoon chopped unsalted raw almonds.

❒ 3 slices whole grain crispbread (such as Wasa crackers)

SNACK

❒ 1 medium apple, sliced

❒ 2 tablespoons all-natural peanut butter

DINNER

❒ Tofu stir-fry: Stir-fry 3 ounces firm tofu (processed with calcium sulfate) and 2 cups mixed vegetables (broccoli, cauliflower, green beans, onion) in 2 tablespoons reduced-sodium stir-fry sauce and 1 tablespoon olive oil. Serve over ⅓ cup cooked brown or wild rice.

SNACK

❒ Stir 1 tablespoon chopped dried fruits and 1 tablespoon chopped unsalted raw nuts into 6 ounces no-sugar-added, fat-free flavored yogurt.

1,600 CALORIES

BREAKFAST

❒ Veggie omelet: Heat 2 teaspoons canola, peanut, or olive oil in a skillet. Add ½ cup egg substitute (or 1 egg white); ½ cup spinach leaves; ½ cup chopped mushrooms, onion, and garlic; and herbs as desired. Cook over low heat until set. Top with 2 tablespoons shredded reduced-fat cheese.

❒ 1 slice whole grain toast spread with 2 teaspoons trans-free canola margarine

❒ 1 cup fat-free milk or low-fat, calcium-enriched soy or rice beverage

LUNCH

❒ Tuna salad: Mix 3 ounces water-packed tuna, drained, with 2 stalks celery, chopped; 4 green olives, chopped; and 1 tablespoon reduced-fat mayonnaise (or 1 teaspoon regular mayonnaise). Add 1 tablespoon seasoned rice vinegar, if desired. Serve on 2 cups mixed dark greens. Top with 1 tablespoon chopped unsalted raw almonds.

❒ 3 slices whole grain crispbread (such as Wasa crackers)

SNACK

❒ 1 medium apple, sliced

❒ 2 tablespoons all-natural peanut butter

DINNER

❒ Tofu stir-fry: Stir-fry 4 ounces firm tofu (processed with calcium sulfate) and 2 cups mixed vegetables (broccoli, cauliflower, green beans, onion) in 2 tablespoons reduced-sodium stir-fry sauce and 1 tablespoon olive oil. Serve over ⅓ cup cooked brown or wild rice.

SNACK

❒ Stir 1 tablespoon chopped dried fruits and 1 tablespoon chopped unsalted raw nuts into 6 ounces no-sugar-added, fat-free flavored yogurt.

HOW DID YOU DO?

BALANCE YOUR BLOOD SUGAR

	TIME	READING
CHECK 1		
CHECK 2		
CHECK 3		
CHECK 4		
CHECK 5		

Keep steadily
before you the fact that
all true success
depends at last upon
yourself.
—THEODORE T. HUNGER

SUCCEED ALL DAY

Have a bit of the best. If you're a chocolate connoisseur, you might feel that chocolate imitations are unacceptable. Get your fix of the good stuff in small (150-calorie) doses. That's two truffles or one snack-size bar.

Leave worries in the dark. If you're tossing and turning, get up and go to another part of the house, but leave the lights off. Usually, anxious thoughts will stop right away, so you can return to bed and fall asleep. This strategy, called stimulus control, also prevents you from associating your bed with anxiety.

PART 4

FULL SPEED AHEAD

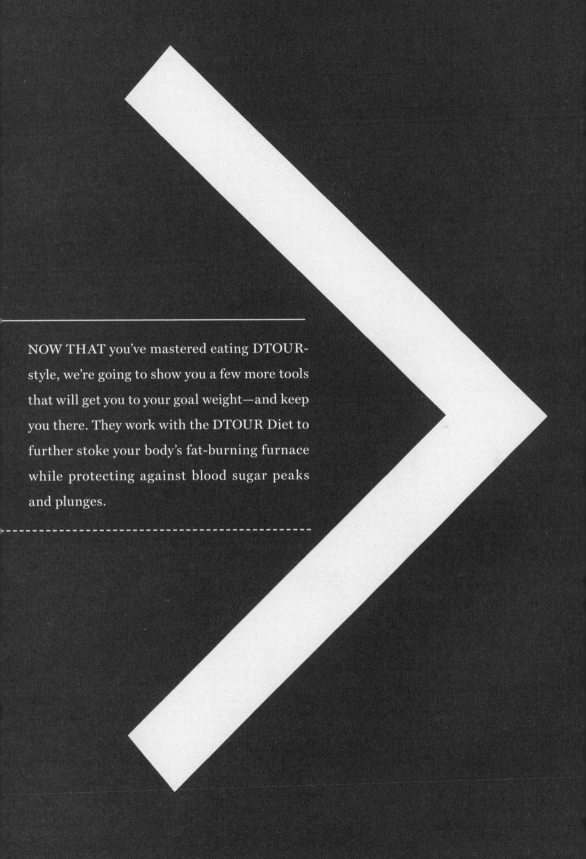

NOW THAT you've mastered eating DTOUR-style, we're going to show you a few more tools that will get you to your goal weight—and keep you there. They work with the DTOUR Diet to further stoke your body's fat-burning furnace while protecting against blood sugar peaks and plunges.

TRANSFORMATION

TOOL #1

GET
FIT

When you think about it, the formula for weight-loss success is pretty simple: Calories burned must be greater than calories consumed. To be more precise, if you expend roughly 3,500 more calories than you take in, you will lose 1 pound.

In theory, you could create this sort of deficit with diet alone. But really, why would you want to? You'd be depriving yourself of one of life's great pleasures—eating! You need food to nourish your soul as well as your body. It's why we took great care to make every one of our Awesome 4some meals and snacks as savory and satisfying as they are healthy. Yes, you're eating fewer calories, but the food is so fabulous that you won't notice the difference!

There is a way to tip the calorie scale in your favor without going hungry. Remember, the idea is to expend more calories than you're eating. You can do that with exercise.

Some experts describe exercise as medicine without the pill, and for good reason. Name just about any chronic health problem, and exercise probably can help control it, if not reverse it. Type 2 diabetes is a perfect example. Time and again, research has shown that regular physical activity helps lower blood sugar because the body uses insulin more efficiently. In fact, people with type 2 who are taking medication are often able to reduce their dosages once they begin a fitness routine. Likewise, those who have type 2 but aren't taking medication may not need it quite so soon, if at all.

Then there's all the other good stuff that exercise can do, such as lower blood pressure and LDL cholesterol (the bad kind), strengthen bones and lubricate joints, boost energy, and alleviate stress. Oh, and we can't forget losing weight! When you combine regular physical activity with a healthy diet, the pounds disappear even faster than they do with diet alone.

For exercise to have any benefit, of course, we need to actually *do* it. And there's the rub. Eating, like breathing, is essential to our survival, and so we make a point of doing it on a fairly regular schedule. Exercise . . . well,

Stop Here

BUY A PAIR OF WALKING SHOES to keep at the office or in your car. You'll be ready to rack up extra miles at a moment's notice, especially during those idle moments—like when your hairstylist is running late or you're waiting for your kid's or grandkid's soccer practice to end.

let's be honest: When our days get hectic—as they do more often than not—our workouts are the first things to go. We tell ourselves, with all sincerity, that we'll pick up where we left off tomorrow, or the next day, or the day after that. Pretty soon we've been away from it for so long that we ask ourselves, Why bother?

Why, indeed. Because, even though we can live without exercise, we risk our long-term health when we do.

For the next 4 weeks of DTOUR, we want you to think of exercise not as an expense, but as an investment. Yes, you're setting aside time that you could be using for something else. But you're buying a stake in your future—in years of good health and independence.

We also encourage you to consider physical activity not as time spent *away* from life, but in the thick of it. Motion is life. Moving your body can be fun. And watching it become slimmer, stronger, and healthier is incredibly rewarding and motivating.

These ideals are at the very core of the DTOUR Workout, which we designed in consultation with diabetes and fitness experts, in addition to using the very latest research. The workout is basic—short, easy-to-remember routines; simple moves; and no gym visits or pricey gear. It's enjoyable because *you* get to define *enjoyable*. It's also customizable; you can adjust it to your changing health and fitness level, as well as to the demands of your schedule. And best of all, it *works*.

SCIENCE-BASED ROUTINE, REAL-WORLD RESULTS

As you might imagine, the science of fitness is growing by leaps and bounds, with researchers regularly announcing fantastic new discoveries about the health effects of various forms of physical activity. We based the DTOUR Workout on the findings of one particularly impressive study—the Diabetes Aerobic and Resistance Exercise (DARE) study, conducted at the University of Ottawa in Canada.

The research team behind DARE determined that both aerobic exercise (also called cardiovascular exercise, or cardio for short) and strength training (that is, lifting weights) can help people with type 2 diabetes lower their blood sugar. What's more, the combination of cardio and strength training controls blood sugar significantly better than either activity alone.

It isn't news that individually, cardio and strength training help prevent or manage type 2 diabetes. Previous studies, for example, have found that aerobic exercise—the kind that elevates the heart rate for a sustained period—helps lower blood sugar and LDL cholesterol while raising HDL cholesterol (the good kind). But the DARE study—published in 2007 in the prestigious medical journal *Annals of Internal Medicine*—was the first to assess the collective effects of both forms of activity on blood sugar.

For this study, the researchers divided 251 people with type 2 diabetes into four groups. Three of the groups worked out for 45 minutes 3 days a week; the

HOW MUCH EXERCISE? HERE'S THE LATEST

How much exercise do you *really* need to lose weight and keep it off? According to a 2008 study at the University of Pittsburgh, the magic number is 275 minutes a week, which works out to about 55 minutes a day 5 days a week.

For this study, researchers recruited 201 women—all of whom were overweight—and divided them into four groups. Two of the groups burned 1,000 calories a week by engaging in moderate- or vigorous-intensity exercise. The third group burned 2,000 calories a week by doing moderate activity, while Group 4 burned 2,000 calories by doing vigorous activity. All of the women reduced their calorie intakes to 1,200 or 1,500 a day, depending on their weight at the start of the study.

According to the study findings, which appeared in the *Archives of Internal Medicine,* all of the women lost 8 to 10 percent of their body weight over 6 months—regardless of exercise intensity.

Two years later, they had successfully kept off 5 percent of their body weight, again with no difference related to exercise intensity.

But the researchers also noticed this: The women who kept off the most weight—10 percent or more—were burning about 1,800 calories a week through physical activity, both at the 6-month mark and again at 2 years. That translates to 275 minutes a week. That's not all. The women also completed more follow-ups with the research team, and they scored higher on a standard test of healthy eating.

The 275-minute finding is almost double the current "official" recommendation of 150 minutes. But it's a reasonable goal. In fact, by Week 4 of the DTOUR Total Transformation, you'll be walking for just over 2 hours a week, plus doing the Metabo Moves and the Belly Blast. By then, you'll be a veritable fat- and calorie-burning machine!

fourth, "control" group did no exercise at all. Group 1 walked on treadmills or rode exercise bikes, both of which qualify as aerobic exercise. Group 2 used weight machines, a form of strength training. Group 3 did both.

Over the course of 6 months, the researchers saw improvements in the blood sugar readings of all the exercise groups. Compared with the control group, Group 1 shaved 0.51 percent off their collective hemoglobin A1c value, while Group 2 showed a reduction of 0.38 percent. Group 3—which did both aerobic exercise and strength training—fared even better: Their collective A1c value fell an additional 0.46 percent over the aerobic-only group and 0.59 percent over the strength-training-only group. Compared to controls, the combination exercisers had a nearly 1 percent lower A1c reading.

This may seem like a modest change, but it comes with huge benefits. Consider this: A 1-point drop in A1c—which, you'll remember, reflects average blood sugar over several months—is associated with a 15 to 20 percent reduction in risk of heart attack and stroke and a 37 percent reduction in diabetes-related complications, such as kidney, eye, and limb damage.

THE DTOUR WORKOUT BLOCKS

Using the DARE findings as our main point of reference, we designed the DTOUR Workout to target a trio of fitness benchmarks: cardiorespiratory fitness (which reflects how well the heart and lungs supply oxygen to the muscles during exercise), muscular strength and endurance, and flexibility. Now, don't break into a sweat just yet; as with all things DTOUR, we're going to make exercise as accessible and doable as we can. In fact, the workout consists of four building blocks—two aerobic, two strength and flexibility—that you interchange. It's really that easy!

FYI

YOU MAY BE ABLE TO REVERSE the earliest symptoms of type 2 diabetes in 1 week just by walking, according to a study at the University of Michigan. When adults who were prediabetic and sedentary began walking for an hour a day, their production of insulin rose by 31 percent over 7 days. In the same period, their sensitivity to insulin improved by 59 percent. Both of these changes are markers of an enhanced ability to regulate blood sugar.

What follows is a short description of each of the four blocks. We'll explore each block in more detail in just a bit. The 4-Week Total Transformation, which begins on page 203, spells out each day's workout for you.

Before we go further, we want to stress the importance of following the DTOUR Workout at your own pace. Your fitness level is going to improve over time, so there's no need to do too much too soon. Also, please be sure to get your doctor's clearance before starting any fitness routine, especially if you have diabetes. Exercise will affect your blood sugar, so it's smart to proceed with care.

BLOCKS A AND B: THE CARDIO WALKS

Brisk walking is an ideal form of aerobic exercise—it's convenient, it's low impact, and it requires no special equipment other than a good pair of walking shoes. According to a 2007 study from the Duke University Medical Center, a brisk, 30-minute walk each day is enough to lower the odds of developing metabolic syndrome, which you'll remember is a major risk factor for type 2 diabetes.

Stop Here

AFTER YOU'VE LIFTED WEIGHTS consistently for a few weeks or months, you may find that you can't seem to progress to heavier weights. This is a sign that your muscles need a new challenge. The solution: Make a change. Try a different exercise to work the same muscles, or lift and lower the weight more slowly.

The DTOUR Workout features two Cardio Walks.

◆ For the Fat-Torch Walk (Block A), you'll maintain a steady, moderate-intensity pace from beginning to end. Research has shown that this style of walking helps to burn body fat. The Fat-Torch walk is slightly longer than the Calorie-Scorch Walk, making it more challenging.

◆ The Calorie-Scorch Walk (Block B) combines a moderate-intensity pace with *intervals*—that is, short bursts of fast walking. Interval training keeps your metabolism in high gear for hours after you finish a workout, so you burn more calories throughout the day.

For the 4 weeks of the Total Transformation, you'll be doing the Cardio Walks 4 to 6 days a week. As your fitness improves, so will the duration of your walks. Your pace will pick up, too—and the faster you move, the more calories you use.

BLOCK C: THE METABO MOVES

This mini-but-mighty strength-training routine delivers a multitude of benefits.

◆ It firms and tones your upper and lower body in just four moves (and one optional move). You can modify each move to make it more or less challenging. Do the version of each move that matches your fitness level.

◆ Strength training builds muscle, which burns more calories than fat does. So the more muscle you have, the more calories you burn, even in your sleep. (Sweet!)

◆ The more muscle you have, the more sensitive to insulin your body becomes. Some studies suggest that strength training enhances cells' insulin response and improves blood sugar just as effectively as diabetes medication does.

◆ As a bonus, strength training is the sort of weight-bearing activity that builds bone density and helps protect against the bone-thinning disease osteoporosis.

You'll perform the Metabo Moves 2 or 3 days a week.

THE DTOUR WORKOUT BASICS

DTOUR makes fitness easy, accessible, and fun! With the combination of aerobic exercise and strength training in this plan, you'll burn calories, melt away fat–and lower your blood sugar, to boot. The 4-Week Total Transformation spells out each day's workout for you; use the guidelines here to get the most from your exercise minutes.

◆ Get your doctor's okay *before* you begin any exercise program.
◆ Perform all workouts at your own pace.
◆ Warm up for 3 minutes before every Cardio Walk, and cool down for 2 minutes afterward. Include these 5 minutes in your total workout time. As for how to warm up and cool down, you needn't do anything elaborate; you might walk at a slower pace or simply march in place.

◆ Do Cardio Walks 4 to 6 times a week.
◆ Do the Metabo Moves and Belly Blast 2 or 3 times a week. The moves in each routine can be modified to increase or reduce the challenge. Choose the version of each move that matches your fitness level.
◆ You may do either the Metabo Moves or the Belly Blast on the same day as a Cardio Walk.
◆ You may do the Metabo Moves and the Belly Blast on the same day. Be sure to allow 1 rest day before your next strength-training session.
◆ Rest at least 1 day each week.

BLOCK D: THE BELLY BLAST

The four moves in this strength-and-flexibility routine zero in on the muscles of your core—that is, the abdominals, lower back, hips, and buttocks. You'll sculpt a tight, trim torso without doing a single crunch! Plus, you'll be targeting belly fat, the kind that contributes to insulin resistance and is a risk factor for metabolic syndrome.

You'll be doing the Belly Blast 2 or 3 days a week. As with the Metabo Moves, you can adjust each move to your fitness level.

WALK RIGHT INTO A SLIMMER, HEALTHIER YOU

Of all the kinds of physical activity we can do, walking comes most naturally. It's so much a part of our lives, in fact, that we tend not to think of it as having any sort of health benefit. But, oh, does it ever!

Dozens of studies have shown that walking can help control and even prevent

COUNT YOUR STEPS

Need a little extra incentive to lace up your walking shoes? Invest in a pedometer. These gadgets—which clip to your waistband and count the number of steps you take—are proving to be effective at convincing people not only to walk, but to go farther than they might otherwise.

For a 2007 meta-analysis, researchers at the Stanford University School of Medicine reviewed 26 studies that examined the use of pedometers as a tool for encouraging people to engage in physical activity. Most of the 2,767 study participants were women who were overweight and inactive before they took up fitness walking. The mean duration of the studies was 18 weeks.

The Stanford team found that the women who used pedometers to monitor their daily activity took about 2,100 more steps every day than the women who didn't count their steps. That's about an extra mile! And it translates to an impressive 27 percent increase in physical activity. The payoff: The women who wore pedometers lowered their blood pressure and lost weight, as well.

GOT DIABETES? BE SMART ABOUT WORKING OUT

There's no doubt that exercise can be a real asset in managing diabetes. It stabilizes blood sugar not only by helping cells use insulin more effectively, but also by burning off excess body fat, which further improves insulin response.

If you have diabetes, you need to be somewhat choosy about how much exercise you get and what kinds. Some activities may not be right for you, especially if you're experiencing complications such as heart disease, kidney disease, or eye or foot problems.

Your doctor can start you on the right path by reviewing the DTOUR Workout with you and suggesting adjustments based on your health status and fitness level. The following pointers can help, too.

If you have diabetes-related eye problems: Too-heavy weights can increase the pressure in the blood vessels of your eyes. Ask your doctor how much you can safely lift.

If nerve damage has made your feet numb: You may want to choose an aerobic activity other than walking, such as bicycling or swimming. Discuss the options with your doctor. If he or she gives you the all-clear to do the Cardio Walks, be sure to wear shoes that fit. And check your feet for any sores, bumps, or redness after every workout.

If you take a diabetes medication that can cause low blood sugar: You may need to adjust your dosage before your workout, or eat a snack if your blood sugar is below 100. Ask your doctor what's best for you.

After your workout: Check your blood sugar. If it's below 70, have *one* of the following immediately:

◆ 3 or 4 glucose tablets *or* 1 serving glucose gel (15 grams carbohydrate)
◆ ½ cup fruit juice
◆ 5 or 6 pieces hard candy
◆ 1 tablespoon sugar or honey

After 15 minutes, check your blood sugar again. If it's still low, go back for another "dose." Repeat until your blood sugar is 70 or higher.

type 2 diabetes. In the landmark Nurses' Health Study, for example, women who worked up a sweat by walking more than once a week reduced their risk of developing diabetes by 30 percent. And Chinese researchers found that people with high blood sugar who engaged in moderate exercise such as walking (among other lifestyle changes) were 40 percent less likely to develop full-blown diabetes.

If you've already been diagnosed with diabetes, a regular walking routine can help slow its progression. And if you're taking insulin or diabetes medication, brisk walking—which helps your body use insulin more efficiently—may reduce the dosage you need.

How about weight loss? Walking definitely can help you shimmy into those smaller-size jeans. According to a study that appeared in the journal *Obesity*, women over age 40 who increased their daily physical activity by 3,520 steps (that's roughly 1³/₄ miles) lost 5 pounds and reduced their belly fat by a whopping 12 percent in 1 year. What makes these results even more impressive is that the women slimmed down without making a single change in their eating habits. So just imagine what the combination of diet and Cardio Walks—à la DTOUR—will do for you!

NOW, STEP IT UP A NOTCH

Just how much benefit you get from walking, especially in terms of weight loss, depends to a large degree on how hard you work it—what exercise physiologists refer to as *intensity*. You might think of intensity as the sum of the pace and duration of your Cardio Walk plus the extra "oomph" that you put into your intervals. In general, the faster and farther you go, and the more you challenge yourself, the more dramatic your results will be.

Most experts describe intensity as *light, moderate,* or *vigorous,* based on the amount of energy or effort expended. You can measure intensity in several ways, but the simplest is the talk test.

PACE GUIDE FOR FAT-TORCH AND CALORIE-SCORCH CARDIO WALKS

This chart can help you gauge the speed and intensity of your Cardio Walks. Remember that what feels like a light workout to one person may be vigorous for another, so use the speeds as guides, not gospel.

	INTENSITY LEVEL	SPEED (MPH)
Warmup and cooldown	Light (you can sing)	3-3½
Fat-Torch Walk	Moderate (you can chat with a friend)	3½-4
Calorie-Scorch Walk, intervals only	Vigorous (you're edging slightly out of your comfort zone)	4+

◆ If you can sing during your workout, you're at a *light* intensity.

◆ If you're breathing hard as you walk, but you can still chat with your exercise buddy or on your cell phone, you're at a *moderate* intensity. (For the Fat-Torch Walk, this is the intensity you want to maintain throughout.)

◆ Going at it too hard to chat? That's *vigorous* intensity. Eventually, you may reach this level when you perform the intervals during the Calorie-Scorch Walk.

As these guidelines suggest, intensity is relative. So, when you're new to exercise, what you perceive as a moderate intensity may feel like a stroll in the park to someone who's been fitness walking for years.

HOW TO DO AN INTERVAL

Our Calorie-Scorch Walk features interval training, which offers a great cardiovascular workout. It's easy to do, once you get the hang of alternating your walking speeds. You will want to wear a watch to time yourself, at least to start out. Eventually your pacing will become second nature.

Regardless of the duration of your interval session, the basic format is the same: moderate-intensity walking intermingled with more vigorous bouts.

We suggest starting out with 1 minute at moderate intensity, followed by 30 seconds at vigorous intensity; then continue switching between the two. As you become more fit, you can increase to 1 minute at moderate intensity and 1-minute intervals. Remember to allow 3 minutes for warming up at the beginning of our workout and 2 minutes for cooling down at the end.

To give an example, here's what a 15-minute Calorie-Scorch Walk would look like:

TIME	INTERVAL	SPEED (MPH)
0:00	Warm-up	3-3.5
3:00	Moderate	3.5-4.0
4:00	Vigorous	4.0+
4:30	Repeat moderate and vigorous intervals until you reach 13 minutes	
13:00	Cooldown	3-3.5

Regardless of your current fitness level, you can increase your workout intensity—and burn more calories—by pushing yourself slightly beyond your comfort zone. For the Fat-Torch Walks, for example, try to step up your pace a bit and notice how you feel. On Calorie-Scorch days, see how much "burst" you can put into the intervals. Just be careful not to overdo. Move at your own pace, and *never* try to maintain a vigorous intensity throughout your entire workout. Just keep walking; your intensity will increase with time.

As it does, the pounds will melt away faster, too. Let's say that you weigh 150 pounds and you walk for 60 minutes four times a week. By increasing your pace from a 20-minute mile (3 miles per hour) to a 15-minute mile (4 miles per hour), you would lose an extra 7 pounds in 1 year!

FYI

STICKING TO A FITNESS ROUTINE over time can double its mood-boosting power, according to a study from the Sacramento VA Medical Center in California. While nonexercisers felt happier and less stressed after a single session, those who worked out 3 times a week for 6 months got those perks plus a bigger energy boost, which improved their mood even more.

MASTERING THE CARDIO WALKS

It's important to learn and maintain good form for your Cardio Walks—not only to maximize your calorie burn, but also to avoid injury. Here's a head-to-toe guide to proper walking technique.

◆ **Head, shoulders, and chest:** Hold your head high, so your neck and the rest of your spine form a straight line. Your chin should be level with the ground; avoid tucking it in toward your neck. Raise your chest and relax your shoulders. An easy way to check your shoulder position on the fly: Take a deep breath every 5 minutes, then exhale strongly. Notice how your shoulders drop? That's how you want to carry them.

◆ **Eyes:** Look well ahead of you—anywhere from 10 to 30 feet, experts say.

◆ **Arms and hands:** Bend your elbows to 90-degree angles and keep them close to your sides. They should move to the rear, but not outward, as you walk. Imagine a shelf extending from your chest and try not to let your hands shoot above it.

◆ **Abdominals and hips:** Your abdominal muscles should be tight. Pull your belly button toward your spine and tuck your pelvis slightly forward. Power your movement from your glutes (that is, your butt) rather than your thighs; let your hips swing.

◆ **Legs:** Taking huge strides actually slows you down. To determine the natural length of your stride, stand straight and extend one foot a few inches in front of you, with your leg straight and your heel not quite touching the ground. Then slowly lean forward; don't worry—your extended heel will hit the ground and stop you from falling. That's how far forward your front foot should go during your stride. (For this test, don't pay attention to the position of your back leg. When you're walking, your back leg will be farther behind you.)

◆ **Feet:** When you step forward, your heel should gently strike the ground before your foot rolls forward and allows you to push off from your toes. Make sure you aren't pounding your feet; if you are, you're not channeling enough energy forward, so you're decreasing your momentum.

It's best to stretch a few minutes into your walk, when your muscles are warm, rather than before you start. You'll find several stretches on page 154.

Stop Here

NOT EVERY PEDOMETER is accurate. When researchers from the University of Tennessee in Knoxville compared 13 brands, they found that some tallied every step twice, while others missed one of every four steps. To check the accuracy of yours, clip it on and walk 100 steps, counting as you go. Then compare your count to the pedometer's reading.

BUILD MUSCLE, BANISH YOUR BELLY, BRING DOWN BLOOD SUGAR

Along with the Cardio Walks, the DTOUR Workout recommends two strength-training routines—one for all-over muscle toning, the other targeting the belly and abdominal muscles. Now, many people, especially women, are not comfortable with the idea of strength training, fearing that they'll bulk up like a bodybuilder. We can promise you that it won't happen, not because the routines aren't effective, but because you really, *really* need to work to get huge. Women in particular just don't have enough testosterone for it.

What *will* happen when you strength train several times a week, as you do on DTOUR, is this: You'll swap jiggly fat for firm muscle. And as you now know, when you have more muscle, you burn more calories, even at rest. How does revving up your metabolic rate by as much as 15 percent sound? Strength training can do just that.

For proof, consider the findings of the 2007 Strong, Healthy, and Empowered (SHE) study conducted at the University of Minnesota. The research team behind this study recruited 164 women, all overweight, and assigned them to one of two groups. The women in Group 1 received a 2-year membership to the YWCA and 4 months of strength-training classes. After the classes concluded, the women were instructed to continue lifting weights twice a week on their own. Those in Group 2, meanwhile, were given brochures that recommended doing 30 to 60 minutes of exercise most days of the week.

After 2 years, the researchers used CT scans to measure the abdominal fat of all the women. Belly fat increased by just 7 percent in the strength-training group, compared with 21 percent in the control group. The strength-trainers also reduced their total body fat by almost 4 percent, while the control group's total body fat didn't decrease at all.

As we mentioned earlier, strength training also supports blood sugar control by improving insulin sensitivity. In other words, insulin is better able to usher blood sugar out of the bloodstream and into cells, where it's used for energy. Strength training is great for heart health, too—and that's important, since high blood sugar can quadruple the risk of heart disease.

Beyond the physical benefits, strength training can do wonders for our emotional health. It's a potent natural remedy for depression, which is fairly common among people with type 2 diabetes. According to some studies, the improvements seen with strength training are on a par with those produced by antidepressants. Strength training also has been shown to boost self-confidence and self-esteem—positive feelings that can spill over into your general quality of life.

But what if you've never picked up a dumbbell before? It doesn't matter! You can start strength training anytime, regardless of your age or fitness level.

MASTERING THE METABO MOVES

For the Metabo Moves, you'll need two pieces of gear: a set of dumbbells (ideally of varying weights) and an exercise mat. You'll be doing this routine 2 or 3 times a week.

The following tips will help guide you through your routine so you'll be doing the moves safely and effectively. Within about a month, you'll notice changes in your body as you replace fat with muscle. Other changes—including a huge surge in energy and an overall improvement in your mood—will happen much sooner. (If you're working with weights for the first time, be sure to get the all-clear from your doctor before diving in.)

◆ A *repetition* (or *rep*, for short) describes 1 complete exercise. A *set* is a specific number of repetitions. Do 2 sets of 8 to 12 repetitions of each exercise. Start with 8 repetitions per set. When you can easily do 12 reps, use a heavier dumbbell.

◆ Choose the right weight. If you can't lift a dumbbell 8 times while maintaining good form, it's too heavy. On the other hand, it's too light if you can easily lift it more than 12 times. Pick a weight that's in between.

◆ Be careful not to hold your breath when you lift, because it can cause your blood pressure to spike. Practice exhaling as you lift the weight, then inhaling as you lower it or return to the starting position.

◆ Perform each move in a slow, controlled manner to help prevent injury. It should take 3 seconds to lift the weight into place and another 3 to return to the starting position, with a 1-second pause in between. Bonus: Because slowly lifting a dumbbell requires more effort, you get more benefit.

◆ Doing the Metabo Moves in precisely the right way—pros call this *good form*—helps you get the most benefit from lifting while avoiding injury. Until you're familiar with the routine, you might want to practice it while standing in front of a mirror so you can monitor your posture and movement. You can use the photos beginning on page 155 for reference. Another

Stop Here

IF YOU HAVE TYPE 2 diabetes and use insulin, ask your doctor how much exercise you can tolerate before you need to replenish your store of carbohydrates. Carry a healthy snack (an apple or a handful of trail mix) with you on your walks for just this purpose.

option: Sign up for a session with a personal trainer, who can observe and correct your form.

◆ That said, don't get so hung up on form that you're petrified to even attempt the moves. Just be patient and work slowly, in a mindful way.

◆ Rest your muscles for at least 1 day between workouts. It's during rest that your muscles grow. Lifting weights causes tiny tears in muscle tissue; as your muscles repair this damage, they become stronger.

◆ You may feel a little sore for a week or so after you begin strength training. That's normal. If you experience outright pain, however, you may be overdoing it. Stop and rest for a day or two before trying again.

WARM UP TO A BETTER WALK

Instead of traditional "static" stretches, try these more active moves. Compared with stationary stretching, they better lubricate your joints, reduce the risk of injury, and get blood flowing to your walking muscles.

Remember to do these a few minutes into your walk, once your muscles have warmed up a bit.

Hurdles: Balance on your right leg, holding on to a bench or wall for support. Bend your left leg so your heel is behind you. Rotate your leg out to your left side and then forward, as if you're drawing a semicircle with your knee. Repeat 15 times, then switch legs.

Windmills: Stand with your arms at your sides. Circle your right arm in front of you, up overhead, and then down behind you— as though you're swimming the back-stroke. Repeat 15 times, then switch arms.

Foot rock-overs: Stand with your right foot about 12 inches behind your left foot. Your right foot should be flat on the floor, while the toes of your left foot should lift off the floor. Shift your weight forward, simultaneously lowering your left toes and rolling onto the ball of your right foot, lifting your right heel. Reverse to the starting position. Repeat 15 times, then switch feet.

Heel raises: Holding on to a bench or wall for support, stand with your feet parallel and hip-width apart. Lift your heels and rise onto your toes for 2 seconds, then lower. Repeat 15 times. Next, do the heel raises with your heels together and your toes pointing outward, and finally with your toes together and your heels pointed outward.

THE METABO MOVES

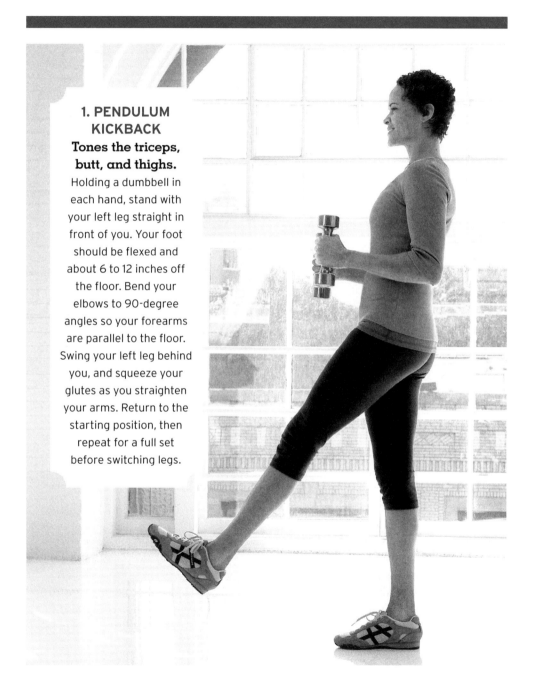

1. PENDULUM KICKBACK

Tones the triceps, butt, and thighs.

Holding a dumbbell in each hand, stand with your left leg straight in front of you. Your foot should be flexed and about 6 to 12 inches off the floor. Bend your elbows to 90-degree angles so your forearms are parallel to the floor. Swing your left leg behind you, and squeeze your glutes as you straighten your arms. Return to the starting position, then repeat for a full set before switching legs.

2. CROUCH AND PULL

Tones the shoulders, upper back, arms, obliques, butt, and thighs. Holding
a dumbbell in each hand, stand with your feet about shoulder-width apart and sit back into
a partial squat. Hinge forward from your hips about 45 degrees, keeping your arms
extended below your shoulders and your palms facing in. With your lower body facing
forward, rotate your torso to the left. Bend your left arm and pull the dumbbell toward your
chest, pointing your elbow toward the ceiling. Return to the starting position, then repeat,
alternating sides. Do 2 full sets per side.
Simplify it: If you have back problems, use one weight at a time and place
the other hand on a chair for support.

3. KNEE-HUGGER CHEST FLY

Tones the chest and abs. Holding a dumbbell in each hand, lie faceup on an exercise mat with your knees bent and your shins parallel to the floor. Your arms should be out to your sides, with your elbows slightly bent and your palms facing the ceiling. Contract your abdominal muscles and lift your hips about 3 inches off the floor. At the same time, squeeze your chest muscles and raise your arms, bringing the dumbbells together over your chest. Lower your hips and arms to the starting position, then repeat.

A

B

4. FIGURE-4 SQUAT CURL

Tones the biceps, butt, and thighs. Hold a
dumbbell in your left hand at your side, with your palm
facing forward. Cross your right ankle over your left
thigh. Bend your left knee and hip and sit back, keeping
your knee behind your toes; as you do, raise the
dumbbell to your left shoulder. Return to the starting
position. Repeat for a full set before switching sides.
Simplify it: Hold on to the back of a chair as shown.

OPTIONAL: LIFTOFF LUNGE

Tones the shoulders, triceps, butt, and thighs.

Stand with your feet hip-width apart. Hold both dumbbells at your shoulders, with your palms facing forward. Step back about 2 feet with your right foot, then bend both knees and lower yourself until your left thigh is about parallel to the floor, keeping your knee over your ankle. Press into your left foot and stand up as you pull your right knee forward so you're balancing on your left leg. Raise the weights overhead. Then, without touching the floor, swing your right leg back into the lunge position as you lower the weights. Repeat for a full set before switching legs.

MASTERING THE BELLY BLAST

The Belly Blast requires no equipment other than an exercise mat. You'll be doing this routine 2 or 3 times a week. As is the case for the Metabo Moves, maintaining good form is crucial. These tips can help.

◆ For maximum results, flatten your belly by pulling your navel toward your spine during each rep.

◆ Focus on keeping your abdominal muscles pulled in and up at all times.

◆ Work slowly and with precision to gain the maximum benefit from each move.

◆ Breathe in through your nose and out through your mouth. This deep inhaling and exhaling rids your lungs of stale air and fills them with fresh, oxygen-rich air, which energizes your entire body.

THE BELLY BLAST

1. TOE DIP
Lie on your back with your feet off the floor and your knees bent (A). Your thighs should be straight up and your calves parallel to the floor. Rest your hands at your sides, with your palms facing down. Contract your abs and press your lower back toward the floor. Inhale and lower your left leg for a count of 2, moving only from your hip (B). Your toes should dip toward the floor without actually touching it. Exhale and raise your leg to the starting position for a count of 2. Repeat with your right leg, then continue alternating until you've done 12 reps with each leg.

2. LEG CIRCLE

Lie on your back with your legs straight and extended along the floor. Your hands should be at your sides, palms facing down. Raise your right leg toward the ceiling, pointing your toes as you do. Hold for 10 to 60 seconds.

Rotate your right leg from the hip to make a small circle on the ceiling with the toes of your right foot. Inhale as you begin the circle and exhale as you finish. Keep your body as still as possible by tightening your abs. Do 6 circles in one direction, then reverse direction for 6 more. Return to the starting position, then repeat with your left leg.

Simplify it: If keeping one leg flat on the floor is uncomfortable, try bending that leg and placing your foot flat on the floor.

A

B

3. CRISSCROSS

For this move, the starting position is the same as for the Toe Dip, only your hands are behind your head and your elbows are out to the sides (A). Curl up to raise your head, neck, and shoulders off the floor.

As you inhale, rotate your torso to the right, bringing your right knee and left shoulder toward each other and extending your left leg toward the ceiling in a diagonal line from your hip (B). As you exhale, rotate to the left, bringing your left knee and right shoulder toward each other and extending your right leg. That's 1 rep. Do 5 more, for a total of 6.

A

B

4. LEG KICK

Lie on your right side with your legs straight and together, so your body forms one long line. Prop yourself up on your right elbow and forearm, lifting your ribs off the floor and your head toward the ceiling. Place your left hand lightly on the floor in front of you for balance. Raise your left leg to hip level and flex your foot so your toes point forward. Exhale as you kick, swinging your left leg forward as far as comfortably possible (A). Pulse for 2 counts (kick, kick). Inhale, point your toes, and swing your leg backward past your right leg (B). That's 1 rep. Do 6 reps without lowering your leg, then switch sides and repeat.

Simplify it: If propping yourself up on your elbow is uncomfortable, extend your right arm along the floor and rest your head on your arm.

ENERGY-BOOSTER WALK

The intensity level of this walk is based on a scale of 1 to 10, with 1 equivalent to how you'd feel standing still and 10 to how you'd feel sprinting. Because the walk is just 10 minutes long, you'll have more energy to give it your all the entire time. You'll burn more fat in the process.

STOPWATCH (IN MINUTES)	ACTIVITY	INTENSITY
0:00	Warmup	4
1:00	Moderate pace: You can talk in short sentences	5
4:00	Picking up the pace	6
7:00	Power-walk pace: Brisk, but you're not breathless	7
9:00	Moderate, slowing to cooldown pace	5-4
10:00	Finish	

THE 10-MINUTE "NO TIME FOR A WORKOUT" WORKOUT

Once you get to the 4-Week Total Transformation (beginning on page 203), you'll see that we've included daily instructions for your DTOUR Workout. Generally, you'll be doing the Cardio Walks and the strength-training routines on alternate days, with 1 rest day each week. We encourage you to follow the workout as we've designed it, unless you already have your own exercise program in place. In that case, by all means, continue what you're doing! What matters most is that you're moving your body in some way every day.

Of course, we all have days when deadlines, appointments, and other obligations conspire to keep us glued to our chairs for hours at a time. You can outfox them with Energy Bursts, mini bouts of movement that fit the bill on days when you can't squeeze in your regular workout. If you can spare 10 minutes, you can burn calories, boost your mood, and reenergize—anytime, anywhere! Just choose two or three activities from the list that follows; Bursts 1 through 5 are easier, while the rest are more challenging.

If you've been advised to ease into exercise, then the Energy Bursts (page 166) are perfect for you. Just show the list to your doctor and ask which moves are okay for you and how many you can do over the course of a day.

DANCE AWAY DIABETES

From mambos and cha-chas to kicks and hip circles, dance workouts such as salsa, jazz, and hip-hop offer a fun way to burn calories and whittle your waistline. In fact, a study from Memorial Hospital of Rhode Island found that dancing provides benefits similar to those you'd get from a walk-jog exercise program.

Many health clubs and community colleges offer dance classes, as do private dance studios. If you're too bashful to bust a move in front of others, check out the dance and fitness DVD collection at your local library or online. We've suggested DVDs for each dance style. If you prefer something more eclectic, check out *Prevention*'s fitness video *Dance Yourself Thin* (www.danceyourselfthin.com).

Belly dancing: As you might imagine, the emphasis of this high-intensity workout is on the belly—specifically, on holding the abs steady while shaking and rocking the hips. Instructors may add jazz and ballet moves such as the relevé, plié, and pirouette to flesh out the dance combinations and tone the entire body.

DVD: *Bellydance for Beginners with Suhaila: Fitness Fusion* series

(www.amazon.com)

Vegas jazz: It's a moderately challenging, showy version of traditional jazz dance, with a focus on stick-straight posture. (That's how those Las Vegas showgirls keep their elaborate headdresses in place!) Pretend you're starring in your own Vegas show as you rehearse short sequences of jazz staples such as high-line kicks and ball steps to classic tunes such as Peggy Lee's "Fever." Then link the moves to make up a complete performance. Your abs, back, butt, and legs get the best of this workout.

DVD: *Musical Theatre Dance* (www.centralhome.com)

Cardio salsa: This low-impact but high-intensity workout combines precise, fast-paced Latin choreography—merengue, mambo, cha-cha, samba—with traditional aerobic dance steps, lunges, and arm raises. Much of the action is centered on the glutes and core.

DVDs: *Crunch: Cardio Salsa; Dance Fitness for Beginners with Joby "Brava": Havana Heat Workout & Latin Dance Instruction;* and *Latin Grooves: Latin Dance Workout* (www.amazon.com)

THE ENERGY BURSTS

1. Walk at your own pace around your neighborhood—5 minutes out, 5 minutes back. Take your dog, if you'd like.

2. When you watch TV, march in place during the commercials, for a total of 10 minutes.

3. Going to your child's or grandchild's baseball or soccer game? Walk around the field while you cheer 'em on.

4. Do yard work—rake leaves or pull weeds.

5. Turn on your favorite music and let loose in your living room!

6. Walk up and down one flight of stairs 3 times at your own pace. Rest if you need to. Work up to 10 times at once.

7. Take our Energy-Booster Walk (page 164). The intensity level varies, but you should go at your own pace.

8. Play catch with a 2- or 3-pound medicine ball, throwing it in the air and catching it. Work your way up to a larger medicine ball (5 to 10 pounds).

9. Do sets of 10 jumping jacks. Go at your own pace, and rest for 30 to 45 seconds between sets.

FYI

FIT HEARTS AND LUNGS squelch diabetes, according to a study from the University of South Carolina in Columbia. When researchers there tracked 6,249 women for 17 years, they found that the women who ranked in the middle or upper third of the group in terms of cardiorespiratory fitness were significantly less likely to develop diabetes than the third who were least fit.

TO MINIMIZE YOUR BELLY, MAXIMIZE YOUR MOTIVATION

Starting any exercise program is relatively easy; sticking with it—well, that's another story. It takes motivation, that special something that compels a person to act. At times, motivation seems almost magical: It materializes suddenly, and can disappear into thin air just as quickly.

Where does motivation come from? Just as important, once you have it, how do you hold on to it? The answer to both questions depends on you.

There are any number of perfectly good reasons to get into exercise. The ones that inspire you are as unique as your fingerprints. You may feel driven by your desire to improve your health, to reduce stress, to find some "quiet time" to be alone with your thoughts, or to fit into last year's swimsuit. All of these are worthy incentives. But any one of them, by itself, probably is not enough to get you going day after day without fail.

If your motivation to get moving changes like the weather, consider its elusiveness an opportunity to learn more about what makes you tick. You need to dig deep to find that thought, emotion, mantra, or goal that resonates most strongly. And once you know what it is, you must encourage it to take root and grow.

True motivation comes from deep within you. It's the little voice that urges you to push through a walk or lift a dumbbell one more time, even though you're tired. The little voice knows that if you can get through your workout, you'll feel as though you've accomplished something. You'll be proud of yourself. You'll be glad you kept going, even though you didn't think you could. Those are the things that propel you to your next workout . . . and the next!

THE DTOUR WORKOUT AT A GLANCE: WEEKS 1 TO 4

Include a 3-minute warmup and a 2-minute cooldown in the total time of your Cardio Walk.

	WEEK 1	WEEK 2	WEEK 3	WEEK 4
Day 1	Fat-Torch Walk, 20 minutes	Fat-Torch Walk, 25 minutes	Fat-Torch Walk, 30 minutes	Fat-Torch Walk, 35 minutes
Day 2	Metabo Moves; Belly Blast	Metabo Moves; Belly Blast	Calorie-Scorch Walk, 25 minutes	Calorie-Scorch Walk, 30 minutes
Day 3	Calorie-Scorch Walk, 15 minutes	Calorie-Scorch Walk, 20 minutes	Metabo Moves; Belly Blast	Metabo Moves; Belly Blast
Day 4	Rest day	Fat-Torch Walk, 25 minutes	Fat-Torch Walk, 30 minutes	Rest day
Day 5	Fat-Torch Walk, 20 minutes	Rest day	Rest day	Fat-Torch Walk, 35 minutes
Day 6	Metabo Moves; Belly Blast	Metabo Moves; Belly Blast	Calorie-Scorch Walk, 25 minutes	Calorie-Scorch Walk, 30 minutes
Day 7	Calorie-Scorch Walk, 15 minutes	Calorie-Scorch Walk, 20 minutes	Metabo Moves; Belly Blast	Metabo Moves; Belly Blast

DTOUR WINNER!

Josi Ferreira-Garcia, 25
POUNDS LOST: 7
INCHES LOST: 3
BLOOD SUGAR: STABLE

BEFORE   **AFTER**

I decided to go on DTOUR because there's a history of heart disease in my family. My dad had high blood pressure and high cholesterol; my grandmother died of a heart attack at a young age. I'm only 25, but I want to have a long, healthy life, so I need to take care of myself now.

My motivation wasn't to lose weight; it was to get to a healthy weight. And I'm on my way. I feel so much more energetic now. Before I started on DTOUR, I got through the day on diet colas and lattes. My energy and mood were up and down all the time. Almost right away on this diet, I felt a difference in my energy level and my mood. That was a nice surprise.

Another surprise is that I can feel satisfied with smaller portions when I choose the right foods. I eat more good fats, like avocados, and more fruits, veggies, and hummus, which I love.

I had to get used to measuring my portions and planning my meals, but after a week or so, it wasn't hard. I'm on the road a lot, so I need to have healthy meals that I can eat in my car. I try to sit down 1 day a week and plan a whole week of meals. Lunch is usually a pita with hummus and veggies. For dinner, I do grilled or roasted veggies.

Sweets are hard to resist, but I feel better when I don't gorge myself on a big slice of cake or pie.

I did slip up once or twice and eat something that wasn't on the menu, but what I learned is that I feel better when I make healthy choices.

I'm much more active now, too. I used to walk my dog for 10 or 15 minutes. Now, we're up to that 45- or 60-minute walk. I enjoy it, and so does he. I also joined a health club that has a boot-camp class. It's a hard workout, but I feel great when I'm done.

Recently, people have started to ask if I've lost weight. Well, I have, and it feels good that it shows. My husband has noticed, too. He's very fit and athletic and is very supportive of the changes I'm trying to make. He didn't follow the diet—he didn't have to—but he eats what I eat.

Normally when I've accomplished a goal, I've rewarded myself with food. I don't have the desire to do that now. I feel like I've turned a corner, and I don't want to go back.

LOST
7
POUNDS!

10

TRANSFORMATION
TOOL #2
SLEEP
BETTER

Mouthwash ads would have you believe that all you need is a good gargle in the morning to leave you feeling refreshed and ready to face the day ahead. But minty-fresh breath can do only so much for your energy level. What really matters, in terms of how well you function during the day, is how well you sleep the night before.

If you're like most Americans, you probably aren't getting as much shut-eye as you should. This downtime is essential for your body to be able to repair damage and restore vital processes. Without it, your health can take a hit in unexpected ways.

Some of the most fascinating research findings of late have turned attention to the effects of sleep—or a lack of it—on weight gain and blood sugar control. Consider the results of a study from the National Center for Health Statistics, which from 2004 through 2006 surveyed 87,000 men and women about their sleep and related risk factors. The data revealed obesity to be most common among participants getting less than 6 hours of sleep a night. A full one-third of them—33 percent—were identified as obese, compared with just 22 percent of those getting between 7 and 8 hours of sleep each night.

Other studies point to a possible link between too little or poor-quality sleep and an increased risk of type 2 diabetes. One explanation for this comes from a 2007 study at the University of Chicago, in which researchers found that suppressing the deepest stage of sleep (called slow-wave sleep) interferes with the body's ability to regulate blood sugar.

So now you have even more reason to get a good night's sleep every night. That's why we've designated sleep as one of your Transformation Tools. Over the next 4 weeks of DTOUR, we'll be passing along lots of expert-recommended tips and techniques for making sure you get the optimal 7 to 8 hours, and that every one of those hours is restful and rejuvenating. Improved sleep translates into better weight and blood sugar control. Kind of gives new meaning to the term *sweet dreams,* doesn't it?

Here's something else that's sweet: Losing weight the DTOUR way just may improve your sleep habits. That was the case for Tom, one of our DTOUR test panelists, anyway. After 6 weeks on our plan, he noticed that he was sleeping more soundly at night and waking up full of energy in the morning. You can, too!

OUTSMART INSOMNIA

Go figure: Women are twice as likely as men to suffer from insomnia. Usually we define this condition as trouble falling asleep, but it's more than that. It can mean frequently waking during the night or waking too early in the morning and then having trouble getting back to sleep.

Insomnia takes two forms: acute and chronic. Acute insomnia lasts from 1 night to several weeks, while chronic insomnia occurs several nights a week for a month or more. The chronic variety, in turn, can be primary or secondary. *Primary* insomnia is not related to any other health problem. *Secondary* insomnia, on the other hand, can be caused by certain medications; stress or depression; or a medical condition such as asthma, arthritis, or cancer.

The first step in treating insomnia is to establish and maintain healthy sleep habits. If that isn't enough to cure your sleeplessness, try a relaxation technique such as yoga or meditation.

For chronic insomnia, cognitive-behavioral therapy (CBT)—which helps you identify and change unhealthy behaviors and thought patterns—has proven beneficial. When Norwegian researchers treated 46 people with chronic insomnia with CBT, a sleep medication, or a placebo, the deep sleep of those in the CBT group increased by 27 percent, more than that of the other groups.

To get a taste of CBT, here's an exercise you can try on your own. First, you'll need to determine the number of hours per night that you actually spend sleeping. If it's 5 hours, then set your alarm for 6:00 a.m. and go to bed at 1:00 a.m. Once you're sleeping for 85 to 90 percent of those 5 hours, extend your sleep time by going to bed 15 to 20 minutes earlier and waking up 15 to 20 minutes later. Over the course of a week or two, you should adjust to the longer rest period.

Another treatment option is sleep medication. It can be effective, but none of the medications available are without risks and side effects, such as morning drowsiness, headaches, and possible withdrawal symptoms when stopping treatment. For this reason, sleep medication should be taken only under medical supervision. Your doctor can help you determine whether and which sleep medication would be best for you.

SKIMPY SLEEP SCHEDULE = BIG BELLY

Forget *Sleepless in Seattle*: From west to east and at all points in between, we Americans are one weary bunch. Just consider how our sleep habits have changed over the past 40 to 50 years. Back in 1960, we averaged 8½ hours of sleep per night. Today, it's more like 6 hours, 40 minutes. That's a lot of lost sleep.

Perhaps not so coincidentally, as our sleep time declined, our waistlines expanded. Between 1960 and today, the rates of overweight and obesity have climbed from 25 percent and 11 percent, respectively, to 66 percent and 32 percent.

FYI

EACH NIGHT, we typically cycle through five stages of sleep. We slip into the light stages of 1 and 2, then progress to the deeper slow-wave sleep (SWS) of stages 3 and 4. Finally, we enter rapid eye movement (REM) sleep, which is when we dream. The sleep cycle lasts between 90 and 120 minutes and usually occurs four times a night; about one-third of this time is spent in SWS.

Sleep researchers are pursuing a number of intriguing theories to explain the apparent correlation between lack of sleep and weight gain. One is that when we're sleep-deprived, we consume more calories than our bodies need, especially in the form of sugary snacks and starches. This was the conclusion of a 2004 study led by sleep scientist Eve Van Cauter, PhD, and a University of Chicago research team. They found that partial sleep deprivation alters blood levels of hunger-regulating hormones, prompting an increase in appetite and a preference for calorie-dense, high-carbohydrate foods.

At about the same time, researchers at Stanford University's Howard Hughes Medical Institute were conducting their own study of the effects of sleep deprivation on these hunger-regulating hormones. They decided to piggyback on the Wisconsin Sleep Cohort Study, which has been tracking the sleep habits of 1,024 men and women since 1989.

For their study, the Stanford team examined data on the sleep duration (both habitual and immediately prior to blood sampling), body mass indexes (BMIs), and pre-breakfast blood hormone levels of the study participants. Among those who were getting less than 8 hours of sleep a night—74 percent of all participants—BMI was inversely proportional to sleep time. In other words, the less sleep, the higher the BMI. Even more intriguing, the researchers found an association between a shortage of sleep and high blood levels of ghrelin, a hormone thought to stimulate food intake. Their conclusion: "In Western societies, where chronic sleep restriction is common and food is widely available, changes in appetite regulatory hormones with sleep curtailment may contribute to obesity."

SLEEP QUALITY COUNTS, TOO

Just as too little sleep can throw the body's finely tuned appetite-control mechanisms out of whack, setting the stage for weight gain, it also can upset the equally sensitive processes responsible for blood sugar balance. Scientists are working to pinpoint precisely how this happens, but the bottom line is that the body must churn out extra insulin to keep blood sugar in check. The risks of developing insulin resistance and diabetes start to climb, as does the likelihood of weight gain, because an elevated insulin level encourages cells to store excess fat instead of burning it. Much of the research so far has focused on the relationship between sleep *quantity* and diabetes. But according to a 2007 study from the University of Chicago Medical Center, sleep *quality* may be an equally important risk factor for the disease.

For the study, researchers recruited nine volunteers, all between ages 20 and 31, all lean and healthy. The men and women spent 5 consecutive nights in the university sleep laboratory. For the first 2 nights, they turned in at 11:00 p.m. and slept undisturbed until 7:30 a.m. They continued this routine for the next 3 nights, but with one key difference: As they began drifting into slow-wave sleep, the researchers played soft sounds through speakers placed by the beds. The sounds were loud enough to reduce slow-wave sleep by 90 percent, though they didn't fully rouse the study participants, who had vague memories of hearing noise from 3 to 15 times the night before. In fact, their sleep was being interrupted between 250 and 300 times a night. No wonder they woke up tired and cranky!

For the researchers, though, the most significant change was not in the volunteers' moods, but in their bloodstreams. Tests revealed that their blood sugar levels had climbed by 23 percent over the 3 nights of disturbed sleep. The researchers concluded that suppressing slow-wave sleep for just this short period had the same negative effect on the body's ability to regulate blood sugar as gaining 20 to 30 pounds!

Because this study was so small, more research is necessary to confirm its findings. Still, it provides the first convincing evidence of the importance of good sleep quality to healthy blood sugar control. As the study's lead author, Esra Tasali, MD, observes, "A profound decrease in slow-wave sleep had an immediate and significant adverse effect on insulin sensitivity and glucose tolerance."

A RECIPE FOR THE PERFECT NIGHT'S SLEEP

The science certainly is impressive, but we'd venture to guess that you don't need a raft of studies to sell you on the health benefits of sleep. After all, you know how fabulous you feel when you get a full 7 to 8 hours of deep, undisturbed slumber. The challenge is to do it consistently, night after night. You can, if you approach it in a systematic way.

We like to compare the process of creating a good night's sleep to that of making a new dish for the first time. To start, you probably follow the recipe to the letter to get the best results. Then, as you become comfortable with it, you tweak it to suit your and your family's tastes—always sticking with the basic recipe, but adding a pinch of this or a dash of that to make it "just right."

There's a basic recipe for sleep, too, and it comes from the National Sleep Foundation. Its staple ingredients are good sleep habits, which include the following:

◆ Use your bed only for sleep and sex.

◆ Try to turn in at the same time each night and get up at the same time each morning.

◆ Finish eating 2 to 3 hours before your regular bedtime.

◆ Exercise regularly, but end your workout at least 3 hours before bedtime. Otherwise, you could have a hard time falling asleep.

◆ Stop caffeinated foods (chocolate) and drinks (coffee, tea, diet cola) 6 to 8 hours before bedtime.

◆ Skip the nightcap before bedtime. Alcohol can interfere with sleep quality and cause you to wake up during the night.

WHEN SNORE MEANS MORE

Your partner saws logs all night long—with a chain saw, from the sound of it. Or does your snoring keep your partner awake?

Either way, loud, start-and-stop snoring (as opposed to quiet, steady snoring)—combined with extreme daytime sleepiness—is a symptom of obstructive sleep apnea (OSA), a serious sleep disorder.

It's serious because people who have OSA are nearly three times more likely to develop type 2 diabetes than those who don't, according to a 2007 study by the Yale Center for Sleep Medicine in New Haven. In fact, 40 percent of patients with OSA have diabetes, while about 23 percent of those with diabetes have OSA. Other research links OSA to obesity, high blood pressure, and heart attack.

People with OSA stop breathing in their sleep for seconds at a time hundreds of times a night. These episodes are caused by the tongue or fatty tissue in the throat blocking the windpipe. As a result, those with OSA drift from the deeper, more restful stages of sleep into the lighter stages. Cheated of deep sleep, they feel exhausted during the day.

They also are prone to weight gain. OSA alters the stages of sleep, and some studies have linked these changes to a reduction in growth hormone, which influences how much fat the body and belly store.

The best treatment for OSA is a CPAP device (CPAP is short for *continuous positive airway pressure*). By way of a face mask, tubes, and a fan, CPAP uses air pressure to push the tongue forward, open the windpipe, and let air inside.

Several studies have found that CPAP helps people with diabetes and OSA sleep better—and improves blood sugar, to boot. In a 2005 study, for example, a research team at the University of Illinois at Chicago evaluated the effects of CPAP treatment on blood sugar in 25 people with diabetes. After 3 months, average blood sugar 1 hour after breakfast fell from 191 to 130 milligrams per deciliter, with similar reductions occurring after other meals.

For another study, German researchers investigated CPAP's effect on insulin resistance by using the device to treat 40 men and women with OSA. After just 2 days, the participants showed improved insulin sensitivity.

Scientists speculate that CPAP lowers blood sugar by reducing insulin resistance. Restless sleep causes a rise in hormones that work against insulin. By improving sleep, CPAP may stabilize hormone levels.

The evidence of a link between loud snoring and diabetes is so strong that the International Diabetes Federation is urging physicians who treat people with one condition to test for the other. Consult your doctor if you (or your partner) experience:

◆ Loud and chronic snoring.
◆ Pauses in snoring, followed by choking or gasping.
◆ Snoring that increases in frequency and gets louder over time.
◆ Dry mouth upon awakening during the night or in the morning.

◆ Establish a relaxing prebedtime routine. Taking a warm bath or sipping a cup of noncaffeinated herbal tea can help you wind down.

◆ Get into bed only when you're tired.

Once you have this recipe down pat, you can tinker with it by adding ingredients that help you create a peaceful, comfortable sleep environment. Things like noise, light (or, rather, darkness), and temperature are to sleep as salt and pepper are to cooking: simple, but vital to the outcome and thoroughly individual. Feel free to pick and choose from the tips in this chapter, as well as those offered throughout the 4-Week Total Transformation. Even one small change can have a big impact on your sleep experience—and that means better weight and blood sugar control.

NOISE

Some of us can sleep through a dripping faucet or the neighbor's barking dog; others wake up at the slightest bump or creak. Some of us need the *whoosh* of a fan to help us nod off; for others, only the familiar screech of sirens or rumble of trains will do the trick.

The point is, each of us has a unique noise threshold that plays an important role in determining how quickly we fall asleep and whether we stay asleep. Experiment with these strategies to find your personal lullaby.

Make some (white) noise. If you combine all of the sound frequencies that are audible to humans (there are about 20,000), you hear the soft hiss of what's called *white noise*. Because white noise contains all frequencies, it masks other sounds.

To make your own white noise, just turn on a fan or air conditioner. It will block out any sounds that disturb you—or fill the silence that keeps you awake. If you prefer something more high-tech, invest in a white-noise machine, also known as a *sound conditioner*. These gadgets come in

FYI

THERE'S A DIFFERENCE between sleepiness and fatigue. Sleepiness is the inability to stay awake even in situations that require you to, such as when you're at work or driving. Fatigue is a state of sustained exhaustion and reduced capacity for physical and mental work that is not relieved by rest. Both conditions can affect your quality of life and safety and should be evaluated for underlying causes so appropriate treatment can be prescribed.

all sizes and styles, but generally they can be programmed to produce either a sleep-promoting hiss or the soothing sounds of nature.

Install sound-absorbent accessories. Hang heavy curtains or drapes in your bedroom, or lay down thick carpet. Both of these absorb slumber-disturbing noises.

Travel with your favorite sleep sound. A small fan, a ticking clock, or a favorite CD can help you get your rest away from home.

Snore-proof your spouse. If your partner's snoring disrupts your sleep (not to mention your sanity), the two of you need to work out a compromise. It's not only your sleep that's at stake, but your partner's health, too. We'll talk more about this later in the chapter.

LIGHT AND DARKNESS

Much of our sleep pattern (i.e., feeling awake during the day and sleepy at night) is regulated by light and darkness. As we awake each morning, the natural light entering our retinas sets our biological clocks for the day. Later on, nightfall prompts the release of melatonin, the hormone that promotes drowsiness and sleep.

Maintaining this cycle, known as circadian rhythm, is vital to sleep quantity and quality. You need to find just the right balance between light and darkness as you go about your daytime and bedtime routines. Here's how.

During the day, get some sun. Bright outdoor light is the most powerful regulator of your biological clock, the master timekeeper in your brain that determines when you feel alert and when you feel sleepy. So head outside for some direct sunlight; even 10 minutes a day will do the trick. (Remember, too, that your body uses sunlight to synthesize vitamin D, one of our all-important Fat-Fighting 4!)

At night, forgo bright overhead lights. Even 30 minutes of exposure to light that's slightly brighter than that in a typical office can suppress melatonin production. Instead, use task lamps with 40- to 60-watt incandescent bulbs when washing dishes, reading, or watching television.

At bedtime, go for blackout conditions. Try wearing an eye mask, or dress your bedroom windows with light-blocking curtains or drapes. If you use a nightlight in your bedroom, equip it with a 7-watt incandescent bulb. It's okay to briefly turn on a low-wattage lightbulb for a bathroom run.

Shed light on middle-of-the-night wake-ups. If you typically awaken earlier than you'd like to, try increasing your exposure to bright light by an hour or two in the evening. It may take you longer to fall asleep, but you'll stay asleep longer in the morning.

TEMPERATURE

Many of us consider a cool, crisp night to be ideal "sleeping weather." Sleep researchers tend to agree. You see, about 4 hours after you fall asleep, your body temperature drops to its lowest daily level. So by keeping your bedroom on the cool side, you mimic your body's internal thermostat. And this, in turn, helps to regulate your body's cycle of alertness and fatigue.

While sleep researchers typically recommend keeping the bedroom between 60° and 70°F, it may take some getting used to—especially if your (or your partner's) internal thermostat runs hotter or colder. These tips can help keep you cozy and comfortable.

In cold weather: You can lock in the heat by using a thick comforter or an electric blanket. Or, wear warmer pajamas. Then, if you get too warm during the night, stick your foot out from under the covers. It's natural climate control!

In hot weather: Sleep is lighter and nighttime awakenings increase, research suggests. But closing the windows and running an air conditioner all night can cause your nose and throat to dry out, which could be just as uncomfortable. Here's a compromise: Use the air conditioner in tandem with a humidifier to moisten your nasal passages and throat.

In any climate: When you sit for most of the day, your core temperature remains low—and you stay wide awake at night when you're supposed to be sleepy. The DTOUR Workout, which you learned all about in Chapter 9, is one surefire way to get moving, but even a brief walk can be beneficial. In one study involving more than 700 men and women, those who walked at least 6 blocks a day at a normal pace were one-third less likely to have trouble sleeping. Those who picked up the pace fared even better.

YOUR MATTRESS AND PILLOW

In the fairy tale *The Princess and the Pea*, the truth of a maiden's claim of being of royal blood is tested by placing a pea under 20 mattresses and 20 feather beds, because the sleep of only a real princess would be disturbed by something so small. Okay, that's overstating the importance of comfort to sleep. Still, your mattress (and pillow) can mean the difference between a good night's sleep and a nightly marathon of tossing and turning. Here are some tips for outfitting your bed for sound snoozing.

Spring for a new mattress. If you wake up achy each morning, or if your

TAP INTO YOUR SENSES FOR BETTER SLEEP

To lull an infant or toddler to sleep, you appeal to their senses. They're soothed by the sound of a ticking clock, the touch and smell of a favorite stuffed animal or blanket, the taste of a bottle of warm milk.

To ease into sleep and turn bedtime into a truly sensual experience, tune in to your senses. These ideas will get you started.

Sight: Make like a movie star. Even a small amount of light can suppress production of melatonin, the hormone that promotes sleep. If you're bothered by the glare of streetlights outside your bedroom window or by your partner's reading light, slip into a satin sleep mask. To sleep even more soundly, invest in a sleep mask or "eye pillow" infused with the sleep-inducing scent of lavender (see below).

Sound: Create an aural oasis. Lull yourself to sleep with a mini-fountain small enough to place on your nightstand, or a "sound conditioner" that generates white noise or recreates the soothing sounds of nature, including rain, chirping crickets, or ocean waves.

Smell: Follow your nose. Sprinkle a few drops of pure lavender essential oil on a tissue and tuck it under your pillow. In a study of 31 men and women, psychologists at Wesleyan University in Middletown, Connecticut, found that the scent of lavender increased slow-wave sleep, the deepest, most restorative stage.

Touch: Invest in cool threads. Wildbleu's pajamas and sheets (www.wildbleu. com) wick away moisture to help ease night sweats and hot flashes, while a body pillow will let you snuggle if you sleep solo. Or, simply ease yourself into the comforting "touch" of a warm bath before bed.

Taste: Nibble a sleepy-time snack. There's evidence that people trying to lose weight wake up frequently and that carbohydrates and dairy products consumed just before bed can reduce the time needed to nod off. Sip a mug of warm, low-fat milk or hot, creamy sugar-free cocoa, or spread a piece of whole grain toast with a tablespoon of all-natural peanut butter. One caveat: If you already have diabetes, follow your doctor's or nutritionist's advice about snacking at bedtime.

mattress is saggy, lumpy, or more than 7 years old, it's time to invest in a new one.

Firm up a squishy bed. For a temporary fix while you're sizing up a replacement mattress, slide a sheet of ³⁄₄-inch plywood between your current mattress and box spring.

Test-drive several models. At the store, lie in your preferred sleep position on each mattress for about 10 minutes. You should feel comfortable and supported, and your back muscles should be relaxed.

Buy for durability. Choose a coil count of at least 400 for a queen mattress and 480 for a king. Make sure that the retailer has an exchange policy; you won't know for several nights whether you've found the right mattress.

Add a pillow to beat back and neck pain. Do you sleep on your back? Tuck an extra pillow under your knees and a smaller one under your lower back. Side sleepers should wedge a flat pillow between their knees; stomach snoozers will want one under their hips.

Get a specialty pillow. A cervical pillow or one made of memory foam is specially contoured to support the neck. Throwing an arm and a leg over a body pillow also can help keep the spine in line. Some medical-supply stores and department stores carry these pillows, as do some specialty linen stores.

Allergy-proof your pillow. Synthetic pillows can hold up to five times as much dust-mite matter as feather pillows, which are encased to prevent feathers from floating away. If you use a synthetic pillow, put it in a plastic cover (underneath your pillowcase) to keep dust mites from aggravating allergy or asthma symptoms.

4 MORE SLEEP-STEALERS—SOLVED!

If your bedroom makeover doesn't produce the desired results, you may need to engage in further sleuthing to figure out just what's hampering your sleep. Experts have identified four situations that can easily keep you from sleeping as well as you should. Do any of these sound familiar?

Your bed is also an entertainment center or workstation. When you habitually work on spreadsheets or watch the 11 o'clock news while propped up on your pillows, your brain learns to associate bed with activity rather than with sleep. It's okay to tune in to TV to relax and unwind, but opt for soothing shows, such as those about nature or animals—and keep your set somewhere other than your bedroom. And definitely shut down your laptop before climbing into bed.

You yak on your cell phone before bed. Turn off your cell and use a landline for nighttime calls. Researchers from Wayne State University, in collaboration with a research team from Sweden, theorize that low-level radiation from cell phones may disrupt production of sleep-inducing melatonin or excite other areas of the brain.

Your pet keeps you awake. While sharing your bed with Fido or Fluffy warms the soul, his or her movements and noises can leave you sleepless. Consider relocating your pooch or kitty to a special sleeping place beside your bed. Don't feel guilty: Once you're well rested, you'll have more energy to give to your pet.

Your partner bugs you in bed. He snores. She tosses, turns, and kicks through the night. If your partner is keeping you awake, you are not alone. According to a 2005 survey administered by the National Sleep Foundation, 38 percent of respondents reported relationship problems related to a partner's sleep disorder.

Snoring is the biggest challenge. You may have tried earplugs; he may have tried nasal strips. The best fix: an honest discussion of the issue and an expression of your concern for his health. Loud snoring—especially if accompanied by choking and gasping—could be a sign of obstructive sleep apnea. (For more on this serious sleep disorder and what to do about it, see page 177.)

If you choose to sleep in another room as a more or less permanent solution, reassure your partner that going solo won't deep-six your sex life. Agree to regular "date nights" in a bed you share.

FYI

JET LAG IS A COMMON SLEEP THIEF: Speeding across time zones disrupts your circadian rhythm, resulting in exhaustion and, paradoxically, trouble falling or staying asleep. A melatonin supplement (available at drugstores) may help you override the urge to stay awake when you should be nodding off. Take 3 milligrams of melatonin 30 minutes before bedtime every night while you're at your travel destination.

CHAPTER 11

TRANSFORMATION TOOL #3

STRESS LESS

Have you seen the stress reduction kit that's making the rounds online? The "kit" consists of a circle bearing the words "Bang head here." The accompanying e-mail instructs you to print out the circle, then take these steps:

1. Place kit on firm surface.
2. Follow directions inside kit.
3. Repeat Step 2 as necessary.

Admit it—that made you smile, didn't it? A dose of humor is an instantaneous antidote to stress, able to defuse just about any tense or upsetting situation. And let's face it: If you're upright and breathing, chances are you're experiencing stress in one form or another.

The thing about stress is, it can do much more than inflict tension headaches and tie your stomach in knots. Studies show that *chronic* stress—the kind that grinds on endlessly, as with a dead-end job or ongoing financial worries—can increase your chances of developing type 2 diabetes, especially if you're genetically susceptible to the disease. If you already have diabetes, chronic stress can fuel the development of complications such as eye and kidney damage. (In contrast to chronic stress, *acute* stress arises from a once-and-done incident, like a fender bender or a long line at the supermarket.)

Getting a handle on stress is vital to controlling your blood sugar. As a bonus, it can help melt away belly fat, which tends to accumulate in the presence of stress hormones. (We'll explore the mechanism behind this in just a bit.) Belly fat, as you'll remember from Chapter 3, is a key risk factor for insulin resistance and diabetes.

So now you know *why* you should keep stress in check. The question is, *how?* In this chapter, and throughout the 4-Week Total Transformation, you'll learn lots of simple strategies to defuse stress on the spot, as well as proven measures to help you stay as stress-free as possible.

The fact is, you can't completely eliminate stress from your life; nor, for that matter, would you want to. There are moments when your body's stress response can work in your favor—when you steer clear of an oncoming car to avoid an accident, for example, or you're giving an important presentation at work. In situations like these, stress helps sharpen your mental and physical performance. It's when stress persists, putting your brain and body on overdrive all the time, that it becomes problematic.

Another fact to keep in mind: Stress arises not from a particular incident or circumstance, but from our *perception of* and *reaction to* it. This is excellent news, actually, because our perceptions and reactions are entirely within our control. In other words, we choose how we react to a situation, even if we're not conscious of doing it. This is why those of us who are generally optimistic and confident that we can handle whatever life throws our way tend to fare better in the face of stress than those who are not. It's a trait known as *resilience,* and it's the closest thing to a stress vaccine that we humans have.

To stay a step ahead of stress, then, you need the skills and tools not only to cope with the stressors that are in your life right now, but also to cultivate the sort of resilient mindset that can keep any stressful situation from getting the best of you. With our C-A-L-M Technique and our Tranquillity Tips, which you'll learn here, you'll be able to shrug off stress—and tighten your control of your blood sugar *and* your weight.

FIGHT-OR-FLIGHT: YOUR BODY ON OVERDRIVE

Now, it's important to remember that not all stress is bad. There's a difference between *eustress*—the positive, butterflies-in-the-belly thrill that accompanies landing a big promotion or even taking a spin on a monster roller coaster—and *distress*, the angst that can manifest as pounding temples, an upset stomach, and sleepless nights. These physical symptoms are characteristic of what's known as the fight-or-flight response.

Hardwired into your brain, fight-or-flight is your body's built-in mechanism for handling a stressful situation. Think of it as an early warning system, sounding the instant it senses imminent danger.

Fight-or-flight originates in the part of the brain called the hypothalamus. When stimulated by a perceived threat, the hypothalamus triggers a sequence of biochemical processes that, in turn, instruct your adrenal glands to secrete cortisol and adrenaline (among other stress hormones) into your bloodstream.

This onslaught of stress hormones puts your body on alert. Your breathing becomes quick and shallow. The blood in your digestive tract is diverted to your muscles and limbs, which need the extra oxygen and nutrients to either defend against the threat or run from it. Your senses sharpen. You prepare—physically and psychologically—to confront or escape danger.

The trouble, especially with chronic stress, is that there usually is no danger. Fight-or-flight would come in handy if we still lived in caves and needed those

TENSE YOUR MUSCLES, SCRAP YOUR STRESS

Richard S. Surwit, PhD, vice-chairman of the department of psychology and neuroscience at Duke University in Durham, North Carolina, pioneered the use of progressive muscle relaxation, or PMR, to lower blood sugar levels in people with diabetes. Among those he's worked with are a woman who was close to losing her eyesight from diabetes and a preacher who used the technique to keep his blood sugar from surging during his Sunday sermons.

PMR—in which you systematically tense and then relax your muscles from head to toe—works by triggering the relaxation response, which counters the fight-or-flight response. By discouraging the release of stress hormones, PMR prevents the liver from releasing too much glucose and allows the pancreas to release the right amount of insulin, thereby controlling blood sugar.

PMR is easy to learn and requires no formal training. The whole process should take about 10 minutes. Try to practice at least once—or, even better, several times—a day.

1. Find a quiet room and lie down on a flat, comfortable surface.

2. Take a few deep breaths.

3. Slowly tighten and relax your body's different muscle groups in succession from head to toe. As you tighten each muscle group, like, say, the muscles in your legs, inhale deeply and hold the tension for several seconds. Then exhale slowly as you relax.

surges of stress hormones to face down a predator. Modern stressors—bills, job worries, and family spats—may keep us awake at night, but they don't threaten our physical survival. Still, our bodies react as if they do.

STRESS AND BLOOD SUGAR: A WEIGHTY LINK

The surging stress hormones activated by fight-or-flight also prompt your liver to make a lot of stored energy (sugar and fat) available to cells so they have the necessary fuel to power the body to react. A healthy pancreas recognizes this rise in blood sugar and secretes the hormone insulin in response.

Not so in a person with type 2 diabetes. Either the pancreas is unable to secrete insulin or cells are unable to respond to the hormone. The result is the same: Blood sugar goes up and stays up.

Researchers who study diabetes continue to ponder whether stress could be a precursor to the disease. Based on the current state of the science, the answer appears to be yes. One 2006 study involving 677 Israeli workers found that those with job burnout were almost twice as likely to develop type 2 diabetes, even when factors such as age, sex, activity level, and obesity were accounted for. In an earlier study, researchers at the University of Washington in Seattle compared 47 people who provided care for spouses with Alzheimer's disease to 77 who were not caregivers. Levels of cortisol, glucose, and insulin turned out to be higher in the caregivers than in the noncaregivers.

Chronic stress not only does a number on your blood sugar, it also widens your waistline—in part because all that cortisol coursing through the bloodstream triggers cravings for high-fat, high-sugar comfort foods. This may help to explain why many of us turn to food when we're stressed out, and why we're likely to choose a brownie rather than a nice bowl of steamed broccoli. (Need we mention that prolonged stress can cause us to ditch our regular workouts, too?)

The continual flood of cortisol that occurs with chronic stress contributes to weight gain in another, more surreptitious way: by instructing the body to store fat around the belly. It's nature's way of ensuring that you have adequate energy reserves to survive a catastrophic event like, say, a famine. Ironic, isn't it? Your body is determined to cling to fat just as you're trying to lose it!

PEACE OUT, SLIM DOWN, CURB BLOOD SUGAR

So, what can you do about stress? A better question might be, What can you do about life? To borrow a line from Buddha, "It is better to travel well than to arrive."

In other words, life is a journey. Enjoy the trip. Once you learn to live in the moment, worrying about neither past nor future, stress recedes and health can thrive. Research bears this out: Learning to cool chronic stress—and you *can* learn—lowers blood sugar and improves diabetes control.

In a landmark 2002 study conducted by Richard S. Surwit, PhD, of Duke University, 108 people with type 2 diabetes attended five diabetes education sessions with or without stress management training. The training involved instruction in a technique called progressive muscle relaxation (see page 188) as well as other stress management strategies. After a year, one-third of the patients in the stress management group had improved their blood sugar levels enough to lower their risk of the most serious diabetes complications, such as heart disease, kidney failure, nerve damage, and vision problems.

More recent studies of a relaxation technique known as mindfulness suggest similar results. The central principle of Buddhist meditation, mindfulness teaches us to achieve tranquillity by living in the moment. You can practice mindfulness anytime, anywhere; all you need to do is focus on the here and now—the sensations in your feet as you walk, the juice that spurts from an orange slice as you bite into it, your rhythm as you sweep the floor.

Back in 1978, pioneering mind/body researcher Jon Kabat-Zinn, PhD, launched the mindfulness-based stress reduction (MBSR) program at the stress reduction clinic he founded at the University of Massachusetts Medical School. Today, MBSR is taught worldwide to help people manage stress, illness, and pain.

Researchers at Jefferson Medical College in Philadelphia decided to investigate whether MBSR could help people with diabetes manage their blood sugar. For a small 2007 pilot study, they recruited 11 men and women with diabetes to follow the program. The group learned a range of mindfulness meditation techniques, such as awareness of breathing and how to walk, eat, and communicate in mindful ways. They practiced these techniques on their own for at least 20 minutes 6 days a week.

After 8 weeks, all 11 participants showed, on average, a 0.48 percent reduction in A1c. Bonus: Their self-reported symptoms of depression, anxiety, and stress declined by 43 percent, 37 percent, and 35 percent, respectively.

FROM THE DTOUR DIETITIAN

If you love the sweet, creamy, stress-relieving power of a cup of hot cocoa, here's some exciting news: Hot chocolate supercharged with natural plant substances called flavonols may help prevent heart disease, which often goes hand in hand with diabetes.

Research has shown that flavonols—found in chocolate and cocoa, as well as red wine and certain fruits and veggies—support heart and blood vessel function. In people with diabetes, unhealthy blood vessels can set the stage for heart attack and stroke.

For a 2008 study published in the *Journal of the American College of Cardiology,* German researchers decided to examine the effect of a specially made flavonol-rich cocoa on people with type 2 diabetes. Their goal: to learn whether flavonols play any role in the ability of blood vessels to relax. This characteristic, called flow-mediated dilation, is a common measure of vascular health.

The researchers randomly assigned 41 men and women with diabetes to drink cocoa that contained either 25 milligrams or 321 milligrams of flavonols per serving. The target "dosage" was 3 servings of cocoa every day for 30 days. The researchers used ultrasound and blood pressure measurements to evaluate blood vessel function at the start of the study and again on Days 8 and 30.

After 30 days, the group who had been drinking the high-flavonol cocoa showed a dramatic, 30 percent improvement in vascular health and function. Not so for those who drank the low-flavonol cocoa.

The high-flavonol cocoa used in the study isn't available in stores, at least not yet. But based on these study findings, we now know that flavonols can be an important part of a healthy diet for people with diabetes, who are at increased risk of heart problems.

—Barbara

And remember how stress—specifically, the stress hormone cortisol—causes your body to hoard fat and store it in your midsection? Well, researchers at the University of California–San Francisco Center for Obesity Assessment, Study, and Treatment recently launched a study to determine whether techniques such as meditation, yoga, and mindful eating could help women shed belly fat and keep it off. It's called the Craving and Lifestyle Management through Mindfulness pilot study, or CALMM, for short. (*Love* it!)

Although the study is ongoing, the researchers are encouraged by the early results. According to the lead author, Elissa Epel, PhD, an assistant professor of psychiatry, "We know that excessive exposure to cortisol can increase belly fat, so it's logical that stress reduction should minimize it."

STRESS CHECK #1: C-A-L-M IN 4 EASY STEPS

As we pointed out earlier, stress isn't so much about a particular incident or circumstance, but rather your perception of and reaction to it. We've devised a simple mental exercise, called C-A-L-M, that you can use whenever you find yourself in a stressful situation. It's intended to help you clear your head and short-circuit the fight-or-flight response. Try it the next time you feel your stress level rising; we promise you'll defrazzle in 5 minutes or less.

Center. Find a quiet, comfortable place without distractions. (If you're at work, close your door or borrow an empty office.) Sit with your back straight; rest your hands in a comfortable position. If you like, ask your higher power, such as God, to help you find your center. Let your eyes rest comfortably downward; gaze softly, but do not focus on anything. Let your breathing become deep and rhythmic. It's okay to let your attention drift a bit, but stay relaxed. If your eyelids get heavy, let them close. Don't worry about doing it right. Just be.

Accept. When you feel centered, open your eyes and formally accept your stressor, whatever it is. Say, silently or out loud, "At this moment, my [job, boss, mother, life] is causing me stress. At this moment, I choose to accept it." Repeat it as many times as you wish as you open yourself to your stress.

Don't fight it. Sit with it. Give yourself permission to relinquish the illusion of control.

Of course, there's a difference between accepting what (or whom) you can't change and being reluctant to change what you can. To help sort that out, consider the stressor. Then ask yourself, "Are the circumstances beyond my control? Have I done all that I can?" If the answer is yes, move to the next step.

Let go. Formally give up control over the person or event that's stressing you. You might literally give yourself a little shake or brush your shoulders as a sign that you've decided to release your worry or frustration.

Often, letting go is accompanied by a sense of relief and release—sometimes subtle, sometimes quite powerful. You might feel your jaw unclench, your shoulders relax, your mind clear, your heart soften. You might even shed a few tears. That's all good.

What if you can't let go? That's okay, too; just keep trying. Letting go is a skill

MEDITATION MADE EASY

Think meditating requires the patience, dedication, and endless free time of a Tibetan monk? Here are three simple ways to work this mind-calming discipline into your daily routine.

Walking meditation. Focus on your breathing as you walk; count your steps. Note how your feet and legs move. Celebrate each movement as a miracle of silent communication between your brain and your body.

Mindfulness break. Whatever you're doing—paperwork, the dishes, driving to the convenience store for milk—focus your attention. Note the smallest sensations and details: the feel of paper between your fingers, the rainbow on a soap bubble, how your fingers close around the cold plastic jug. Consider each element of the activity as if you are moving in slow motion. If other thoughts interrupt, gently bring your mind back to your task.

Mantra. In Sanskrit, *man* means mind and *tra* means deliverance. Repeating a mantra—a word, phrase, or sound—creates a vibration that can deliver you from worldly cares. Choose a prayer, word, or sound that invokes a spiritual feeling. Sit comfortably and breathe deeply as you chant it silently.

that takes a lifetime of practice to learn, so we're all perpetual students. But it does get easier with time.

Move on. Get on with your day. With your *life*. This minivisualization can help: Imagine an old-fashioned English garden with a cobblestone path winding its way through the lush and fragrant space. Then see your stressors—your boss, your broken dishwasher, even your diabetes—as cobblestones in that path. Those rough stones lead through some breathtaking scenery, don't they? That's the lesson here: Life is what you make it. So is stress.

STRESS CHECK #2:
BANK TRANQUILLITY POINTS

The C-A-L-M Technique is perfect for dealing with the sorts of stressors that seem to loom large over your home or work life. But what about the more everyday variety of stress—the broken appliances, the unexpected bills, the lost dry cleaning? Sure, they're minor events in the grand scheme of things. But by repeatedly triggering the fight-or-flight response, they, too, can take a toll on your blood sugar and your waistline.

We have the solution—or, rather, 50 solutions! They're called Tranquillity Points—50 simple, fast-working strategies that not only provide instant relaxation but also help build your "immunity" to stress, so you're ready whenever life decides to take a swing at you. We're talking things like making a paper airplane, waving to the stranger in the next car, and chomping bubble gum. (When was the last time you blew a bubble?)

Your mission is to accumulate as many Tranquillity Points as you can throughout the day. No need to aim for a specific number; after all, you're under enough pressure already! Just enjoy doing as many as you can. You may be surprised by how easily you can squeeze pleasure and relaxation into your daily routine. (Note that the three exercises in "Meditation Made Easy" on page 193 count as Tranquillity Points, too.)

1. Belt out a show tune in the shower.
2. Tickle a baby.

3. Buy a bottle of soap bubbles, the kind you used to blow with a wand as a kid, and keep it in your car. Blow when you're stuck in traffic.

4. Snuggle up with your dog or cat.

5. Go to a local pet store and coo at the puppies and kitties in the window.

6. Make faces in the mirror in the restroom at work. (Best to do this when alone.)

7. On your daily walk, break into a skip for a spell.

8. Teach a kid to fly a kite or operate a remote-control car.

9. Buy yourself a fake-glasses-and-nose set. Wear it around the house when life just feels too hard. Get a few pairs for your family, too.

MEN MAY WORRY THEMSELVES INTO DIABETES

Men who are chronically stressed or depressed may have another worry to contend with: They're more likely to develop type 2 diabetes. That's according to a 2008 Swedish study that found that psychological distress—including anxiety and depression—more than doubles a man's diabetes risk.

For the study, researchers at the Karolinska Institute in Stockholm recruited 2,127 men and 3,100 women, all with normal blood sugar levels at the outset. The volunteers were screened for signs of distress, such as anxiety, sleeplessness, apathy, and depression. Then, 8 to 10 years later, they were tested for diabetes.

The study data showed that men with high levels of distress were 2.2 times more likely than those with the lowest levels to have developed diabetes in the intervening decade. That's even after accounting for other diabetes risk factors, such as age, family history, and body mass index.

Interestingly, the women in the study—even those with the most distress—showed no change in diabetes risk. They were, however, slightly more likely to have developed prediabetes.

Why the different outcomes for men and women? The researchers theorize that it may have something to do with how the sexes cope with distress. While women are more inclined to share their emotions with others, men tend to conceal feelings and instead turn to unhealthy behaviors—such as eating too much—to cope.

10. Sing in the rain.
11. Buy a box of Mr. Bubble bubble bath and invite your partner to a tub party.
12. Knit baby hats and booties for a local charity.
13. Ask a friend for a hug.
14. Spread a blanket on your lawn and look at the clouds. Or the stars.
15. Buy a cheap extra umbrella. On the next rainy day, offer it to a stranger.
16. Learn to whistle.
17. Try your luck at yodeling.
18. Reread one of the books you loved as a child.
19. Buy yourself a bouquet of daisies.
20. Plant a seed—any seed—and watch it sprout.
21. Feed the birds.
22. Buy special pens and doodle.
23. Memorize a joke.
24. Buy a Mad Libs book and ask your child or partner to play.
25. Make and throw a paper airplane.
26. Buy a few pieces of bubble gum. Sharpen your bubble-blowing skills.
27. Clean out a closet.
28. Play peekaboo with the baby in the cart in front of you while waiting in the supermarket checkout line.
29. Plan and go on an old-fashioned, honest-to-goodness picnic with someone special.
30. Take a different route to work.
31. Sneak out of work early and go to a matinee.
32. Hang a pretty air freshener in your car.
33. Send a card to someone you haven't seen in years.
34. Go to a kids' peewee baseball game and cheer for everyone.
35. Dine by candlelight.
36. Compliment a surly co-worker.
37. Drag out your high school yearbook and laugh at your senior picture.
38. Buy a coloring book and crayons.
39. During your next argument with your spouse, let him or her win. Giggle to yourself.

40. Ambush your spouse with a Nerf gun.

41. Challenge your kid or grandkid to a lightning round of whatever—checkers, Battleship, Uno.

42. Learn one magic trick from start to finish.

43. If the above tip stresses you out, try a card trick.

44. Buy a collection of cheap 100- or 200-piece jigsaw puzzles. When you're feeling panicked, assemble one. Voilà—instant gratification.

45. Challenge yourself to a game of jacks.

46. Buy a Barrel of Monkeys. Creating a colorful chain of chimps can calm you right down.

47. Tired of high-maintenance manicures? Buff your nails to a high shine.

48. Browse local used-book stores, some of the most relaxing places on the planet.

49. Ditto for tiny, local antiques stores or junk shops.

50. Buy a special candle. Light it and thank your higher power, or the universe, for three things in your life.

By the way, you're welcome to add to this list! Think of the things that make your toes curl or that simply take you outside of the same-old, same-old. Often the most profound sources of pleasure and relaxation are those that grow out of living in the moment, as kids do. These are the Hershey's Kisses of life: You need just one or two a day to feel completely satisfied.

DTOUR WINNER!

Courtney Matthews, 39
POUNDS LOST: 8
INCHES LOST: 3
BLOOD SUGAR: STABLE

BEFORE

AFTER

I developed gestational diabetes when I was pregnant with my daughter, who is now 1½. It was an extreme case; I couldn't control it with diet, so I had to use insulin.

The condition went away after I delivered, but my fasting blood sugar is still high. Half the women who experience gestational diabetes will develop full-blown diabetes within 5 years, so when I got the opportunity to join the DTOUR group, I took it. Now is the time for me to change my eating habits so I don't end up being one of those women. I want to be healthy for my children.

When I started DTOUR, I was a little bit hungry, but the snacks helped me make it to my next meal. Now, I'm not hungry between meals at all. I feel like I've definitely hit a rhythm.

I've really enjoyed trying new foods and eating familiar foods in new ways. My absolute favorite is the fish tacos. I never much liked fish, but when I saw fish tacos on the menu, I dutifully prepared them; I was very committed to following through with the plan. Surprise, surprise—I loved them! Now, every Sunday, my whole family sits down to fish tacos. And I love having apples and peanut butter for dessert.

I'm very lucky because my entire family got on board. My husband does all the cooking, and my whole family—even my 6-year-old—eats what I eat. I just eat the right quantity, and my family eats their regular portions. I've had no complaints at all. Everyone seems to enjoy our meals. I've also been exercising, and I'll continue to.

Obviously, the plan has helped drive home the importance of portion control. And the benefits are huge. I have more energy. My mood is more even—I'm happier during the day. I get fewer head-aches. And, of course, my clothes fit better. My entire wardrobe used to be so tight and uncomfortable.

My long-term goals are to lose more weight and get my choles-terol down a bit more. DTOUR has helped a lot, but I still want to improve those numbers. At my age, you don't want to be going to the doctor with health issues you think will come up way in the future, only for him to tell you that you have them now.

Change is hard, but the benefits of changing your lifestyle are worth the challenge.

I feel great. I'm eating healthier, but, just as important, so is my family. We've all benefited, and we'll all continue to follow DTOUR, more or less, going forward.

LOST
8
POUNDS!

PART 5

CRUISE CONTROL: KEEP LOSING

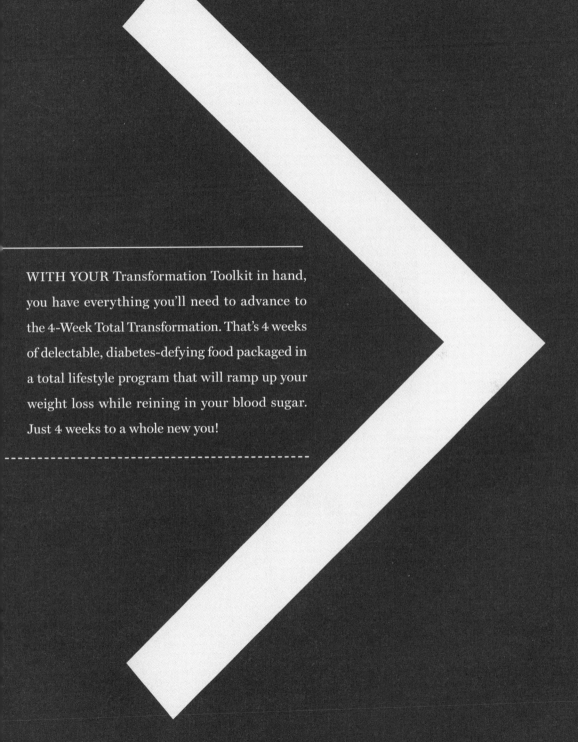

WITH YOUR Transformation Toolkit in hand, you have everything you'll need to advance to the 4-Week Total Transformation. That's 4 weeks of delectable, diabetes-defying food packaged in a total lifestyle program that will ramp up your weight loss while reining in your blood sugar. Just 4 weeks to a whole new you!

CHAPTER

12

THE 4-WEEK

TOTAL

TRANSFORMATION

So you've got the first 2 weeks of DTOUR behind you. Way to go! If you're like our DTOUR test panelists, your pants are fitting a little looser, your tummy is looking a little flatter, and you're feeling a little more energized and focused. These are fabulous changes; they show that you're not only losing weight, you're stabilizing your blood sugar, too. With every pound gone, with every blood sugar point down, you're one step closer to staying diabetes free or—if you already have diabetes—to avoiding medications and complications.

Your success so far is just a hint of what's to come over the next 4 weeks. For this phase of DTOUR, which we call the Total Transformation, we're going to mix things up a bit with fresh menu choices plus "helper" lifestyle strategies to add on as you wish. The Total Transformation is meant to be a little more flexible and customizable than the 2-Week Fast Start to help you continue to learn the new habits that will keep you fit and healthy for life.

Let's start with the food—because DTOUR is all about food! For the Total Transformation, you'll be building your own daily menus from a selection of breakfasts, lunches, dinners, and snacks. As you'll see, each menu option comes in a 1,400-calorie version and a 1,600-calorie version. You'll choose the one that matches your daily calorie target. We've done all of the nutritional calculations for you, so no matter how you mix and match, you'll be within range for all of your key nutrients, including the Fat-Fighting 4. How easy is that?

If you're feeling more adventurous or you just love to cook, feel free to swap any meal or snack for one of the DTOUR recipes beginning on page 287. They require a bit more preparation, though they're by no means complicated. They adhere to the same nutritional standards as the rest of the DTOUR menu items, so you can seamlessly slip them into your daily eating plan.

Between the recipes and the menu options below, you have more than 100 meals and snacks to choose from. You can go for days, or even weeks, without eating the same meal twice! On the other hand, if you find a few favorites—and we're certain you will—you can eat them as often as you'd like. We do recommend varying your daily menus a bit so you get a good mix of nutrients beyond the Fat-Fighting 4.

The Total Transformation has a few other bells and whistles that can boost your results over the next 4 weeks. One is the DTOUR Workout, which we introduced in Chapter 9. Six days a week, you'll be doing either one of the Cardio Walks (the Fat-Torch or the Calorie-Scorch) or the strength-training routines (the Metabo Moves and the Belly Blast). The workouts are designed to grow with you, increasing in duration and intensity as you become slimmer and fitter.

Throughout the Total Transformation, we give you tips and techniques for reducing stress and improving sleep—both of which enhance weight loss and blood sugar control, as you'll remember from Part 4. As in the 2-Week Fast Start, there's space to record your daily blood sugar readings as well as your weekly weigh-ins and monthly waist measurements. You can use the journal block (called "How Did You Do?") to write down anything noteworthy about a particular day, whether it's a recipe you liked, a workout that you breezed through, or a challenging situation that you handled with ease.

You can use these extra tools to customize the Total Transformation to your unique needs and lifestyle. If you'd rather stick with just the diet, as in the 2-Week

DTOUR AT A GLANCE:
THE 1,400-CALORIE PLAN

Nutrition information for the Fat-Fighting 4 is in **bold.**

Nutrient Goals per Meal
◆ Calories: 300-350
◆ Protein: 15-25 grams
◆ Carbohydrates: 30-40 grams
◆ Total fat: 10 grams
◆ Saturated fat: less than 3 grams
◆ **Fiber: 5-10 grams**
◆ **Calcium: 300 milligrams**
◆ **Vitamin D: 80 IU**
◆ **Omega-3s:**
　◆ Alpha-linolenic acid (ALA): 0.22 gram
　◆ EPA/DHA: 0.15 gram

Nutrient Goals per Snack
◆ Calories: 150-200
◆ Protein: 5-10 grams
◆ Carbohydrates: 10-30 grams
◆ Total fat: 5 grams
◆ Saturated fat: less than 2 grams
◆ **Fiber: 5 grams**
◆ **Calcium: 200 milligrams**
◆ **Vitamin D: 80 IU**
◆ **Omega-3s:**
　◆ Alpha-linolenic acid (ALA): 0.22 gram
　◆ EPA/DHA: 0.15 gram

Fast Start, that's okay, too. Do what feels right for you; you can always add other activities as you go along. Remember, this phase of DTOUR is about more than losing weight and reining in your blood sugar—though you'll definitely be doing both of those things! It's about laying the foundation for a lifestyle that's going to put you in control of your health and whether or not diabetes has a place in it.

YOUR AWESOME 4SOMES

Building your daily menus is super-easy. Just read through the following lists and choose one breakfast, one lunch, one dinner, and two snacks. One important note: If you've been advised to watch your salt intake, be sure to stick with the lower-sodium meal and snack choices. In general, we recommend limiting sodium consumption to no more than 2,300 milligrams per day.

DTOUR AT A GLANCE: THE 1,600-CALORIE PLAN

Nutrition information for the Fat-Fighting 4 is in **bold**.

Nutrient Goals per Meal
- Calories: 400-450
- Protein: 25-30 grams
- Carbohydrates: 40-45 grams
- Total fat: 15-20 grams
- Saturated fat: less than 3 grams
- **Fiber: 5-10 grams**
- **Calcium: 300 milligrams**
- **Vitamin D: 80 IU**
- **Omega-3s:**
  - **Alpha-linolenic acid (ALA): 0.32 gram**
  - **EPA/DHA: 0.15 gram**

Nutrient Goals per Snack
- Calories: 200-250
- Protein: 10-15 grams
- Carbohydrates: 20-35 grams
- Total fat: 5-10 grams
- Saturated fat: less than 3 grams
- **Fiber: 5 grams**
- **Calcium: 200 milligrams**
- **Vitamin D: 80 IU**
- **Omega-3s:**
  - **Alpha-linolenic acid (ALA): 0.32 gram**
  - **EPA/DHA: 0.15 gram**

BREAKFASTS

Breakfast 1

❑ Good Lox Bagel: Spread $\frac{1}{2}$ whole grain bagel (2 ounces) with mixture of 2 table-spoons low-fat cream cheese and 2 ounces canned drained salmon

❑ $\frac{1}{2}$ cup fat-free milk or low-fat, calcium-enriched soy or rice beverage

351 calories, 32 g protein, 33 g carbohydrates, 10 g fat (4 g saturated fat), 61 mg cholesterol, 538 mg sodium

1,600-calorie plan: Use 3 ounces salmon and drink 1 cup fat-free milk or low-fat, calcium-enriched soy or rice beverage.

397 calories, 39 g protein, 33 g carbohydrates, 12 g fat (4 g saturated fat), 80 mg cholesterol, 648 mg sodium

Breakfast 2

❑ Get Up and Go Veggie Omelet: In a pan, heat 2 teaspoons canola, peanut, or olive oil. Add $\frac{1}{4}$ cup egg substitute (or 1 egg white); $\frac{1}{2}$ cup chopped spinach; $\frac{1}{2}$ cup chopped mushrooms, chopped onion, and finely chopped garlic; and chopped herbs as desired. Cook until set. Top with $\frac{1}{4}$ cup shredded reduced-fat cheese.

❑ 1 slice reduced-calorie whole grain toast spread with 1 tablespoon fat-free or 1% cottage cheese

❑ 1 cup fat-free milk or low-fat, calcium-enriched soy or rice beverage

347 calories, 25 g protein, 30 g carbohydrates, 16 g fat (5 g saturated fat), 26 mg cholesterol, 552 mg sodium

1,600-calorie plan: Use $\frac{1}{2}$ cup egg substitute (or 2 egg whites), add 1 additional slice (2 slices total) reduced-calorie whole grain toast, and use 2 tablespoons fat-free or 1% cottage cheese.

427 calories, 33 g protein, 43 g carbohydrates, 17 g fat (5 g saturated fat), 27 mg cholesterol, 803 mg sodium

Breakfast 3

❑ Top $\frac{1}{2}$ cup cooked oatmeal with $\frac{1}{4}$ cup chopped pecans. Sprinkle with ground cinnamon and/or sugar substitute to taste.

❑ $\frac{1}{2}$ cup fat-free or low-fat milk or low-fat, calcium-enriched soy or rice beverage

357 calories, 14 g protein, 30 g carbohydrates, 22 g fat (2 g saturated fat), 5 mg cholesterol, 112 mg sodium

1,600-calorie plan: Use 1 cup cooked oatmeal and 3 tablespoons chopped pecans (about 15) and drink 1 cup fat-free or low-fat milk or low-fat, calcium-enriched soy or rice beverage.

393 calories, 16 g protein, 43 g carbohydrates, 19 g fat (2 g saturated fat), 5 mg cholesterol, 117 mg sodium

Breakfast 4

❑ On-the-Run Peanut Butter–Banana Toast: Spread 1 slice reduced-calorie whole grain toast with $1\frac{1}{2}$ tablespoons all-natural peanut butter and $\frac{1}{2}$ medium sliced banana.

❑ Starbuck's Tall Skinny Latte (made with fat-free or low-fat milk or low-fat, calcium-enriched soy or rice beverage and sugar-free syrup) or 1 cup coffee and 1 cup fat-free milk or low-fat, calcium-enriched soy or rice beverage

351 calories, 18 g protein, 42 g carbohydrates, 13 g fat (2 g saturated fat), 5 mg cholesterol, 289 mg sodium

1,600-calorie plan: Use 2 tablespoons all-natural peanut butter.

404 calories, 20 g protein, 44 g carbohydrates, 17 g fat (3 g saturated fat), 5 mg cholesterol, 301 mg sodium

Breakfast 5

❑ 1 ounce whole grain, flaxseed-enriched cereal (Note: 1 ounce equals the serving size on the Nutrition Facts label.)

❑ 1 cup fat-free milk or low-fat, calcium-enriched soy or rice beverage

❑ 2 tablespoons walnut pieces (about 7 halves)

321 calories, 17 g protein, 41 g carbohydrates, 12 g fat (1 g saturated fat), 5 mg cholesterol, 108 mg sodium

continued . . .

Breakfast 5

1,600-calorie plan:
Use 1 ounce walnut halves (about 14).

411 calories, 19 g protein, 43 g carbohydrates, 21 g fat (2 g saturated fat), 5 mg cholesterol, 108 mg sodium

Breakfast 6

❐ Breakfast smoothie: In a blender, combine 1 cup fat-free milk or low-fat, calcium-enriched soy or rice beverage; ³⁄₄ cup (6 ounces) fat-free plain yogurt; ¹⁄₂ cup sliced strawberries, banana, or other fresh fruit; 2 tablespoons walnuts; and 2 tablespoons flaxseed meal. Add ground cinnamon and/or sugar substitute to taste. Blend for 15 seconds.

344 calories, 22 g protein, 37 g carbohydrates, 14 g fat (1 g saturated fat), 5 mg cholesterol, 224 mg sodium

1,600-calorie plan: Use 1 cup (8 ounces) fat-free plain yogurt.

371 calories, 25 g protein, 42 g carbohydrates, 14 g fat (1 g saturated fat), 5 mg cholesterol, 262 mg sodium

Breakfast 7

❐ Fancy French Toast: Dip 2 slices reduced-calorie whole grain bread into mixture of 1 beaten egg (or ¹⁄₄ cup egg substitute); ¹⁄₄ cup fat-free milk or low-fat, calcium-enriched soy or rice beverage; and ¹⁄₂ teaspoon cinnamon. Melt 1 teaspoon canola oil and 1 teaspoon trans-free canola margarine in hot pan; add bread and grill on both sides until golden brown. Top with 2 tablespoons sugar-free syrup or 1 tablespoon low-calorie syrup. Serve with 1 slice (1 ounce) Canadian-style bacon and ¹⁄₂ cup fat-free milk or low-fat, calcium-enriched soy or rice beverage.

368 calories, 22 g protein, 37 g carbohydrates, 16 g fat (3 g saturated fat), 204 mg cholesterol, 777 mg sodium

1,600-calorie plan: Use 1 whole egg + 1 egg white or ¹⁄₂ cup egg substitute.

420 calories, 29 g protein, 42 g carbohydrates, 17 g fat (4 g saturated fat), 390 mg cholesterol, 830 mg sodium

Breakfast 8

❐ Breakfast in a Hurry: 1 can (8 ounces) low-sugar meal-replacement drink, such as Glucerna, Boost Glucose Control, or No Sugar Added Carnation Instant Breakfast

❐ 1 medium orange

❐ 1 tablespoon walnuts or other nuts

364 calories, 12 g protein, 46 g carbohydrates, 15 g fat (1.5 g saturated fat), 2.5 mg cholesterol, 217 mg sodium

1,600-calorie plan: Use 2 tablespoons walnuts or other nuts.

380 calories, 13 g protein, 47 g carbohydrates, 18 g fat (2 g saturated fat), 2.5 mg cholesterol, 217 mg sodium

Breakfast 9

❐ Super White Eggs: Heat 2 teaspoons canola oil in a small skillet. Add 1 whole egg, then 1 egg white around the outside of the whole egg. Cook over low heat until set. Top with 2 tablespoons chopped tomato or salsa. Serve with 1 slice reduced-calorie, high-fiber whole grain toast spread with 1 teaspoon trans-free canola margarine.

❐ 1 cup fat-free milk or low-fat, calcium-enriched soy or rice beverage

351 calories, 21 g protein, 28 g carbohydrates, 19 g fat (3 g saturated fat), 216 mg cholesterol, 620 mg sodium

1,600-calorie plan: Use 1 whole egg, 2 egg whites, ¹⁄₂ teaspoon canola oil, and ¹⁄₂ teaspoon trans-free canola margarine; and eat 2 slices reduced-calorie, high-fiber whole grain toast spread with 1 teaspoon trans-free canola margarine. Serve with ³⁄₄ cup fat-free milk or low-fat, calcium-enriched soy or rice beverage.

383 calories, 27 g protein, 40 g carbohydrates, 15 g fat (2.5 g saturated fat), 216 mg cholesterol, 817 mg sodium

Breakfast 10

❐ Spread 3 buckwheat or whole wheat pancakes (6" diameter) with 1 teaspoon trans-free canola margarine and ¹⁄₄ cup unsweetened applesauce or 2 tablespoons sugar-free syrup, if desired.

❐ 1 ounce Canadian-style bacon

❐ 8 ounces fat-free milk or low-fat, calcium-enriched soy or rice beverage

340 calories, 18 g protein, 36 g carbohydrates, 14 g fat (3 g saturated fat), 54 mg cholesterol, 738 mg sodium

1,600-calorie plan: Eat 4 buckwheat or whole wheat pancakes (6" diameter) spread with 2 teaspoons trans-free canola margarine and ¼ cup unsweetened applesauce or 2 tablespoons sugar-free syrup, if desired, and add 2 ounces Canadian-style bacon.

398 calories, 24 g protein, 41 g carbohydrates, 16 g fat (3.5 g saturated fat), 80 mg cholesterol, 1173 mg sodium

Breakfast 11

❐ Egg Muffin Olé: Toast 1 whole grain English muffin and top with 1 slice (1 ounce) reduced-fat cheese and 1 egg or ¼ cup egg substitute scrambled in 1 teaspoon canola or olive oil. Flavor with ¼ cup chopped tomato, onion, and/or salsa.

❐ ½ cup fat-free milk or low-fat, calcium-enriched soy or rice beverage

335 calories, 25 g protein, 39 g carbohydrates, 11 g fat (4 g saturated fat), 17 mg cholesterol, 1039 mg sodium

1,600-calorie plan: Use ½ cup egg substitute, and drink 1 cup fat-free milk or low-fat, calcium-enriched soy or rice beverage.

407 calories, 35 g protein, 46 g carbohydrates, 11 g fat (3.5 g saturated fat), 20 mg cholesterol, 1206 mg sodium

Breakfast 12

❐ Good-Morning Blend: Stir 2 tablespoons dried fruit; 2 tablespoons flaxseed meal; and 2 tablespoons chopped unsalted raw almonds, walnuts, or pecans into 1 cup fat-free or low-fat plain yogurt (no sugar added). Add ground cinnamon and/or sugar substitute to taste.

345 calories, 20 g protein, 38 g carbohydrates, 14 g fat (1 g saturated fat), 5 mg cholesterol, 214 mg sodium

1,600-calorie plan: Use 4 tablespoons chopped nuts.

403 calories, 16 g protein, 34 g carbohydrates, 26 g fat (3 g saturated fat), 10 mg cholesterol, 140 mg sodium

Breakfast 13

❐ Spread ¼ cup fat-free or 1% cottage cheese on 2 slices toasted reduced-calorie, high-fiber bread. Top with 2 tablespoons chopped dates or other dried fruit and ½ ounce (about 2 tablespoons) chopped unsalted raw walnuts or other nuts.

342 calories, 23 g protein, 45 g carbohydrates, 11 g fat (1.5 g saturated fat), 4.5 mg cholesterol, 752 mg sodium

1,600-calorie plan: Use ½ cup fat-free or 1% cottage cheese and 3 tablespoons chopped walnuts or other nuts.

400 calories, 25 g protein, 46 g carbohydrates, 16 g fat (1.5 g saturated fat), 4.5 mg cholesterol, 753 mg sodium

Breakfast 14

❐ Breakfast Burrito: Cook ½ cup chopped onions; 1 clove garlic, finely chopped; and ½ cup chopped green, yellow, or red bell pepper in 1 teaspoon olive or canola oil. Add ½ cup egg substitute (or 1 egg white) and cook until set. Place mixture in 1 whole grain tortilla (8"–10" diameter). Sprinkle with 2 tablespoons shredded reduced-fat cheese, 2 tablespoons salsa, and 1 tablespoon reduced-fat sour cream.

364 calories, 20 g protein, 20 g carbohydrates, 14.5 g fat (3.5 g saturated fat), 12 mg cholesterol, 900 mg sodium

1,600-calorie plan: Use 1 cup chopped green, yellow, or red bell pepper, 1 tablespoon olive or canola oil, and 2 tablespoons reduced-fat sour cream.

409 calories, 22 g protein, 47 g carbohydrates, 16 g fat (4.5 g saturated fat), 16 mg cholesterol, 1034 mg sodium

LUNCHES

Lunch 1

❒ Grilled Ham-and-Cheese Reuben: Spread 2 slices reduced-calorie whole grain bread with 1 tablespoon Dijon mustard. Pile 1 ounce (1 slice) reduced-fat Swiss cheese, 1 ounce lean ham, and $\frac{1}{2}$ cup shredded cabbage on top. Spread $\frac{1}{2}$ teaspoon trans-free canola margarine on each outer side. Brown each side in hot pan until cheese melts.

❒ 1 cup (8 ounces) fat-free milk or low-fat, calcium-enriched soy or rice beverage

380 calories, 28 g protein, 41 g carbohydrates, 13 g fat (3.5 g saturated fat), 37 mg cholesterol, 1373 mg sodium

1,600-calorie plan: Use 3 ounces lean ham.

414 calories, 32 g protein, 41 g carbohydrates, 15 g fat (4.5 g saturated fat), 48 mg cholesterol, 1641 mg sodium

Lunch 2

❒ Tuna pita pocket: Place sliced tomatoes inside pocket of $\frac{1}{2}$ whole grain pita. Combine 2 ounces water-packed tuna, drained, with 1 tablespoon reduced-fat mayonnaise (or 1 teaspoon regular mayonnaise); 1 tablespoon fat-free plain yogurt; 1 tablespoon chopped celery; 8 black olives, chopped; and 1 tablespoon chopped onion. Season with salt-free herbs and spices as desired. Add mixture to pita. Top with $\frac{1}{2}$ cup fat-free plain yogurt.

324 calories, 26 g protein, 38 g carbohydrates, 9 g fat (1.5 g saturated fat), 19 mg cholesterol, 829 mg sodium

1,600-calorie plan: Use 3 ounces water-packed tuna, drained; and 2 tablespoons reduced-fat mayonnaise (or 2 teaspoons regular mayonnaise).

400 calories, 32 g protein, 37 g carbohydrates, 15 g fat (1.5 g saturated fat), 30 mg cholesterol, 1120 mg sodium

Lunch 3

❒ D'lightful Sub Salad: Add 2 ounces deli ham and turkey to 3 cups fresh spinach and other salad greens. Add 1 tomato, chopped; sliced red onion; and $\frac{1}{4}$ avocado, sliced. Top with 2 tablespoons low-calorie salad dressing and $\frac{1}{4}$ cup shredded reduced-fat cheese.

❒ 2 rye crisp crackers

346 calories, 22 g protein, 31 g carbohydrates, 17 g fat (3.5 g saturated fat), 34 mg cholesterol, 1148 mg sodium

1,600-calorie plan: Use 3 ounces deli ham and turkey.

400 calories, 28 g protein, 32 g carbohydrates, 20 g fat (5 g saturated fat), 61 mg cholesterol, 1647 mg sodium

Lunch 4

❒ On-the-Go Vegetable Wrap: Spread 1 whole grain or high-fiber (at least 5 grams dietary fiber per serving) vegetable-based tortilla wrap (8"-10" diameter) with $\frac{1}{3}$ cup hummus. Add 2 ounces turkey breast, $\frac{1}{2}$ cup shredded cabbage and/or spinach leaves, and $\frac{1}{4}$ cup shredded or |finely chopped carrots. Sprinkle with 1 tablespoon seasoned rice vinegar and roll up tightly.

367 calories, 22 g protein, 45 g carbohydrates, 15 g fat (1.5 g saturated fat), 24 mg cholesterol, 1480 mg sodium

1,600-calorie plan: Use 8 green olives, chopped; and 3 ounces turkey breast.

396 calories, 27 g protein, 46 g carbohydrates, 16 g fat (2 g saturated fat), 36 mg cholesterol, 1867 mg sodium

Lunch 5

❒ High-fiber antioxidant mix: Mix 1 cup cooked or canned red, white, pinto, or black beans; $\frac{1}{4}$ cup chopped scallions; and 2 tablespoons light Italian dressing. Serve over 2 cups mixed salad greens. Sprinkle with $\frac{1}{4}$ cup shredded reduced-fat cheese.

363 calories, 20 g protein, 49 g carbohydrates, 9 g fat (3 g saturated fat), 15 mg cholesterol, 736 mg sodium

1,600-calorie plan: Add 2 tablespoons chopped unsalted raw nuts.

416 calories, 22 g protein, 50 g carbohydrates, 15 g fat (3.5 g saturated fat), 15 mg cholesterol, 726 mg sodium

Lunch 6

❏ Easy Cheesy Quesadilla: Layer 2 ounces shredded chicken and 2 tablespoons shredded reduced-fat cheese on 1 corn tortilla (6" diameter). Place another tortilla on top and cook in a small pan over medium heat until cheese melts and quesadilla is browned on both sides. (You can also microwave on medium for 30 to 45 seconds.) Cut into 4 wedges and garnish with 1/4 cup salsa. Serve with 2 cups mixed green salad topped with 2 tablespoons mashed avocado mixed with 1 tablespoon reduced-fat sour cream.

368 calories, 29 g protein, 39 g carbohydrates, 12 g fat (4 g saturated fat), 62 mg cholesterol, 591 mg sodium

1,600-calorie plan: Use 3 ounces shredded chicken.

415 calories, 38 g protein, 39 g carbohydrates, 13 g fat (4 g saturated fat), 86 mg cholesterol, 612 mg sodium

Lunch 7

❏ Banana Split Salad: Split 1 small banana in half lengthwise. Top with 1/2 cup 1% or fat-free cottage cheese and 1/4 cup unsalted raw chopped almonds or other nuts.

❏ 1/2 cup fat-free milk or low-fat, calcium-enriched soy or rice beverage.

360 calories, 24 g protein, 41 g carbohydrates, 13 g fat (2 g saturated fat), 7 mg cholesterol, 572 mg sodium

1,600-calorie plan: Use 3/4 cup 1% or fat-free cottage cheese and add 1 whole grain crispbread cracker. Skip the milk or soy or rice beverage.

389 calories, 28 g protein, 44 g carbohydrates, 14 g fat (2 g saturated fat), 7 mg cholesterol, 739 mg sodium

Lunch 8

❏ Chicken salad: Top 2 cups mixed greens, 1/2 cup chopped tomato, 1/2 cup sliced cucumber, and 1/4 cup chopped carrot with 2 ounces chicken breast. Drizzle with avocado-yogurt dressing (1/4 cup mashed avocado, 1/3 cup fat-free plain yogurt, and vinegar and/or herbs to taste).

❏ 1 whole grain crispbread cracker

355 calories, 27 g protein, 33 g carbohydrates, 14 g fat (3 g saturated fat), 53 mg cholesterol, 221 mg sodium

1,600-calorie plan: Use 3 cups mixed greens, 1 cup chopped tomato, and 3 ounces chicken breast. For the dressing, use 1/2 cup mashed avocado.

408 calories, 36 g protein, 34 g carbohydrates, 15 g fat (3 g saturated fat), 77 mg cholesterol, 247 mg sodium

Lunch 9

❏ Tuna Toss: Mix 3 ounces water-packed tuna, drained, with 2 stalks celery, chopped; 4 green olives, chopped; and 1 tablespoon reduced-fat mayonnaise (or 1 teaspoon regular mayonnaise). Add 1 tablespoon seasoned rice vinegar, if desired. Serve on 2 cups mixed dark greens. Top with 1 tablespoon chopped unsalted raw almonds or other nuts.

❏ 5 whole grain crackers (about 1 ounce)

❏ 1 cup fat-free milk or low-fat, calcium-enriched soy or rice beverage

329 calories, 36 g protein, 19 g carbohydrates, 12 g fat (2 g saturated fat), 46 mg cholesterol, 719 mg sodium

1,600-calorie plan: Use 2 tablespoons reduced-fat mayonnaise (or 2 teaspoons regular); and 3 cups mixed dark greens.

407 calories, 38 g protein, 21 g carbohydrates, 19 g fat (2.5 g saturated fat), 48 mg cholesterol, 751 mg sodium

Lunch 10

❏ Hearty Burger: 3 ounces cooked lean hamburger (or soy vegetable patty), lettuce, tomato, mustard, and 1 tablespoon ketchup on a whole grain bun

❏ 8 baby carrots dipped in 1 tablespoon reduced-fat ranch dressing

❏ 12 ounces light lemonade or diet soda (look for a product with less than 5 calories per serving)

372 calories, 29 g protein, 39 g carbohydrates, 12 g fat (3.5 g saturated fat), 67 mg cholesterol, 703 mg sodium

continued . . .

Lunch 10

1,600-calorie plan: Use 2 tablespoons reduced-fat ranch dressing.

401 calories, 29 g protein, 38 g carbohydrates, 15 g fat (4 g saturated fat), 69 mg cholesterol, 845 mg sodium

Lunch 11

❏ Bean tostada: Bake 1 corn tortilla (6" diameter) in a hot oven (400°F) until dry. Spread with ¼ cup cooked or canned pinto beans (rinsed) and 2 tablespoons shredded reduced-fat Mexican-blend cheese. Return to oven for 5 to 10 minutes or microwave on medium for 30 to 45 seconds until cheese melts. Top with ¼ cup salsa.

❏ Cabbage salad: Mix 1 cup shredded cabbage with 1 chopped tomato and 2 tablespoons light salad dressing.

288 calories, 9 g protein, 43 g carbohydrates, 11 g fat (3 g saturated fat), 17 mg cholesterol, 1191 mg sodium

1,600-calorie plan: Use ½ cup cooked or canned pinto beans (rinsed). Add 2 ounces cooked lean ground beef.

407 calories, 25 g protein, 47 g carbohydrates, 14 g fat (4.5 g saturated fat), 60 mg cholesterol, 1350 mg sodium

Lunch 12

❏ Easy Mix-Up Salad: Toss 3 cups mixed salad greens, ½ cup 1% cottage cheese, 1 tangerine or small orange

divided into sections, and 2 tablespoons light Italian dressing. Top with 1 tablespoon unsalted raw chopped almonds or walnuts.

❏ 5 whole grain crackers (such as Triscuits)

337 calories, 19 g protein, 35 g carbohydrates, 14 g fat (2 g saturated fat), 5 mg cholesterol, 835 mg sodium

1,600-calorie plan: Use 1 cup 1% cottage cheese.

418 calories, 33 g protein, 38 g carbohydrates, 15 g fat (3 g saturated fat), 9 mg cholesterol, 1294 mg sodium

Lunch 13

❏ Taco No Taco: Mix 2 ounces grilled fish, chicken, or lean beef; ⅓ cup brown rice; and ½ cup cooked red, black, or pinto beans. Top with 2 tablespoons shredded reduced-fat cheese. Top with ¼ cup salsa and 1 tablespoon reduced-fat sour cream. Serve over 2 cups mixed lettuce greens.

370 calories, 30 g protein, 41 g carbohydrates, 9 g fat (3 g saturated fat), 54 mg cholesterol, 548 mg sodium

1,600-calorie plan: Use 3 ounces grilled fish.

422 calories, 38 g protein, 41 g carbohydrates, 12 g fat (3.5 g saturated fat), 74 mg cholesterol, 564 mg sodium

Lunch 14

❏ Pesto pizza: Split and toast a whole grain English muffin. Spread with 1 tablespoon basil pesto sauce (such as Buitoni

brand). Top each half with 1 slice tomato (or ½ cup canned tomatoes) and ½ slice reduced-fat cheese. Broil or bake until cheese melts.

❏ ½ cup fat-free milk or low-fat, calcium-enriched soy or rice beverage

354 calories, 20 g protein, 40 g carbohydrates, 14 g fat (6 g saturated fat), 27 mg cholesterol, 840 mg sodium

1,600-calorie plan: Use 2 tablespoons basil pesto sauce.

428 calories, 22 g protein, 42 g carbohydrates, 21 g fat (7 g saturated fat), 32 mg cholesterol, 980 mg sodium

DINNERS

Dinner 1

❏ 3 ounces grilled lean beef top round or sirloin

❏ Cheesy mashed cauliflower: Mash 1 cup cooked cauliflower with ¼ cup fat-free milk or low-fat, calcium-enriched soy or rice beverage and 2 tablespoons shredded reduced-fat cheese. Season with Mrs. Dash or other salt-free herbal seasoning.

❏ 2 cups mixed green salad with 2 tablespoons light salad dressing

❏ 1 rye crisp cracker

363 calories, 40 g protein, 20 g carbohydrates, 14 g fat (4 g saturated fat), 88 mg cholesterol, 491 mg sodium

1,600-calorie plan: Have 2 rye crisp crackers and add ½ cup fat-free milk or low-fat, calcium-enriched soy or rice beverage.

435 calories, 45 g protein, 33 g carbohydrates, 15 g fat (4 g saturated fat), 90 mg cholesterol, 592 mg sodium

Dinner 2

❐ Grilled Tomato Melt: Place 1 ounce (1 slice) fat-free mozzarella cheese on 1 slice high-fiber, reduced-calorie bread. Add 2 thick slices fresh tomato and several leaves of fresh basil or spinach. Top with another slice bread. Spread ½ teaspoon trans-free canola margarine on outside of each bread slice. Place sandwich in hot skillet over medium heat and cook until both sides are browned and cheese is melted.

❐ 1 cup fat-free milk or low-fat, calcium-enriched soy or rice beverage

322 calories, 21 g protein, 42 g carbohydrates, 10 g fat (4 g saturated fat), 23 mg cholesterol, 622 mg sodium

1,600-calorie plan: Add 1 ounce deli chicken or turkey and 2 tablespoons mashed avocado.

400 calories, 27 g protein, 46 g carbohydrates, 15 g fat (4.5 g saturated fat), 35 mg cholesterol, 908 mg sodium

Dinner 3

❐ 3 ounces grilled salmon

❐ 1 large steamed artichoke or 2 cups broccoli drizzled with mixture of 1 tablespoon reduced-calorie mayonnaise (or 1 teaspoon regular mayonnaise) and 1 tablespoon lemon juice

❐ Garlic toast: Toast 1 slice sourdough bread and spread with mixture of 1 teaspoon olive oil and 1 clove garlic, finely chopped. Place in hot oven or under broiler until browned.

372 calories, 28 g protein, 31 g carbohydrates, 16 g fat (2.5 g saturated fat), 62 mg cholesterol, 309 mg sodium

1,600-calorie plan: Eat 4 ounces grilled salmon.

423 calories, 36 g protein, 31 g carbohydrates, 18 g fat (3 g saturated fat), 82 mg cholesterol, 325 mg sodium

Dinner 4

❐ 3 ounces grilled chicken breast, seasoned with lemon pepper or other salt-free seasoning mix

❐ ½ oven-baked potato (about 3 ounces): Slice potato lengthwise, drizzle cut side with 1 teaspoon olive oil, and bake, cut side down, in a 400°F oven for 30 minutes.

❐ Garlic roasted asparagus or green beans: Preheat oven to 400°F. Toss 10 medium (5-7" long) asparagus spears or 2 cups green beans in 1 teaspoon olive oil and finely chopped garlic to taste. Roast for 20 minutes.

358 calories, 35 g protein, 30 g carbohydrates, 12 g fat (2 g saturated fat), 72 mg cholesterol, 78 mg sodium

1,600-calorie plan: Eat 1 whole oven-baked potato (6 ounces).

438 calories, 37 g protein, 48 g carbohydrates, 13 g fat (2 g saturated fat), 72 mg cholesterol, 86 mg sodium

Dinner 5

❐ Tofu stir-fry: Stir-fry 3 ounces tofu, 1 cup broccoli florets, ¾ cup chopped cauliflower, ½ cup sliced carrot, 2 slices scallion, and 2 cloves garlic in 2 tablespoons reduced-sodium stir-fry sauce and 2 teaspoons olive oil. Serve over ⅓ cup cooked brown rice.

335 calories, 15 g protein, 38 g carbohydrates, 16 g fat (2 g saturated fat), 0 mg cholesterol, 610 mg sodium

1,600-calorie plan: Use 4 ounces tofu and ½ cup cooked brown rice.

392 calories, 18 g protein, 46 g carbohydrates, 18 g fat (2.5 g saturated fat), 0 mg cholesterol, 614 mg sodium

Dinner 6

❐ 3 ounces fish, such as haddock or cod, seasoned with lemon and other salt-free seasonings

❐ Preheat oven to 400°F. Toss ½ cup sliced mushrooms, ½ cup sliced onion,

continued ...

1 cup chopped zucchini and/or yellow squash, ½ cup chopped bell pepper, and ½ cup chopped red potato in 2 teaspoons olive oil. Sprinkle with Mrs. Dash or other salt-free herb seasoning. Bake for 30 minutes or until browned and tender.

❏ ½ cup fat-free milk or low-fat, calcium-enriched soy or rice beverage

326 calories, 30 g protein, 30 g carbohydrates, 10 g fat (1.5 g saturated fat), 65 mg cholesterol, 146 mg sodium

1,600-calorie plan: Eat 4 ounces fish and have 1 cup fat-free milk or low-fat, calcium-enriched soy or rice beverage.

399 calories, 41 g protein, 36 g carbohydrates, 11 g fat (1.5 g saturated fat), 89 mg cholesterol, 222 mg sodium

Dinner 7

❏ 3 ounces roast beef or pork tenderloin

❏ 2 cups spinach salad with chopped red bell peppers, 1 tablespoon slivered almonds, and 2 tablespoons light Italian dressing

❏ ⅔ cup wild rice

336 calories, 23 g protein, 33 g carbohydrates, 13 g fat (1.5 g saturated fat), 40 mg cholesterol, 784 mg sodium

1,600-calorie plan: Eat 4 ounces roast beef or pork tenderloin and 1 cup wild rice.

422 calories, 30 g protein, 45 g carbohydrates, 15 g fat (2 g saturated fat), 54 mg cholesterol, 954 mg sodium

Dinner 8

❏ Grilled fish tacos: Tuck 2 ounces grilled fish and 1 cup shredded cabbage sprinkled with seasoned rice vinegar into 1 corn tortilla (6" diameter). Top with 1 tablespoon reduced-fat sour cream.

❏ Grilled or roasted vegetables: Marinate 1 cup chopped eggplant, ½ cup chopped mushrooms, ½ cup green beans, and 2 tablespoons chopped onion in 2 tablespoons light Italian dressing and 1 teaspoon olive oil. Grill or roast at 400°F for 30 to 45 minutes or until lightly browned.

367 calories, 23 g protein, 35 g carbohydrates, 16 g fat (2.5 g saturated fat), 45 mg cholesterol, 305 mg sodium

1,600-calorie plan: Eat 3 ounces grilled fish and 2 corn tortillas. For the vegetables, use 1 tablespoon light Italian dressing.

449 calories, 31 g protein, 45 g carbohydrates, 17 g fat (3 g saturated fat), 65 mg cholesterol, 218 mg sodium

Dinner 9

❏ ½ cup cooked whole wheat spaghetti tossed in finely chopped garlic to taste and 1 teaspoon olive oil

❏ 3 ounces lean meatballs (made with turkey, chicken, or soy)

❏ 1 teaspoon grated Parmesan cheese

❏ Cucumber Salad: On bed of 1 cup mixed greens, arrange 1 cup cucumber slices; 10 cherry tomatoes, halved; and ¼ cup chopped red onion. Drizzle with 2 tablespoons light Italian dressing.

351 calories, 15 g protein, 41 g carbohydrates, 16 g fat (3 g saturated fat), 24 mg cholesterol, 580 mg sodium

1,600-calorie plan: Eat 4 ounces lean meatballs (made with turkey, chicken, or soy) and add ½ cup fat-free milk or low-fat, calcium-enriched soy or rice beverage.

423 calories, 21 g protein, 48 g carbohydrates, 18 g fat (3.5 g saturated fat), 34 mg cholesterol, 733 mg sodium

Dinner 10

❏ 1 cup Progresso Healthy Classics or Campbell's Healthy Request canned beef barley or bean soup

❏ Spinach salad: Toss 2 cups fresh spinach with 1 tablespoon olive oil and balsamic vinegar dressing. Top with 1 tablespoon shredded reduced-fat mozzarella cheese and 1 tablespoon slivered unsalted raw almonds or other nuts.

334 calories, 17 g protein, 22 g carbohydrates, 20 g fat (3.5 g saturated fat), 24 mg cholesterol, 620 mg sodium

1,600-calorie plan: Eat 1½ cups soup.

402 calories, 23 g protein, 31 g carbohydrates, 21 g fat (4 g saturated fat), 34 mg cholesterol, 884 mg sodium

Dinner 11

❒ Grilled chicken Caesar salad: 2 cups romaine or other mixed lettuce greens, 2 ounces grilled chicken, and 2 tablespoons reduced-fat Caesar dressing (or 1 tablespoon regular Caesar dressing).

❒ 1 ounce whole grain crackers

❒ 8 ounces fat-free milk or low-fat, calcium-enriched soy or rice beverage

337 calories, 29 g protein, 32 g carbohydrates, 10 g fat (2 g saturated fat), 53 mg cholesterol, 514 mg sodium

1,600-calorie plan: Use 3 cups romaine or other mixed lettuce greens and 3 ounces grilled chicken.

394 calories, 39 g protein, 34 g carbohydrates, 12 g fat (2 g saturated fat), 77 mg cholesterol, 539 mg sodium

Dinner 12

❒ Oven-fried chicken: Preheat oven to 350°F. Toss 3 ounces raw chicken breast in 1 tablespoon light Italian dressing. Coat with 2 tablespoons seasoned bread crumbs; spray lightly with canola cooking spray. Place on lightly oiled cookie sheet. Bake for 30 minutes

or until browned and no longer pink inside.

❒ Perky Tomato Salad: Toss together 1 cup coarsely chopped tomatoes, 1 cup torn red or green leaf lettuce, and 1 tablespoon fresh basil (or 1 teaspoon dried basil). Drizzle with a mixture of 1 teaspoon olive oil and 1 teaspoon balsamic vinegar. Top with 1 tablespoon toasted pine nuts.

343 calories, 23 g protein, 19 g carbohydrates, 20 g fat (2.5 g saturated fat), 49 mg cholesterol, 433 mg sodium

1,600-calorie plan: Use 4 ounces raw chicken breast, 4 tablespoons seasoned bread crumbs, and 2 tablespoons toasted pine nuts.

428 calories, 33.5 g protein, 29 g carbohydrates, 20 g fat (2.5 g saturated fat), 73 mg cholesterol, 718 mg sodium

Dinner 13

❒ Lazy Chef Salad: Toss together 2 cups mixed salad greens; 2 ounces water-packed canned tuna or salmon, drained; ¼ cup cooked chickpeas; 2 tablespoons shredded reduced-fat cheese; and 2 tablespoons reduced-fat ranch dressing.

❒ 1 rye crisp cracker

❒ ½ cup fat-free milk or low-fat, calcium-enriched soy or rice beverage

349 calories, 28 g protein, 33 g carbohydrates, 11 g fat (3 g saturated fat), 34 mg cholesterol, 839 mg sodium

1,600-calorie plan: Use 3 cups mixed salad greens and 3 ounces canned water-packed tuna or salmon, drained. Drink 1 cup fat-free milk or low-fat, calcium-enriched soy or rice beverage.

430 calories, 39 g protein, 40 g carbohydrates, 12 g fat (3.5 g saturated fat), 45 mg cholesterol, 991 mg sodium

Dinner 14

❒ Grilled fajitas: Heat 1 teaspoon olive oil in a skillet. Add 2 ounces chicken breast, pork, or beef tenderloin; ½ cup sliced onion; 1 cup chopped green and red bell peppers; ½ cup sliced carrots; and 2 cloves garlic, and sauté. Serve on 1 corn tortilla.

❒ ½ cup fat-free milk or low-fat, calcium-enriched soy or rice beverage

359 calories, 25 g protein, 40 g carbohydrates, 11 g fat (3 g saturated fat), 55 mg cholesterol, 147 mg sodium

1,600-calorie plan: Use 3 ounces chicken breast, pork, or beef tenderloin.

417 calories, 33 g protein, 40 g carbohydrates, 14 g fat (4 g saturated fat), 80 mg cholesterol, 164 mg sodium

SNACKS

Snack 1

❒ Mix together ⅓ cup fat-free or 1% cottage cheese and ½ cup chopped peaches (fresh or canned in water or juice, drained). Top with 2 tablespoons chopped unsalted raw almonds, walnuts, or other nuts.

177 calories, 12 g protein, 21 g carbohydrates, 6 g fat (0.5 g saturated fat), 3 mg cholesterol, 284 mg sodium

1,600-calorie plan: Use ½ cup fat-free or 1% cottage cheese and 1 cup chopped peaches.

205 calories, 17 g protein, 24 g carbohydrates, 6 g fat (0.5 g saturated fat), 5 mg cholesterol, 430 mg sodium

Snack 2

❒ 3 tablespoons unsalted walnuts or other raw nuts

❒ 1 tablespoon mixed dried fruits (blueberries, cherries, cranberries, and/or raisins)

168 calories, 4 g protein, 10 g carbohydrates, 14 g fat (1.5 g saturated fat), 0 mg cholesterol, 9 mg sodium

1,600-calorie plan: Eat 2 tablespoons dried fruits.

193 calories, 4 g protein, 16 g carbohydrates, 14 g fat (1.5 g saturated fat), 0 mg cholesterol, 18 mg sodium

Snack 3

❒ 1 ounce reduced-fat cheese

❒ 1 medium apple

152 calories, 7 g protein, 20 g carbohydrates, 6 g fat (3.5 g saturated fat), 20 mg cholesterol, 241 mg sodium

1,600-calorie plan: Use 1 tablespoon natural peanut butter and cut the apple into slices (about ½ cup.

177 calories, 4 g protein, 22 g carbohydrates, 8 g fat (1 g saturated fat), 0 mg cholesterol, 61 mg sodium

Snack 4

❒ ⅔ cup fat-free or low-fat yogurt (6 ounces)

❒ ½ cup fresh or frozen blueberries

❒ 1 tablespoon chopped unsalted raw nuts

169 calories, 10 g protein, 26 g carbohydrates, 5 g fat (0.5 g saturated fat), 0 mg cholesterol, 116 mg sodium

1,600-calorie plan: Use 2 tablespoons chopped nuts.

217 calories, 11 g protein, 26 g carbohydrates, 10 g fat (1 g saturated fat), 0 mg cholesterol, 116 mg sodium

Snack 5

❒ 2 fig cookies

❒ 1 cup fat-free milk or low-fat, calcium-enriched soy or rice beverage

193 calories, 9 g protein, 34 g carbohydrates, 3 g fat (0.5 g saturated fat), 5 mg cholesterol, 218 mg sodium

1,600-calorie plan: Same as above.

Snack 6

❒ ½ cup light ice cream

❒ 1 tablespoon reduced-fat chocolate syrup

❒ 1 tablespoon chopped unsalted raw nuts

190 calories, 4 g protein, 25 g carbohydrates, 9 g fat (2.5 g saturated fat), 36 mg cholesterol, 67 mg sodium

1,600-calorie plan: Same as above.

Snack 7

❒ 6 cups reduced-fat popcorn sprinkled with 2 tablespoons grated Parmesan cheese

❒ 12 ounces diet soda or sugar-free beverage

165 calories, 8 g protein, 25 g carbohydrates, 6 g fat (1.5 g saturated fat), 9 mg cholesterol, 435 mg sodium

1,600-calorie plan: Add 1 ounce beef jerky.

165 calories, 8 g protein, 25 g carbohydrates, 6 g fat (1.5 g saturated fat), 9 mg cholesterol, 435 mg sodium

Snack 8

❒ 1 ounce mozzarella string cheese

❒ 2 fresh or dried figs

200 calories, 8 g protein, 28 g carbohydrates, 6 g fat (4 g saturated fat), 20 mg cholesterol, 240 mg sodium

1,600-calorie plan: Add 7 walnut halves.

200 calories, 8 g protein, 28 g carbohydrates, 6 g fat (4 g saturated fat), 20 mg cholesterol, 240 mg sodium

Snack 9

❐ 4 tablespoons hummus or 1 tablespoon natural peanut butter

❐ 2 whole grain crispbread crackers

173 calories, 4 g protein, 26 g carbohydrates, 6 g fat (0 g saturated fat), 0 mg cholesterol, 373 mg sodium

1,600-calorie plan: Have 3 whole grain crispbreads.

210 calories, 4 g protein, 35 g carbohydrates, 6 g fat (0 g saturated fat), 0 mg cholesterol, 399 mg sodium

Snack 10

❐ 2 tablespoons walnut halves or other nut halves

❐ 3 fresh apricots or 6 dried apricot halves

146 calories, 4 g protein, 14 g carbohydrates, 10 g fat (1 g saturated fat), 0 mg cholesterol, 1.5 mg sodium

1,600-calorie plan: Have 2 tablespoons walnut halves and 4 fresh apricots or 8 dried apricot halves.

163 calories, 4 g protein, 18 g carbohydrates, 10 g fat (1 g saturated fat), 0 mg cholesterol, 1.5 mg sodium

Snack 11

❐ Turkey or chicken sandwich: Spread 1 slice reduced-calorie whole grain bread with 1 tablespoon reduced-fat mayonnaise (or 1 teaspoon regular mayonnaise). Cut bread in half and pile 2 ounces sliced turkey or chicken breast and ¼ cup shredded lettuce on one side. Top with other half of bread.

❐ ½ cup cherry tomatoes

164 calories, 13 g protein, 20 g carbohydrates, 5 g fat (1 g saturated fat), 28 mg cholesterol, 795 mg sodium

1,600-calorie plan: Use 2 slices reduced-calorie whole grain bread.

220 calories, 15 g protein, 32 g carbohydrates, 6 g fat (1 g saturated fat), 28 mg cholesterol, 938 mg sodium

Snack 12

❐ Bone-Soothing Hot Chocolate: Mix ⅓ cup fat-free powdered milk with 1 tablespoon cocoa powder and 1 teaspoon sugar substitute. Add 8 ounces boiling water and stir. Top with 1 regular-size marshmallow.

❐ 3 small no-sugar-added gingersnap cookies (serving size not to exceed 15 grams total carbohydrates; Murray Sugar Free is one brand)

170 calories, 10 g protein, 31 g carbohydrates, 3 g fat (1 g saturated fat), 4 mg cholesterol, 181 mg sodium

1,600-calorie plan: Have 4 small no-sugar-added gingersnap cookies.

129 calories, 10 g protein, 34 g carbohydrates, 4 g fat (1 g saturated fat), 4 mg cholesterol, 199 mg sodium

Snack 13

❐ 3 graham cracker squares spread with 1 teaspoon all-natural peanut or other nut butter

❐ ½ cup fat-free or low-fat milk or low-fat, calcium-enriched soy or rice beverage

174 calories, 7 g protein, 26 g carbohydrates, 5 g fat (1 g saturated fat), 2.5 mg cholesterol, 202 mg sodium

1,600-calorie plan: Use 2 teaspoons all-natural peanut or other nut butter.

209 calories, 8 g protein, 27 g carbohydrates, 8 g fat (1 g saturated fat), 2.5 mg cholesterol, 210 mg sodium

Snack 14

❐ 1 cup raw fresh sugar snap peas

❐ 2 tablespoons reduced-fat ranch dressing

❐ 1 ounce string cheese

195 calories, 12 g protein, 16 g carbohydrates, 10 g fat (4.5 g saturated fat), 23 mg cholesterol, 527 mg sodium

1,600-calorie plan: Eat 1½ cups sugar snap peas.

191 calories, 8 g protein, 25 g carbohydrates, 7 g fat (1 g saturated fat), 5 mg cholesterol, 503 mg sodium

Your Awesome 4somes

BREAKFAST

LUNCH

SNACK 1

DINNER

SNACK 2

Your DTOUR Workout

☐ Fat-Torch Walk (page 144), 20 minutes

> All glory comes from daring to begin.
> —WILLIAM SHAKESPEARE

HOW DID YOU DO?

BALANCE YOUR BLOOD SUGAR

	TIME	READING
CHECK 1		
CHECK 2		
CHECK 3		
CHECK 4		
CHECK 5		

MEASURE YOURSELF

Starting weight: _____ pounds

Starting waistline: _____ inches

SUCCEED ALL DAY

Try iPod therapy. Create an upbeat playlist on your MP3 player to help you deal with cravings. When you're blindsided by a yen for pizza, ice cream, or chocolate, crank up those tunes. The music will distract you and provide the emotional release you'd get from indulging your craving.

Give yourself some props. It's more challenging to start a fitness program—or start one again—than to continue one. It takes more determination, planning, encouragement—and a major shot of courage. On Day 1, give yourself credit for tackling such a demanding task.

Your Awesome 4somes

BREAKFAST

LUNCH

SNACK 1

DINNER

SNACK 2

Your DTOUR Workout

☐ Metabo Moves (page 155)
☐ Belly Blast (page 160)

> It's always fun to do the impossible.
> —WALT DISNEY

HOW DID YOU DO?

BALANCE YOUR BLOOD SUGAR

	TIME	READING
CHECK 1		
CHECK 2		
CHECK 3		
CHECK 4		
CHECK 5		

SUCCEED ALL DAY

Hang with optimists. Who do you know who's relentlessly cheerful and optimistic? A parent at your child's soccer game? Your sister? Whoever it is, make an effort to spend more time with him or her. Call her to chat. Invite him out for coffee. It's hard to fret when you're bathing in positive vibes.

Imagine a good night's sleep. Focusing your mind on a repetitive action can help your brain to shut down and drift off. Try this: Imagine walking down an endless stairwell.

Your Awesome 4somes

BREAKFAST

LUNCH

SNACK 1

DINNER

SNACK 2

Your DTOUR Workout

☐ Calorie-Scorch Walk (page 144), 15 minutes

> Your future is created by what you
> do today, not tomorrow.
> —ROBERT KIYOSAKI

HOW DID YOU DO?

BALANCE YOUR BLOOD SUGAR

	TIME	READING
CHECK 1		
CHECK 2		
CHECK 3		
CHECK 4		
CHECK 5		

SUCCEED ALL DAY

Walk off winter cravings. Seasonal affective disorder (SAD), a reaction to reduced sunlight during the winter months, creates cravings for highly refined carbohydrates. If you suspect SAD is at the root of your cravings, soak up natural light on daily walks until the longer days of spring arrive.

Learn to say "The world won't end." This phrase is an all-purpose stress reliever, and it will help you put your life in perspective. The car didn't get washed this weekend? The world won't end.

DAY
4

Your Awesome 4somes

BREAKFAST

LUNCH

SNACK 1

DINNER

SNACK 2

Your DTOUR Workout
☐ Rest Day

> If you really want something,
> you can figure out how to make it happen.
> —CHER

HOW DID YOU DO?

BALANCE YOUR BLOOD SUGAR

	TIME	READING
CHECK 1		
CHECK 2		
CHECK 3		
CHECK 4		
CHECK 5		

SUCCEED ALL DAY

Set specific goals. What it really boils down to is, *What type of exercise will you do, when, and where?* A specific goal might be "I will do 3 Cardio Walks at 6:45 a.m. before work and 2 on the weekends, and the Belly Blast and Metabo Moves before dinner on Mondays, Wednesdays, and Fridays."

Question your medication. Certain over-the-counter and prescription medications, particularly those that treat colds and allergies, heart disease, high blood pressure, and pain, can keep you awake. If you take prescription medication routinely, ask your doctor about the side effects. If she suspects the drug could be interfering with your sleep, she may be able to substitute another medication or change the time of day you take it.

Your Awesome 4somes

BREAKFAST

LUNCH

SNACK 1

DINNER

SNACK 2

Your DTOUR Workout

☐ Fat-Torch Walk (page 144), 20 minutes

> It is hard to fail, but it is worse never
> to have tried to succeed.
> —THEODORE ROOSEVELT

HOW DID YOU DO?

BALANCE YOUR BLOOD SUGAR

	TIME	READING
CHECK 1		
CHECK 2		
CHECK 3		
CHECK 4		
CHECK 5		

SUCCEED ALL DAY

Replace images of food with other pleasant images. Imagining a steaming, gooey slice of pizza? Instead, imagine walking on the beach in a flattering bathing suit. Swapping images may work better than trying to quash a particular craving.

Resist the urge to sleep in. Late night? Get up within an hour of your usual rising time. It's fine to catnap for 30 minutes to make up for lost slumber. Nap longer than that, however, and you may have trouble getting to sleep come bedtime.

Your Awesome 4somes

BREAKFAST

LUNCH

SNACK 1

DINNER

SNACK 2

Your DTOUR Workout

☐ Metabo Moves (page 155)
☐ Belly Blast (page 160)

> People often say that motivation
> doesn't last. Well, neither does bathing—
> that's why we recommend it daily.
> —ZIG ZIGLAR

HOW DID YOU DO?

BALANCE YOUR BLOOD SUGAR

	TIME	READING
CHECK 1		
CHECK 2		
CHECK 3		
CHECK 4		
CHECK 5		

SUCCEED ALL DAY

Nag via sticky notes. Visual reminders to work out can help, but only if you notice them. You might overlook a sticky note reminding you to go to the gym if you place it on your magnet- and photo-cluttered fridge door, but you can't miss it on the steering wheel of your car.

Make time for a morning hug. Before you head out the door, take 10 seconds to hold your partner in your arms. That simple embrace can help you stay calmer throughout the entire day, researchers at the University of North Carolina at Chapel Hill found.

Your Awesome 4somes

BREAKFAST

LUNCH

SNACK 1

DINNER

SNACK 2

Your DTOUR Workout

☐ Calorie-Scorch Walk (page 144), 15 minutes

> ## What would you attempt to do if you knew you would not fail?
> —ROBERT SCHULLER

HOW DID YOU DO?

BALANCE YOUR BLOOD SUGAR

	TIME	READING
CHECK 1		
CHECK 2		
CHECK 3		
CHECK 4		
CHECK 5		

MEASURE YOURSELF

Starting weight: _____ pounds

Starting waistline: _____ inches

SUCCEED ALL DAY

Silence your sweet tooth. To block a craving for sweets, rinse your mouth with 30 drops of a tincture of the Indian herb gymnema mixed with water, suggests Andrew Weil, MD. You'll find gymnema in health-food stores.

Set realistic goals. They should be challenging, but doable. If a goal is too hard (like wanting to run 10 miles when you have yet to run 1), you'll get discouraged. If it's too easy, you won't feel much satisfaction when you achieve it.

Your Awesome 4somes

BREAKFAST

LUNCH

SNACK 1

DINNER

SNACK 2

Your DTOUR Workout

☐ Fat-Torch Walk (page 144), 25 minutes

> Smooth seas do not make skillful sailors.
> —AFRICAN PROVERB

HOW DID YOU DO?

BALANCE YOUR BLOOD SUGAR

	TIME	READING
CHECK 1		
CHECK 2		
CHECK 3		
CHECK 4		
CHECK 5		

SUCCEED ALL DAY

Tame stress together. Chances are that life is stressful for your partner, too. Start a discussion aimed at helping you both recognize and defuse each other's stressors. How about a shared glass of wine or mutual foot rub? Discuss how you might share chores—you cook dinner while he runs the vacuum, for example, or you pay the bills while he folds the laundry.

Play sleuth to your sleeplessness. Keep a sleep log for a week to identify possible causes of insomnia. Record what times you go to bed and wake up, the total number of hours of sleep you get, whether you awaken during the night and what you do (toss and turn, watch TV), how much and when you ingest caffeine and/or alcohol, your emotional state, and at what time and dosage you took any over-the-counter or prescription medications.

Your Awesome 4somes

BREAKFAST

LUNCH

SNACK 1

DINNER

SNACK 2

Your DTOUR Workout

☐ Metabo Moves (page 155)
☐ Belly Blast (page 160)

> If you can't make a mistake,
> you can't make anything.
> —MARVA COLLINS

HOW DID YOU DO?

BALANCE YOUR BLOOD SUGAR

	TIME	READING
CHECK 1		
CHECK 2		
CHECK 3		
CHECK 4		
CHECK 5		

SUCCEED ALL DAY

Refuel every 4 hours. Regular eating keeps blood sugar stable, which prevents you from feeling famished. If you're hungry between meals, a 150-calorie snack should hold you over. Pack healthful, portable snacks such as string cheese, fruit, and unsalted raw nuts in your bag or glove compartment.

Turn unknowns into knowns. If your stress is caused by unknown dangers, choose education over anxiety. Make reasonable plans to take precautions, then live your life. Turn off the television and radio if the news increases your anxiety. Plan activities that are familiar and rewarding—doing a hobby or yard work, cleaning out the attic or garage, taking a long walk or hike.

Your Awesome 4somes

BREAKFAST

LUNCH

SNACK 1

DINNER

SNACK 2

Your DTOUR Workout

☐ Calorie-Scorch Walk (page 144), 20 minutes

> That some achieve great success, is proof to all that others can achieve it as well.
> —ABRAHAM LINCOLN

HOW DID YOU DO?

BALANCE YOUR BLOOD SUGAR

	TIME	READING
CHECK 1		
CHECK 2		
CHECK 3		
CHECK 4		
CHECK 5		

SUCCEED ALL DAY

Be alert to prime dropout time. About half of new exercisers quit within the first few months, research has shown. If you struggle with exercise, find (or start) a walking or fitness group. If you're goal focused, sign up to participate in an event that's a few months away, like a 5- or 10-K walk.

Hit the sack *later*. If you often lie awake at night, spending less time in bed can help break that cycle. You'll fatigue your body and start to associate bedtime with sleep instead of tossing and turning. Track your night's sleep. If you typically get 5 hours a night, set your alarm for that. Once you're sleeping for most of that time, go to bed 15 minutes earlier until you reach the recommended 8 hours a night.

DAY
11

Your Awesome 4somes

BREAKFAST

LUNCH

SNACK 1

DINNER

SNACK 2

Your DTOUR Workout

☐ Fat-Torch Walk (page 144), 25 minutes

> Remember: Success is nothing but luck.
> Just ask any failure.
> —AUTHOR UNKNOWN

HOW DID YOU DO?

BALANCE YOUR BLOOD SUGAR

	TIME	READING
CHECK 1		
CHECK 2		
CHECK 3		
CHECK 4		
CHECK 5		

SUCCEED ALL DAY

Push back breakfast. If you can't stomach an early-morning meal, eat it at 9:00, 10:00, or even 11:00 a.m. It will help you stay in control later in the day.

Launch a mite raid. If nighttime coughing, sneezing, and snuffling disrupt your sleep and you don't have a cold, you could be allergic to dust mites. (Their residue can trigger mild to severe allergies.) To reduce allergens, vacuum and dust regularly. If you can, replace your mattress if it's more than 10 years old, and wash your pillow every week or put a miteproof plastic cover under your regular pillowcase. Crack the windows and doors, too. Increasing a room's airflow is one of the most effective ways to reduce mites.

Your Awesome 4somes

BREAKFAST

LUNCH

SNACK 1

DINNER

SNACK 2

Your DTOUR Workout

☐ Rest Day

> Your future depends on many
> things, but mostly on you.
> —FRANK TYGER

HOW DID YOU DO?

BALANCE YOUR BLOOD SUGAR

	TIME	READING
CHECK 1		
CHECK 2		
CHECK 3		
CHECK 4		
CHECK 5		

SUCCEED ALL DAY

Sign up for a race. It doesn't matter whether you're fast or slow, or even if you come in last. The idea is to set a goal. It gives you a tangible reason to put your sneakers on—you're in training. Making that commitment can be really motivating, because you'll want to do well on race day. Choose a race that's happening 8 to 10 weeks from today.

Rediscover the joy of cooking. Good nutrition helps short-circuit the effects of stress. If you're often too tired to cook after work, reframe the activity as a way to unwind rather than a chore. Choose healthy recipes and shop over the weekend, so you'll have everything you need. Pour a glass of wine, put on some smooth jazz, and hum as you chop, stir, and taste.

DAY
13

Your Awesome 4somes

BREAKFAST

LUNCH

SNACK 1

DINNER

SNACK 2

Your DTOUR Workout

☐ Metabo Moves (page 155)
☐ Belly Blast (page 160)

> Who dares, wins. —WINSTON CHURCHILL

HOW DID YOU DO?

BALANCE YOUR BLOOD SUGAR

	TIME	READING
CHECK 1		
CHECK 2		
CHECK 3		
CHECK 4		
CHECK 5		

SUCCEED ALL DAY

Nap cravings away. Fatigue can trigger food cravings. If you're tired at work, shut your office door, close your eyes, and reenergize. If you're at home, take a 15-minute catnap (but no longer than that).

Seek instant gratification. If you find it tough to wait for weeks to see the results of your efforts, fitness gadgets can provide right-now motivation. A heart rate monitor can tell you whether to increase or reduce the intensity of your workout, and a pedometer can boost your resolve to move more during the day.

DAY 14

Your Awesome 4somes

BREAKFAST

LUNCH

SNACK 1

DINNER

SNACK 2

Your DTOUR Workout

☐ Calorie-Scorch Walk (page 144), 20 minutes

Leap and the net will appear.
—JULIA CAMERON

HOW DID YOU DO?

BALANCE YOUR BLOOD SUGAR

	TIME	READING
CHECK 1		
CHECK 2		
CHECK 3		
CHECK 4		
CHECK 5		

MEASURE YOURSELF

Starting weight: _____ pounds

Starting waistline: _____ inches

SUCCEED ALL DAY

Set your alarm 15 minutes early. Those 900 extra seconds are a cushion against that inevitable morning chaos—making lunches, finding your car keys, arranging drop-offs and pickups for your kids.

Sip serenity now. The flower, vine, and leaves of the passionflower herb contain substances that have proven, gentle sedating qualities. Recommended by herbalists as a top treatment for insomnia, it's especially helpful when sleep is disturbed by anxiety. Use 1 teaspoon of dried herb per cup of boiling water.

Your Awesome 4somes

BREAKFAST

LUNCH

SNACK 1

DINNER

SNACK 2

Your DTOUR Workout

☐ Fat-Torch Walk (page 144), 30 minutes

> If you are in a hurry, you will never get there.
> —CHINESE PROVERB

HOW DID YOU DO?

BALANCE YOUR BLOOD SUGAR

	TIME	READING
CHECK 1		
CHECK 2		
CHECK 3		
CHECK 4		
CHECK 5		

SUCCEED ALL DAY
Instead of trying to ignore the craving, admit to it. This technique (cognitive diffusion) works on the same principle as getting the hots for a co-worker when you're happily partnered: Recognizing that you'll always be attracted to cute guys (or yummy foods) prevents you from acting on the feeling when it arises.

Prepare for the a.m. in the p.m. Make everyone's lunch for the next day the night before. Put out the clothes you plan to wear, and have your kids do it, too.

Your Awesome 4somes

BREAKFAST

LUNCH

SNACK 1

DINNER

SNACK 2

Your DTOUR Workout

☐ Calorie-Scorch Walk (page 144), 25 minutes

> The greater the obstacle,
> the more glory in overcoming it.
> —MOLIÈRE

HOW DID YOU DO?

BALANCE YOUR BLOOD SUGAR

	TIME	READING
CHECK 1		
CHECK 2		
CHECK 3		
CHECK 4		
CHECK 5		

SUCCEED ALL DAY

Hire a personal trainer for a workout or two. It's Day 16. Do you know where your motivation is? A few sessions with a pro can help ensure that you make it to the gym, perfect your technique, and boost your motivation.

Make breakfast your heaviest meal of the day. Digesting food takes energy, so if you eat a heavy meal late in the day, your body will be working hard to digest it when you're trying to go to sleep. Many people sleep better if they have protein at breakfast and lunch and then some carbohydrates at a light dinner.

Your Awesome 4somes

BREAKFAST

LUNCH

SNACK 1

DINNER

SNACK 2

Your DTOUR Workout

☐ Metabo Moves (page 155)
☐ Belly Blast (page 160)

HOW DID YOU DO?

BALANCE YOUR BLOOD SUGAR

	TIME	READING
CHECK 1		
CHECK 2		
CHECK 3		
CHECK 4		
CHECK 5		

SUCCEED ALL DAY

Feed a fantasy, starve a craving.
Occupying your senses with a vivid nonfood
fantasy can help stifle a craving, researchers at
Flinders University in Australia found. Think
about what some hot Hollywood actor looks
like in nothing but a towel. You might forget all
about those chips.

Go toward the light. Get outside when
it's sunny, or at least turn on the lights at home
in the morning. This will help you reset your
awake-sleep cycle.

Your Awesome 4somes

BREAKFAST

LUNCH

SNACK 1

DINNER

SNACK 2

Your DTOUR Workout

☐ Fat-Torch Walk (page 144), 30 minutes

> Who has never tasted what is bitter
> does not know what is sweet.
> —GERMAN PROVERB

HOW DID YOU DO?

BALANCE YOUR BLOOD SUGAR

	TIME	READING
CHECK 1		
CHECK 2		
CHECK 3		
CHECK 4		
CHECK 5		

SUCCEED ALL DAY

Cut a high-energy soundtrack. Upbeat music makes a workout seem easier and go by faster, according to research conducted at the University of Scranton in Pennsylvania. That's because high-tempo music helps block out the sensations associated with pain and effort.

Got garden? Go dig. Researchers in the United Kingdom found that mice that inhaled bacteria commonly found in soil tried harder to solve a stressful problem (escaping from a pool of water); mice who didn't gave up more easily. The soil-loving bugs are thought to stimulate the release of mood-enhancing brain chemicals.

Your Awesome 4somes

BREAKFAST

LUNCH

SNACK 1

DINNER

SNACK 2

Your DTOUR Workout

☐ Rest Day

> One's best success comes
> after their greatest disappointments.
> —HENRY WARD BEECHER

HOW DID YOU DO?

BALANCE YOUR BLOOD SUGAR

	TIME	READING
CHECK 1		
CHECK 2		
CHECK 3		
CHECK 4		
CHECK 5		

SUCCEED ALL DAY

Forgo crash diets. It's common sense: The more restrictive your diet, the more likely you'll binge in rebellion. Consume a minimum of 1,200 calories a day, diet experts recommend.

If you splurge, get up—and active. Snarfing a pint of ice cream won't doom your weight loss if you don't let guilt derail your workout. In a French study, obese exercisers who bicycled for 45 minutes 3 hours after a high-fat meal metabolized more stored belly fat than those who cycled on an empty stomach. The upshot: All is not lost when you stray from your diet—in fact, your body may even kick it up a gear to help with damage control.

Your Awesome 4somes

BREAKFAST

LUNCH

SNACK 1

DINNER

SNACK 2

Your DTOUR Workout

☐ Calorie-Scorch Walk (page 144), 25 minutes

> Surround yourself with only people
> who are going to lift you higher.
> —OPRAH WINFREY

HOW DID YOU DO?

BALANCE YOUR BLOOD SUGAR

	TIME	READING
CHECK 1		
CHECK 2		
CHECK 3		
CHECK 4		
CHECK 5		

SUCCEED ALL DAY

Indulge in a before- or after-work "dog-tail." For a few minutes before or after work, chase your pup around your backyard. He'll love the companionship and exercise. You'll love feeling like a 10-year-old again.

Cool out night sweats. If night sweats disrupt your sleep, keep your bedroom cool. A lower body temperature promotes sleep. Also, consider a low-dose oral contraceptive to even out hormone levels, especially if you also experience irregular menstrual cycles.

Your Awesome 4somes

BREAKFAST

LUNCH

SNACK 1

DINNER

SNACK 2

Your DTOUR Workout

- ☐ Metabo Moves (page 155)
- ☐ Belly Blast (page 160)

> There are no shortcuts to any place worth going.
> —BEVERLY SILLS

HOW DID YOU DO?

BALANCE YOUR BLOOD SUGAR

	TIME	READING
CHECK 1		
CHECK 2		
CHECK 3		
CHECK 4		
CHECK 5		

SUCCEED ALL DAY
Try an ex-smoker's craving buster. Suck a cinnamon stick or flavored toothpick, or chomp on sugarless gum.
Do unpleasant tasks first. Need to see your accountant? Get your teeth cleaned? Get the car inspected? Schedule any un-fun task for early in the day and get it over with. The rest of your day will be free of anxiety.

MEASURE YOURSELF
Starting weight: _____ pounds
Starting waistline: _____ inches

Your Awesome 4somes

BREAKFAST

LUNCH

SNACK 1

DINNER

SNACK 2

Your DTOUR Workout

☐ Fat-Torch Walk (page 144), 35 minutes

> Kites rise highest against the wind—not with it.
> —WINSTON CHURCHILL

HOW DID YOU DO?

BALANCE YOUR BLOOD SUGAR

	TIME	READING
CHECK 1		
CHECK 2		
CHECK 3		
CHECK 4		
CHECK 5		

SUCCEED ALL DAY

Take a picture. Slip into a swimsuit and take a photo. Place it somewhere where you'll see it constantly. Take a new photo every 4 weeks—and get stoked as your body transforms before your eyes.

Create a sleep schedule and stick to it. You may not be able to go to bed at the same time every night, but you can establish a regular wake-up time. Get up at the same time every morning, even on weekends.

Your Awesome 4somes

BREAKFAST

LUNCH

SNACK 1

DINNER

SNACK 2

Your DTOUR Workout

☐ Calorie-Scorch Walk (page 144), 30 minutes

> It is not because things are difficult
> that we do not dare, it is because we
> do not dare that they are difficult.
>
> —SENECA

HOW DID YOU DO?

BALANCE YOUR BLOOD SUGAR

	TIME	READING
CHECK 1		
CHECK 2		
CHECK 3		
CHECK 4		
CHECK 5		

SUCCEED ALL DAY

Make a reward list. List ways you can reward yourself for making it through another chocolate-chip-cookie craving. Buy yourself a new lipstick or rent a favorite video, for example.

Try magnesium. According to some naturopaths, this mineral helps the body make serotonin, which in turn produces melatonin, the brain chemical that sets your body clock and helps the brain's inhibitory neurotransmitters (the ones that help us relax) work more efficiently. Take 200 to 300 mg of magnesium citrate daily with dinner. Because it works best when balanced with calcium (which aids absorption), also take 400 mg of calcium daily with lunch.

Your Awesome 4somes

BREAKFAST

LUNCH

SNACK 1

DINNER

SNACK 2

Your DTOUR Workout

☐ Metabo Moves (page 155)
☐ Belly Blast (page 160)

> Always bear in mind that your own resolution to succeed is more important than any one thing.
> —ABRAHAM LINCOLN

HOW DID YOU DO?

BALANCE YOUR BLOOD SUGAR

	TIME	READING
CHECK 1		
CHECK 2		
CHECK 3		
CHECK 4		
CHECK 5		

SUCCEED ALL DAY

Go on the defensive. If you need more inspiration to exercise than simply slimming down, consider a self-defense class. You'll learn a skill that can potentially save your life as you burn calories and build muscle.

Spot-check your posture. Stooping and slumping can lead to muscle tension and increased stress, so throughout the day, check your posture. Hold your head high and your spine and shoulders straight.

Your Awesome 4somes

BREAKFAST

LUNCH

SNACK 1

DINNER

SNACK 2

Your DTOUR Workout

☐ Rest Day

> The creation of a thousand
> forests is in one acorn.
> —RALPH WALDO EMERSON

HOW DID YOU DO?

BALANCE YOUR BLOOD SUGAR

	TIME	READING
CHECK 1		
CHECK 2		
CHECK 3		
CHECK 4		
CHECK 5		

SUCCEED ALL DAY

Stay hydrated. Drink at least eight 8-ounce glasses of water a day. Water is nature's appetite suppressant: It keeps your stomach full and prevents dehydration, which can lead to cravings and hunger.

Watch the rut. Every 4 to 6 weeks, switch up your workout routine (try a different walking route or new strength moves). You'll keep your motivation strong and your muscles challenged.

Your Awesome 4somes

BREAKFAST

LUNCH

SNACK 1

DINNER

SNACK 2

Your DTOUR Workout

☐ Fat-Torch Walk (page 144), 35 minutes

> Your body is your vehicle for life. As long as you are here, live in it. Love, honor, respect and cherish it, treat it well and it will serve you in kind.
>
> —SUZY PRUDDEN

HOW DID YOU DO?

BALANCE YOUR BLOOD SUGAR

	TIME	READING
CHECK 1		
CHECK 2		
CHECK 3		
CHECK 4		
CHECK 5		

SUCCEED ALL DAY

Turn wait time into found time. Lines at the grocery store, bank, or post office are a fact of life. Plan for them. Tuck a paperback in your bag. Your "stressful" wait will turn into an oasis of calm.

De-stress with a good "book." Are you a worrier? Buy a small journal to use as a worry book. Choose a time during the day to regularly jot down concerns that keep you awake at night (anything from bills to world affairs). The idea is to worry *before* the lights go out—and to brainstorm potential solutions you can act on.

Your Awesome 4somes

BREAKFAST

LUNCH

SNACK 1

DINNER

SNACK 2

Your DTOUR Workout

☐ Calorie-Scorch Walk (page 144), 30 minutes

> Learn from yesterday, live
> for today, hope for tomorrow.
> —AUTHOR UNKNOWN

HOW DID YOU DO?

BALANCE YOUR BLOOD SUGAR

	TIME	READING
CHECK 1		
CHECK 2		
CHECK 3		
CHECK 4		
CHECK 5		

SUCCEED ALL DAY

Eat balanced meals. Eating meals that are very high in refined carbohydrates, such as pasta, can trigger cravings for more carbs and sugar. Balancing your meals with protein and a bit of healthy fat can dramatically reduce cravings.

Make three extra car and/or house keys. If you're constantly misplacing your keys, make a slew of spares. Carry a duplicate car key in your wallet. Hide a house key in a toolbox in the garage.

Your Awesome 4somes

BREAKFAST

LUNCH

SNACK 1

DINNER

SNACK 2

Your DTOUR Workout

☐ Metabo Moves (page 155)
☐ Belly Blast (page 160)

> # Do or do not. There is no try.
> ## —YODA

HOW DID YOU DO?

BALANCE YOUR BLOOD SUGAR

	TIME	READING
CHECK 1		
CHECK 2		
CHECK 3		
CHECK 4		
CHECK 5		

MEASURE YOURSELF

Starting weight: _____ pounds

Starting waistline: _____ inches

SUCCEED ALL DAY

Treat yourself. To celebrate your commitment to fitness, treat yourself to a little something at the end of each workout week: a new lipstick, a pedicure, a new skin-care product.

Calm down with chamomile. A bright, daisylike flower, chamomile has an age-old reputation for calming nerves and gently aiding sleep. Drinking 1 or 2 cups of tea before bedtime will help soothe you into sleep.

DTOUR WINNER!

Therese Ciesinski, 47
POUNDS LOST: 7
INCHES LOST: 5½
BLOOD SUGAR: STABLE

BEFORE

AFTER

I decided to try DTOUR because, although I don't have diabetes, I wasn't feeling so great. I have hypoglycemia, which means that I get shaky if I don't eat regularly. I also have celiac disease, and heart disease runs in my family.

I was at my highest weight ever— 144 pounds—and I always felt tired and sluggish. Although I was eating a relatively healthy diet, my portions were too large, and I ate way too much sugar and salt—lots of granola and granola bars and gluten-free waffles and doughnuts, which are all loaded with fat and sugar. So I looked forward to eating healthy whole foods.

At first, it was a challenge to prepare my own meals; I was used to grabbing junk food because it's fast and easy. Now I know that cooking for myself is an important part of losing weight and keeping it off. I try to prepare my week's meals on the weekend, which isn't that hard. Yogurt with fruit, granola, and flaxseed isn't tough to whip up in the morning, and I love snacking on nuts and hummus. Dinner is more of a challenge, but I'll get there.

Portion sizes were definitely a wake-up call for me. The first day or two, I thought, *I get ⅓ cup of cooked rice? That can't be right*. I mean, I was used to eating 2 cups at a time.

Now I realize that I can eat in a way that actually helps control hunger and cravings. Before I started this plan, I was afraid I'd be hungry and my life would center around waiting for my next meal. That didn't happen. Once I started eating more good fats and fiber—nuts, peanut butter, hummus, fruits—that panicky "I've got to eat now or I may faint" feeling went away. That was a big change.

It's amazing how good I feel. I have more energy. I'm more alert. I don't get the up-and-down swings that I now realize must have been related to my blood sugar. I don't want to take a nap in the afternoon.

I'd like to lose 5 or 6 more pounds, so I plan to continue this way of eating for now, then tweak it to maintain my goal weight. That probably involves physical activity. I wasn't able to do the exercise part of the program because I was recovering from an illness. Now that I feel better and have more energy, it will be easier to get moving. But even without exercise, I lost weight, especially off my belly, which is where you want to lose it. I lost only 7 pounds, but my waistline shrank almost 6 inches. I'm very pleased.

LOST

5

INCHES!

13

STAY ON THE
ROAD TO
SUCCESS

Congratulations—you did it! You finished the full 6 weeks of DTOUR. Before you do anything else, take time to acknowledge what you've accomplished. You might even treat yourself with a visit to a day spa, an evening out with friends, or a brand-new outfit to show off your trim and toned physique. You've achieved a lot over these past 6 weeks; you've proven that you can win the battle of the bulge and conquer high blood sugar, too. Now you deserve to celebrate!

Whether you're at your goal weight or you have a few more pounds to lose, you can stay the course by continuing to use the tools and techniques you've learned so far. We'll wager that you've gotten quite good at recognizing food sources of the Fat-Fighting 4 nutrients; at gauging portion sizes; at timing your meals to prevent spikes and dips in your blood sugar. You're more aware of how physical activity, sleep, and stress management can ramp up weight loss and blood sugar control. You've formed habits and behaviors that will tip the proverbial scale away from diabetes and its complications and toward a long, healthy, vital life.

So keep up the good work! We're confident that you can do it. To help, we've put together a short to-do list of sorts—a collection of strategies that capture the key principles and guidelines of DTOUR. Review the list, memorize it, live by it. The payoff: long-term, lasting weight-loss success. (Remember, too, that you can always find insight, advice, and support at www.dtour.com.)

FOUR RULES TO LIVE BY

If you've followed DTOUR faithfully, these four rules may be second nature to you by now. Nevertheless, they're important enough that we'll take time to review them here. Stick with them, and you can't go wrong!

1. PICK YOUR CALORIE RANGE

You can continue using the DTOUR menus and recipes for as long as you'd like. We're sure you have your favorites! Feeling more adventurous? Then by all means expand your dietary horizons by creating your own meals. Just be sure to pay attention to your daily calorie intake.

- *To continue losing weight:* Stick with your current benchmark of 1,400 or 1,600 calories per day.

- *If you've reached your goal weight on the 1,400-calorie plan:* Increase to 1,600 calories a day and see how you fare. If you start to regain, cut back on calories—or burn more with exercise.

- *If you've reached your goal weight on the 1,600-calorie plan:* Add an extra 200-calorie snack every day.

For most women, 1,600 calories a day is enough to maintain energy, immune function, and muscle mass, but not enough to regain belly fat. Men should aim for at least 1,700 calories per day once at their goal weight.

2. EAT EVERY 3 TO 4 HOURS

Having meals and snacks at regular intervals is vital to keeping your blood sugar on an even keel. Did you notice a difference while eating this way over the past 6 weeks? If you're like our DTOUR panelists, you felt more energized, more focused, and less hungry during the day. That's what optimal blood sugar control can do for you!

- *To continue losing weight:* Aim for three meals of approximately 350 to 400 calories each, plus two snacks of 175 to 200 calories each. (If you're eating 1,400 calories per day, you'll want to be at the lower end of these ranges; at 1,600 calories per day, you can go toward the higher end.)

- *If you've reached your goal weight and you want to maintain it:* Try for 400 calories at breakfast, lunch, and dinner, along with 200 calories at each snack. (Remember that you're adding a snack if you've been following the 1,600-calorie plan.)

3. STAY FAITHFUL TO THE FAT-FIGHTING 4

They've been your loyal allies for the past 6 weeks, helping you to whittle your waistline and balance your

FYI

ACCORDING TO DATA from the National Weight Control Registry, a database of over 5,000 people who've maintained a weight ioss of at least 30 pounds for at least 1 year, those who succeed in staying slim find the first 2 years most challenging . Eventually, though, they become quite comfortable with their new, right-sized lifestyles.

blood sugar. So why mess with a good thing? The FatFighting 4 will continue to serve you well, provided you're getting enough of them. That means:

- At least 20 to 25 grams per day of fiber, both soluble and insoluble
- Two or 3 servings per day of low-fat dairy products fortified with vitamin D
- Between 2.5 and 2.7 grams per day of omega-3s from good sources such as fish (if you like it) or ground flaxseed or flaxseed oil, canola oil, or walnuts or walnut oil (if you don't)

4. SCORCH, TORCH, LIFT, AND SQUEEZE

Exercise isn't mandatory on DTOUR, but it definitely can enhance your results. You'll burn more calories not just during your workouts but all day long, as you

DTOUR WHEN YOU DINE OUT, TOO

Eating out is one of life's pleasures. On DTOUR, you can have a wonderful meal at a favorite restaurant without guilt! Just do a little planning ahead, and you'll be set.

Have a snack before you go. Won't it spoil your dinner? In a way, that's the idea. At least you won't be going to the restaurant on an empty stomach, which is a surefire recipe for overeating. Not that you want to gorge, mind you. A slice of low-fat cheese or a small piece of fruit should be enough to take the edge off your hunger. It'll be far easier to make wise choices once you're looking at that big menu.

Follow the Fat-Fighting 4 formula. Good choices: low-fat yogurt with berries for breakfast, fish broiled without butter for lunch and dinner, a fruit cup for dessert. Instead of french fries, request a double order of steamed veggies, or pay a bit extra for a salad—dressing on the side, of course.

Splurge responsibly. If you're anticipating a special-occasion indulgence—for a birthday or anniversary celebration, for example—ask your doctor or dietitian for guidance on adjusting the rest of your day's meals and snacks accordingly. You can manage your portion sizes by splitting that slice of cake with your spouse or boxing up half to take home.

Match your meds with your meal. If you take diabetes medication or insulin, you need to think about when you'll eat as well as what you'll eat. Make a reservation so that you aren't kept waiting for a table. You want to be eating your meal at about your usual time. If you know that it will be late, have a piece of fruit or a serving of starch in place of your regular meal.

build muscle and lose fat. You'll feel better, too—thanks in part to endorphins, those feel-good brain chemicals that contribute to a sense of well-being.

◆ *To continue losing weight:* Follow the DTOUR Workout as presented in the 4-Week Total Transformation, gradually stepping up the intensity and duration as you feel comfortable.

◆ *If you've reached your goal weight:* Your weekly exercise regimen should include at least one 30-minute Calorie-Scorch Walk, two 60-minute Fat-Torch Walks, and two sessions of the Metabo Moves and Belly Blast routines. Be sure to allow at least a day between strength-training sessions so your muscles have a chance to recover.

FOUR MORE STRATEGIES FOR STAYING SLIM

If the above rules are the foundation of DTOUR, then think of the following strategies as the reinforcements. Though not essential to the plan, they give it a bit more flexibility and *oomph*. Use them as you wish!

1. TAKE ADVANTAGE OF MEAL REPLACEMENTS

Despite your best-laid plans, you occasionally will find yourself confronted with very un-DTOUR-like food choices and portion sizes. You could give in and vow to do better tomorrow. But before you do, consider whether you really want to spend calories on a feast that you may not enjoy anyway. If the answer is no, you do have another option: meal replacements—shakes, bars, and other packaged, calorie-controlled meals.

Research has shown that trading a meal or snack for one of these products on a daily basis really can promote weight loss or weight maintenance. In some studies, participants have used meal replacement drinks for as long as 4 to 5 years with impressive

Stop Here
STAY WITHIN A 5-POUND "SAFE ZONE." Continue to monitor your weight after you've reached your goal. If you start to regain, immediately rein in your diet and—if you've stopped working out—get moving again. According to researchers at Brown University in Providence, the safety zone around weight maintenance is about 5 pounds. If you slip out of this range, you need to immediately reverse course before all is (un)lost.

results. In one study, which appeared in the *Archives of Internal Medicine* in 2000, people with type 2 diabetes experienced significant weight loss and improvement in blood sugar levels after 1 year of using prepared meals.

Certain meal replacements are formulated especially for people with diabetes; you can find them in the supplement aisle of your local supermarket or pharmacy. While these products can be high in carbohydrates, they're often lower in carbs than the meal or snack they're replacing. If you take oral diabetes medications or use insulin, however, talk with your doctor before swapping a sit-down meal for an on-the-go shake or bar. You'll likely need to adjust your dosage.

2. CONTINUE TO ACCUMULATE TRANQUILLITY POINTS

To stay trim and fit for life, you need to stick with the habits and behaviors that support weight loss and blood sugar control. To do that, you should be in a good place emotionally. That means finding ways to blow off stress when you need to and making time every day to do at least one thing that you love. Your long-term health depends on it!

Tranquillity Points, which we first talked about in Chapter 11, are like daisies in a field: easy to gather, easy to enjoy. So blow bubbles in traffic jams, go polka dancing, stomp in puddles like you did as a kid. These are the sorts of things that keep agita at bay. And the less agita you have in your life, the less likely you are to stray from your eating plan. Your blood sugar will thank you!

3. KEEP UP WITH YOUR JOURNAL

Studies have shown that those who are most successful at losing and maintaining their weight practice a technique called *self-monitoring*. Journals are a powerful self-monitoring tool. They allow you to explore your thoughts and feelings, brainstorm fresh goals and strategies, acknowledge your challenges, and celebrate your successes. This healthy—and private—form of self-expression can be the first step in a long-running personal dialogue about your relationship with food, exercise, and even your body.

Hopefully, you took advantage of the "How Did You Do?" sections of the 2-Week Fast Start and the 4-Week Total Transformation to get in the habit of documenting your DTOUR experience. You needn't write pages and pages each day; just jot down a paragraph or two, several times a week, about your thoughts, feelings, and behaviors. The more aware you are of how you're doing, the more likely you are to stay on track.

4. STEP OUTSIDE FOR AT LEAST 10 MINUTES A DAY

As you learned in Chapter 5, your body makes vitamin D when your skin absorbs the sun's ultraviolet B (UVB) rays. It doesn't take much sunlight to do the trick—just 10 to 15 minutes twice a week of direct exposure to your face, hands, arms, or back.

In most areas of the United States, however, the sun is not strong enough from November through February for the body to make its own vitamin D. Wearing sunscreen will prevent this process, as well. So for most of the year, you need to depend on foods and supplements for adequate amounts of this vitamin.

But don't stretch 10 minutes to an hour: Long-term, unprotected exposure to sunlight is a risk factor for skin cancer. When you're going to be outdoors for more than 10 to 15 minutes at a time, follow the American Cancer Society's "Slip, Slap, Slop" rule: Slip on a shirt, slap on a hat, and slop on the sunscreen. Do this even on cool or cloudy days.

FYI

THE RESEARCH IS CLEAR: Those who lose weight and keep it off have people around them for support and encouragement. Your cheering section might include your family or colleagues, a personal trainer or workout buddy, or even an online weight-loss community.

4 WAYS TO PUSH PAST A PLATEAU

It happens to almost everyone who's trying to lose weight: The number on the scale steadily declines, then suddenly gets stuck for no apparent reason. It's frustrating and discouraging, for sure—but it's no reason to give up. To help troubleshoot your efforts, consider these four reasons that you may have stopped losing weight. Then try the accompanying strategies to get back on track.

You're not eating enough. Flush with success on DTOUR, did you cut your calories even more to lose weight even faster? Not a good idea. Your body needs a minimum number of calories every day to carry out its normal biological functions and to maintain its muscle mass. If your calorie intake falls below this threshold, your body kicks into survival mode, slowing its metabolism to a snail's pace in an effort to conserve fuel. So bump up your calories to the recommended 1,400 to 1,600 a day. Just like that, the scale should start moving again.

You're eating more than you think. Are you filching chocolate kisses from

IN CASE OF BINGE, BREAK GLASS: 5 WAYS TO STOP OVEREATING COLD

To keep off the weight you've lost, you need to anticipate hunger-induced overeating traps and have a plan in place to neutralize each one. Here's what to do.

Problem: There's no time in the morning for breakfast, so you grab a muffin or doughnut.

Solution: Zap a packet of oatmeal (such as Quaker's High Fiber Instant Oatmeal). Splash with fat-free milk. Take bites between showering, dressing, and packing your briefcase. Crunch an apple on your way to work.

Problem: It's late afternoon, you're crashing, and the office vending machine is calling your name.

Solution: Stash single-serving packages of unsalted almonds in your desk. Plan to munch a few hours after lunch, when your hunger is still in control.

Problem: You've planned a late dinner

with friends, but it's only 5 o'clock and you're already starved.

Solution: Eat a 150- to 200-calorie snack, such as a light yogurt or celery with 2 tablespoons of peanut butter, about 2 hours before your dinner date.

Problem: You underestimated how long your errands would take; now you're ready for lunch but stuck in traffic.

Solution: Dig into your glove compartment for the high-fiber, protein-packed bar you keep there for just such emergencies. When you reach your destination, eat a lighter-than-normal lunch to compensate for the extra calories.

Problem: It's past your normal bedtime and your stomach is growling.

Solution: Grab a fiber-filled apple or pear instead of diving into the cookie jar. Or have a cup of warm, fat-free milk jazzed up with a drop of vanilla and a dash of cinnamon to help you sleep.

the jar on your co-worker's desk or polishing off the leftover french fries from your child's or grandchild's Happy Meal? If so, you may be taking in more calories over the course of a day than you realize. This is when keeping a food diary of some kind can come in handy: You can spot those situations where you're prone to nibble. True, a few extra calories here and there won't hurt, but they can add up over time.

You're easing up on exercise. Slowing up on your Cardio Walks? Skipping your Metabo Moves sessions? That may be why the scale has become stuck. Metabolism slows with age, especially after 35; if you're not exercising regularly, you may have a harder time getting to your goal weight. The DTOUR Workout provides a fat-melting mix of heart-pumping aerobic activity and muscle-building strength training—but if it's not for you, feel free to do something else. As long as you're moving at a moderate intensity, you're burning calories.

You're stuck in a workout rut. As you lose weight, your body won't need to work as hard simply because there's less of you to move around. That means you won't burn as many calories during your workouts. Let's say you started out at 180 pounds and you've lost 35. You'll burn about 100 fewer calories in an hour-long Calorie-Scorch Walk.

To continue to lose weight, you need to challenge your body in new ways. Ask your doctor if you're healthy enough to walk longer, harder, or more often. Even replacing one activity with another can help. The trick is to keep your body guessing so it's forced to adapt.

So, what if you try these strategies but still can't unstick a stubborn scale? Just stay true to the DTOUR Diet, be patient—and be philosophical. This plateau, too, shall pass.

PART 6

THE AWESOME 4SOME RECIPES

HUNGRY FOR MORE DTOUR? Just turn the
page! You'll find more than 60 fabulous meals
and snacks tailor-made for the Diabetes DTOUR
Diet. We call them Awesome 4some recipes
because they contribute to your daily quotas of
the Fat-Fighting 4. Each dish follows our sensible, dietitian-recommended guidelines for

calories, carbohydrates, and total and saturated fats. And, of course, they taste fabulous. (We know because we tested every one!)

Feel free to swap an Awesome 4some recipe for a meal or snack in the 4-Week Total Transformation. (We do recommend sticking with the menus in the 2-Week Fast Start as you get accustomed to eating DTOUR-style.) Most of the recipes require a bit more prep time than your other menu options, though they're by no means complicated. They're perfect if you love to cook, or you have a special occasion that requires a special dish, or you just want to treat your taste buds to something different.

We've organized this mini-cookbook by recipe category: breakfast, salads, soups and sandwiches, dinner, and snacks. But if you'd rather have the Chicken and Cheese Panini for breakfast or the Breakfast Taco Skillet for dinner, there's no reason you can't. So be adventurous! Our only caveat is that you stick with the snacks for your appointed snack times, as their calorie and nutritional values have been adjusted accordingly.

For a handful of recipes, we recommend pairing the finished dish with a glass of milk. That way, you'll boost your daily intake of calcium and vitamin D. (As you'll remember, it's challenging to get enough vitamin D from foods alone, which is why we also recommend a multivitamin or a single D supplement.)

As you'll see, we've flagged recipes that are higher in sodium. If you're watching your sodium intake, you may want to choose these dishes only on occasion. When you do eat them, be sure to watch your sodium consumption at the rest of your meals that day. Even if sodium isn't an issue for you, we recommend limiting your intake to 2,300 milligrams a day.

Remember to keep track of your meals and snacks in the journal pages for the 4-Week Total Transformation, beginning on page 000. You'll also find the Awesome 4some recipes online at www.dtour.com.

Enjoy!

RECIPES

Cream of Wheat with Maple Walnuts and Cranberries

PREP TIME: 5 MINUTES ◆ TOTAL TIME: 8 MINUTES

½ cup fat-free evaporated milk
2 tablespoons whole grain cream
   of wheat cereal or Wheatena
1 tablespoon ground flaxseed
½ teaspoon vanilla extract

1 tablespoon chopped walnuts
1 teaspoon maple syrup
1 tablespoon dried cranberries

FAT-FIGHTING 4

5 g fiber
- - - - - - - - -
388 mg
calcium
- - - - - - - - -
102 IU
vitamin D
- - - - - - - - -
700 mg
omega-3s
- - - - - - - - -

1 Combine the milk and cream of wheat or Wheatena in a 4-cup microwaveable bowl or mixing cup. Whisk with a fork. Microwave on high power for 2 minutes. Whisk again. Microwave in 30-second intervals, whisking after each interval, for about 60 seconds, or until thickened. Stir in the flaxseed and vanilla extract. Spoon into a cereal bowl. Set aside.

2 Coat a small microwaveable plate with cooking spray. Spread the walnuts on the plate. Drizzle them with syrup. Microwave on high power for about 45 seconds, or until sizzling. Using a spatula, scatter the glazed walnuts over the cereal mixture. Top with the cranberries.

PER SERVING: 300 calories, 15 g protein, 42 g carbohydrates, 9 g fat (1 g saturated fat), 5 mg cholesterol, 150 mg sodium

Makes 1 serving

Coconut Rice Pudding with Raspberries

PREP TIME: 5 MINUTES ◆ TOTAL TIME: 18 MINUTES

¼ cup instant brown rice
   (such as Uncle Ben's)
¾ cup water
2 tablespoons nonfat dry milk
1 teaspoon honey

⅛ teaspoon coconut extract
½ cup fresh or loose-pack frozen
   and thawed raspberries

1 Combine the rice and water in a microwaveable mixing bowl or 8-cup glass measuring cup. Stir. Cover with plastic wrap, leaving a small vent for steam to escape. Microwave on high power for 5 minutes. Reduce the power to medium and cook for 3 minutes longer.

2 Remove from the microwave and allow to sit for 5 minutes so the rice softens. Carefully remove the plastic. Stir in the dry milk, honey, and coconut extract. Gently fold in the raspberries. Spoon into a cereal bowl.

PER SERVING: 170 calories, 6 g protein, 35 g carbohydrates, 1 g fat (0 g saturated fat), 0 mg cholesterol, 60 mg sodium

Makes 1 serving

FAT-FIGHTING
4

5 g fiber
----
135 mg calcium

0.5 IU vitamin D
----
80 mg omega-3s

Peanut–Oats Breakfast Pudding

PREP TIME: 5 MINUTES ◆ TOTAL TIME: 13 MINUTES

¼ cup nonfat dry milk
1½ tablespoons omega-3-enriched
peanut butter
½ cup water

¼ cup rolled oats
1 tablespoon fat-free plain yogurt
1 teaspoon finely chopped peanuts

FAT-
FIGHTING
4

4 g fiber
----
266 mg
calcium
----
6 IU
vitamin D
----
750 mg
omega-3s
----

1 Whisk 2 tablespoons of the dry milk with the peanut butter in a 4-cup microwaveable bowl or mixing cup until creamy. While whisking, gradually add the water and the remaining dry milk and whisk until the mixture is smooth. Stir in the oats.

2 Cover with plastic wrap, leaving a small vent for steam to escape. Microwave on high power for 1 minute. Reduce the power to medium and cook for about 90 seconds or until creamy. Remove and allow to sit for 5 minutes.

3 Spoon the mixture into a cereal bowl. Top with the yogurt and peanuts.

PER SERVING: 318 calories, 16 g protein, 30 g carbohydrates, 16 g fat (2 g saturated fat), 3 mg cholesterol, 190 mg sodium

Makes 1 serving

Open-Faced Broiled Egg, Spinach, and Tomato Sandwich

PREP TIME: 10 MINUTES ◆ TOTAL TIME: 2 MINUTES

½ whole wheat English muffin
¼ cup fresh spinach, cooked and
squeezed dry (about 4 ounces)
1 slice tomato
1 hard-boiled egg, sliced widthwise

1 tablespoon omega-3-enriched
mayonnaise
Salt-free seasoning blend (such as
Mrs. Dash)

FAT-FIGHTING 4

1 Set the muffin half on a toaster oven pan or double sheet of foil. Top with the spinach and tomato. Lay on the egg slices in an overlapping spiral. Dollop on the mayonnaise and swirl slightly to partially cover the egg slices. Sprinkle on seasoning to taste.

2 Place under the broiler for 2 to 3 minutes, watching carefully, until the mayonnaise is lightly browned.

PER SERVING: 210 calories, 11 g protein, 20 g carbohydrates, 10 g fat (1 g saturated fat), 185 mg cholesterol, 398 mg sodium

Makes 1 serving

4 g fiber

----

188 mg
calcium

----

18 IU
vitamin D

----

790 mg
omega-3s

Herb Breakfast Scramble

PREP TIME: 12 MINUTES ◆ TOTAL TIME: 22 MINUTES

2 tablespoons canola oil
1 small red onion, finely chopped
1 container (14 ounces) soft tofu
    packed in calcium sulfate,
    drained
¼ teaspoon salt

⅛ teaspoon pepper
⅛ teaspoon turmeric
1 cup shredded reduced-fat
    Cheddar cheese
2 tablespoons chopped fresh basil
1 tablespoon chopped fresh thyme

FAT-
FIGHTING
4

3 g fiber
----
604 mg
calcium
----
100 IU
vitamin D
----
260 mg
omega-3s
----

1 Heat the oil in a large skillet over medium heat. Cook the onion for 5 minutes or until tender. Crumble the tofu into the pan. Sprinkle with the salt, pepper, and turmeric. Cook for 5 minutes, stirring frequently, until firm and lightly browned.

2 Remove from the heat. Add the cheese, basil, and thyme and stir until the cheese melts.

3 Serve with 1 slice of whole grain toast and a glass of fat-free milk.

PER SERVING: 387 calories, 27 g protein, 30 g carbohydrates, 18 g fat (5 g saturated fat), 23 mg cholesterol, 673 mg sodium*

∗ Limit saturated fat to 10 percent of total calories—about 17 grams per day for most women—and sodium intake to less than 2,300 milligrams.

NOTE: This dish works well as leftovers. Simply refrigerate in an airtight container and reheat in the microwave on medium power for 45 seconds. Don't overcook.

Makes 4 servings

Chinese Egg Pancakes

PREP TIME: 15 MINUTES ◆ TOTAL TIME: 35 MINUTES

2 cups thinly sliced brussels sprouts (about 8 ounces)
³/₄ cup thinly sliced scallions (10-12 thin)
³/₄ cup shredded carrots
¹/₄ teaspoon salt

4 omega-3-enriched eggs
2 omega-3-enriched egg whites
1 tablespoon grated fresh ginger
2 tablespoons water
6 teaspoons ground flaxseed

1 Coat a large nonstick skillet with cooking spray. Add the brussels sprouts, scallions, carrots, and salt. Toss to mix. Cover and cook over medium heat, tossing occasionally, for 7 to 10 minutes or until the vegetables are wilted and lightly browned. Reduce the heat slightly if the vegetables are browning too fast.

2 Meanwhile, beat the eggs, egg whites, ginger, and water with a fork in a mixing bowl.

3 Heat a 9" nonstick omelet pan over medium-high heat. Turn the heat off and coat the surface with cooking spray. Turn the heat back on, to medium. Ladle one-quarter of the egg mixture (5 tablespoonfuls) into the pan. Cook for 20 to 30 seconds or until the edges start to set. Using a silicone spatula, carefully lift the edges, tipping the pan to allow runny mixture to get underneath. When the eggs are almost set and just shimmering on top, about 1 minute, sprinkle on 1¹/₂ teaspoons flaxseed and ¹/₂ cup of the reserved vegetable mixture. Cook for about 30 seconds or until the eggs are completely set. Slide the pancake onto a dinner plate or roll the pancake like a jelly roll before sliding onto the plate.

4 Repeat for the remaining 3 pancakes.

PER SERVING: 140 calories, 11 g protein, 11 g carbohydrates, 6 g fat (1 g saturated fat), 180 mg cholesterol, 273 mg sodium

NOTE: To prepare 1 large pancake instead of 4 individual ones, after the vegetables are wilted in Step 1, remove them to a plate. Wipe the skillet with a paper towel. Continue with the recipe, using the large skillet instead of the 9" omelet pan and adding all the ingredients at once. Cooking time will increase slightly. To serve, cut into 4 wedges or slide the whole pancake onto a work surface, roll like a jelly roll, and cut into 4 spirals.

Makes 4 servings

FAT-FIGHTING **4**

4 g fiber
----
69 mg calcium
----
18 IU vitamin D
----
150 mg omega-3s

Breakfast Taco Skillet

PREP TIME: 10 MINUTES ◆ TOTAL TIME: 20 MINUTES

5 soft corn tortillas (6" diameter)
6 scallions, chopped
1 red bell pepper, chopped
1 small jalapeño chile pepper, seeded and finely chopped (optional), wear plastic gloves when handling
1 clove garlic, minced
1 teaspoon ground cumin
1 can (15 ounces) reduced-sodium black beans, rinsed and drained

4 cups baby spinach (about 4 ounces)
1 large tomato, chopped
1 cup shredded reduced-fat Cheddar cheese
4 tablespoons reduced-fat sour cream
Sprigs fresh cilantro

FAT-FIGHTING 4

8 g fiber
----
206 mg calcium
----
0 IU vitamin D
----
60 mg omega-3s
----

1 Preheat the oven to 350°F. Stack the tortillas on a large piece of foil, sprinkle the top one with water, and wrap in the foil. Heat for 10 minutes.

2 Meanwhile, heat a large nonstick skillet coated with olive oil cooking spray over medium-high heat. Add the scallions and bell pepper and cook for 5 minutes or until lightly browned. Add the jalapeño chile pepper (if using), garlic, and cumin. Cook for 2 minutes or until lightly browned. Stir in the beans, spinach, and tomato. Cook for 2 minutes or until heated through. Spread the mixture evenly in the skillet.

3 Remove from the heat and sprinkle with the cheese. Let stand until melted. Top with dollops of the sour cream and sprinkle with the cilantro.

4 Cut the warmed tortillas into quarters or strips. Serve immediately with the taco skillet.

PER SERVING: 236 calories, 13 g protein, 37 g carbohydrates, 5 g fat (2 g saturated fat), 12 mg cholesterol, 428 mg sodium

NOTE: It's important to heat the tortillas properly, or they will fall apart. Follow the steps given above to keep them soft.

Makes 4 servings

Peanut Butter and "Jelly" Pancake

PREP TIME: 5 MINUTES ◆ TOTAL TIME: 2 MINUTES

**1 frozen Whole Wheat Pancake
  (page 298)**
1 teaspoon honey
¼ teaspoon cornstarch

**¼ cup fresh or loose-pack frozen
  and thawed blueberries**
**2 tablespoons omega-3-enriched
  peanut butter**

1 Heat the pancake in a toaster oven to desired crispness.

2 Meanwhile, combine the honey and cornstarch in a small microwave-able bowl, and stir until smooth. Add the blueberries and stir. Microwave on high power for about 90 seconds or until bubbling and thickened.

3 Spread the peanut butter on the pancake. Top with the blueberry mixture.

PER SERVING: 325 calories, 10 g protein, 26 g carbohydrates, 20 g fat (3 g saturated fat), 16 mg cholesterol, 307 mg sodium

NOTE: If you don't have a homemade pancake, a store-bought frozen pancake works fine.

Makes 1 serving

FAT-FIGHTING 4

4 g fiber
----
27 mg calcium
----
0 IU vitamin D

1,220 mg omega-3s

Whole Wheat Pancakes

PREP TIME: 10 MINUTES ◆ TOTAL TIME: 14 MINUTES

1 cup white whole wheat flour
(such as King Arthur) or whole
wheat pastry flour
6 tablespoons buttermilk powder
(such as SACO)
¼ cup ground flaxseed
1 teaspoon baking powder

1 teaspoon baking soda
½ teaspoon ground cinnamon
Pinch of salt
1 omega-3-enriched egg
1½ cups water
2 tablespoons canola oil

FAT-
FIGHTING
4

1 g fiber
----
26 mg
calcium
----
0 IU
vitamin D
----
210 mg
omega-3s
----

1 Combine the flour, buttermilk powder, flaxseed, baking powder, baking soda, cinnamon, and salt in a mixing bowl. Stir to mix in another mixing bowl. Beat the egg with a fork or whisk. Whisk in the water and oil. Add the flour mixture. Whisk just until combined. Do not beat. Allow to sit for 5 minutes.

2 Heat a griddle over medium-high heat. Turn off the heat and coat the griddle with cooking spray. Turn the heat back on to medium-high. Ladle ¼ cup of the batter onto the griddle to make each pancake. Cook for 1 to 2 minutes or until the bottoms are browned and bubbles form on the top, adjusting the heat as needed.

Flip and cook for about 2 minutes or until cooked through. Reduce the heat if the bottoms are browning too fast. Repeat until all the pancakes are cooked. Serve right away or place on a rack to cool for freezing.

PER PANCAKE: 80 calories, 3 g protein, 10 g carbohydrates, 4 g fat (0 g saturated fat), 20 mg cholesterol, 200 mg sodium

NOTE: To freeze the pancakes, place each pancake between squares of waxed paper. Store in a resealable plastic freezer bag or plastic freezer container for up to 3 months.

Makes 12 (4½" diameter;
about 2 ounces each)

Lemon-Blueberry Scones

PREP TIME: 20 MINUTES ◆ TOTAL TIME: 32 MINUTES

1¼ cups whole grain pastry flour
1 cup ground whole oats
½ cup nonfat dry milk
2 tablespoons ground flaxseed
2 teaspoons baking powder
½ teaspoon baking soda
½ teaspoon salt

1 cup low-fat plain yogurt
¼ cup honey
2 tablespoons canola oil
2 tablespoons lemon juice
1 teaspoon lemon zest
1 cup blueberries

1 Preheat the oven to 400°F. Lightly coat a baking sheet with cooking spray.

2 Whisk together the flour, oats, dry milk, flaxseed, baking powder, baking soda, and salt in a large bowl.

3 Stir together the yogurt, honey, oil, lemon juice, and lemon zest in a measuring cup.

4 Make a well in the center of the flour mixture and stir in the yogurt mixture. Add the blueberries and stir just until blended.

5 Drop the batter onto the prepared baking sheet using a large (¼ cup) ice cream scoop to make 10 scones. Bake for 12 to 15 minutes or until lightly browned and firm. Serve with a glass of fat-free milk.

PER SERVING: 260 calories, 15 g protein, 40 g carbohydrates, 5 g fat (0 g saturated fat), 5 mg cholesterol, 420 mg sodium

Makes 10

FAT-FIGHTING 4

3 g fiber
----
402 mg calcium
----
100 IU vitamin D
----
260 mg omega-3s

Ginger-Mango Smoothie

PREP TIME: 10 MINUTES

1 cup low-fat vanilla yogurt
1 cup peeled and chopped mango
   (about ½)
4 ounces soft tofu
2 tablespoons ground flaxseed

1 teaspoon finely chopped
   crystallized ginger
1 teaspoon flaxseed oil
Pinch of cardamom

FAT-FIGHTING 4

3 g fiber
----
282 mg
calcium
----
0 IU
vitamin D

1,380 mg
omega-3s

Combine the yogurt, mango, tofu,
flaxseed, ginger, oil, and cardamom
in a blender. Puree until smooth.

PER SERVING: 239 calories,
12 g protein, 30 g carbohydrates,
9 g fat (2 g saturated fat), 6 mg
cholesterol, 87 mg sodium

Makes 2 servings

Roasted Pepper Pasta Salad

PREP TIME: 20 MINUTES

**7 ounces (about ¹/₂ box) multigrain
    pasta**
**2 jarred roasted red peppers,
    drained and patted dry**
1 clove garlic, halved
1 tablespoon flaxseed oil

1 tablespoon balsamic vinegar
¹/₂ cup low-fat plain yogurt
¹/₄ cup fresh basil leaves
4 cups baby arugula
**2 ounces Parmesan cheese,
    shaved**

1 Prepare the pasta according to package directions. Rinse with cold water and drain.

2 Meanwhile, puree the peppers, garlic, oil, and vinegar in a blender until smooth. Add the yogurt and pulse until blended. Place in a large bowl. Cut the basil into thin strips. Add the pasta and basil to the yogurt mixture, tossing to coat.

3 Arrange the arugula on 4 salad plates. Top each plate with one-quarter of the pasta mixture. Top each with one-quarter of the cheese.

PER SERVING: 303 calories, 17 g protein, 39 g carbohydrates, 9 g fat (3 g saturated fat), 12 mg cholesterol, 323 mg sodium

Makes 4 servings (4 cups)

FAT-
FIGHTING
4

4 g fiber
- - - - - - - - -
273 mg
calcium
- - - - - - - - -
0 IU
vitamin D
- - - - - - - - -
1,900 mg
omega-3s
- - - - - - - - -

Warm Lentil Salad with Roasted Asparagus and Goat Cheese

PREP TIME: 20 MINUTES ◆ TOTAL TIME: 45 MINUTES

³/₄ cup green lentils
1 small red onion, chopped
1 carrot, chopped
1 rib celery, chopped
1 pound asparagus, trimmed
2 tablespoons balsamic vinegar
1 teaspoon honey

¹/₂ teaspoon Dijon mustard
1 tablespoon extra-virgin olive oil
1 tablespoon flaxseed oil
1 large bunch frisée
4 ounces reduced-fat goat cheese, crumbled

FAT-FIGHTING 4

13 g fiber
----
167 mg calcium
----
0 IU vitamin D

1,870 mg omega-3s
----

1 Preheat the oven to 450°F.

2 Bring 2 cups of water to a boil in a medium saucepan over high heat. Add the lentils, onion, carrot, and celery. Reduce the heat to low, cover, and simmer for 15 to 20 minutes or until the lentils are tender. Drain.

3 Meanwhile, place the asparagus on a baking sheet and coat it on all sides with cooking spray. Tilt the sheet to roll the asparagus to coat it underneath. Roast for 10 to 15 minutes or until tender-crisp and browned. (Time varies depending on the thickness of the asparagus.)

4 Whisk together the vinegar, honey, and mustard in a medium bowl. Whisk in the olive oil and flaxseed oil. Stir in the lentil mixture, tossing to coat.

5 Arrange the frisée on 4 plates. Mound one-quarter of the lentil mixture in the center of each plate. Arrange the asparagus on or around the lentil mixture. Sprinkle each plate with one-quarter of the cheese.

PER SERVING: 290 calories, 16 g protein, 37 g carbohydrates, 11 g fat (3 g saturated fat), 5 mg cholesterol, 170 mg sodium

Makes 4 servings

Moroccan Bean and Couscous Salad on Greens

PREP TIME: 15 MINUTES ◆ TOTAL TIME: 27 MINUTES

1 cup Israeli couscous

2 tablespoons lime juice

1 tablespoon extra-virgin olive oil

1 tablespoon flaxseed oil

1/4 teaspoon salt

1/4 teaspoon ground cumin

1/4 teaspoon ground coriander

1/8 teaspoon smoked paprika

1 can (15 1/2 ounces) chickpeas, rinsed and drained

2 carrots, sliced diagonally

1 red bell pepper, chopped

4 cups baby romaine lettuce

1 Bring 4 cups of water to a boil in a medium saucepan over high heat. Add the couscous and reduce the heat to low. Cover and simmer for 8 to 10 minutes or until tender, stirring occasionally. Drain and rinse under cold water.

2 Meanwhile, whisk together the lime juice, olive oil, flaxseed oil, salt, cumin, coriander, and paprika in a large bowl. Add the couscous, chickpeas, carrots, and pepper. Toss to coat.

3 Line each of 4 salad plates with 1 cup lettuce. Top each with one-quarter of the salad.

PER SERVING: 280 calories, 9 g protein, 45 g carbohydrates, 8 g fat (1 g saturated fat), 0 mg cholesterol, 260 mg sodium

Makes 4 servings

FAT-FIGHTING 4

7 g fiber

- - - - - - - - -

56 mg calcium

- - - - - - - - -

0 IU vitamin D

- - - - - - - - -

1,890 mg omega-3s

- - - - - - - - -

Asian Slaw with Salmon

PREP TIME: 25 MINUTES ◆ TOTAL TIME: 30 MINUTES

1½ tablespoons rice wine vinegar
2 teaspoons sesame oil
1½ teaspoons reduced-sodium
    soy sauce
¼ teaspoon ground ginger
3 cups shredded Napa cabbage
1 carrot, shredded (about 1 cup)
1 red bell pepper, cut into thin
    strips

1 pouch or can (6–7 ounces)
    wild pink boneless, skinless
    salmon, drained
1 egg white, beaten
½ cup panko
¼ cup fat-free plain yogurt
2 scallions, minced
1 tablespoon lime juice
½–1 teaspoon wasabi paste

FAT-FIGHTING 4

5 g fiber
----
397 mg calcium
----
0 IU vitamin D

1,970 mg omega-3s
----

1 Whisk together the vinegar, oil, soy sauce, and ginger in a medium bowl. Stir in the cabbage, carrot, and pepper, tossing to coat. Set aside.

2 Mash the salmon with a fork in a medium bowl. Add the egg white, panko, yogurt, scallions, lime juice, and wasabi paste. Stir to blend. Shape into 2 burgers.

3 Coat a nonstick skillet with cooking spray. Cook the burgers over medium heat, turning once, until browned and crisp, about 6 minutes.

4 Divide the slaw between 2 plates. Top each with a salmon burger.

PER SERVING: 350 calories, 30 g protein, 29 g carbohydrates, 12 g fat (2 g saturated fat), 65 mg cholesterol, 480 mg sodium

Makes 2 servings

Greek Shrimp Salad

PREP TIME: 20 MINUTES ◆ TOTAL TIME: 40 MINUTES

1 medium russet potato, cut
   into 1" cubes
2 teaspoons finely chopped fresh
   oregano or $\frac{1}{2}$ teaspoon dried
6 teaspoons lemon juice
2 tablespoons olive oil
$\frac{1}{2}$ teaspoon flaxseed oil
1 small clove garlic, minced

$\frac{1}{2}$ pound cooked, peeled, and
   deveined large shrimp
$\frac{1}{2}$ small English cucumber, halved
   lengthwise and sliced
1 cup cherry tomatoes, halved
$\frac{1}{2}$ small red onion, sliced
3 cups shredded romaine lettuce

FAT-
FIGHTING
4

4 g fiber
- - - - - - - - -
106 mg
calcium
- - - - - - - - -
0 IU
vitamin D
- - - - - - - - -
1,170 mg
omega-3s
- - - - - - - - -

1 Preheat the oven to 425°F.

2 Place the potato on a baking sheet with sides. Sprinkle with 1 teaspoon of the fresh oregano (or $\frac{1}{4}$ teaspoon of the dried) and 1 teaspoon of the lemon juice and coat with canola cooking spray; toss to coat. Roast for 15 to 20 minutes, turning once, or until tender.

3 Meanwhile, whisk together the olive oil, flaxseed oil, garlic, the remaining 1 teaspoon fresh oregano (or $\frac{1}{4}$ teaspoon dried), and the remaining 5 teaspoons lemon juice in a medium bowl. Pour half of the dressing into another bowl.

4 Add the shrimp to the dressing in one bowl. Add the cucumber, tomatoes, and onion to the dressing in the other bowl. Toss to coat. Let stand for about 10 minutes.

5 Divide the lettuce between 2 plates. Divide and arrange the shrimp, vegetable mixture, and potatoes in separate piles on the lettuce.

PER SERVING: 340 calories, 28 g protein, 23 g carbohydrates, 16 g fat (3 g saturated fat), 220 mg cholesterol, 270 mg sodium

Makes 2 servings

Tuna Salad on Bed of Greens

PREP TIME: 15 MINUTES ◆ TOTAL TIME: 20 MINUTES

2 slices whole grain bread, cut into 1" cubes
¼ cup low-fat plain yogurt
1 tablespoon omega-3-enriched mayonnaise
1 tablespoon lemon juice
¼ teaspoon lemon zest
1 can (6 ounces) low-sodium water-packed white tuna, drained

¼ small red onion, finely chopped
2 tablespoons chopped parsley leaves
2 teaspoons capers, rinsed, drained, and chopped
3 cups mesclun or spring mix
1 large carrot, peeled into long strips
1 tomato, halved lengthwise and sliced

FAT-FIGHTING 4

5 g fiber
- - - - - - - - -
154 mg calcium
- - - - - - - - -
0 IU vitamin D
- - - - - - - - -
270 mg omega-3s
- - - - - - - - -

1 Preheat the oven to 400°F. Place the bread on a baking sheet with sides and coat with canola cooking spray. Toss to coat all sides of the cubes. Bake for 5 minutes or until toasted, tossing once to toast all sides. Set aside.

2 Stir together the yogurt, mayonnaise, lemon juice, and lemon zest in a large bowl. Add the tuna, onion, parsley, and capers.

3 Divide the mesclun, carrot, and tomato between 2 plates. Top with the tuna mixture. Sprinkle with the croutons.

PER SERVING: 302 calories, 31 g protein, 23 g carbohydrates, 10 g fat (2 g saturated fat), 49 mg cholesterol, 398 mg sodium

NOTE: To add more flavor to the croutons, sprinkle them with a pinch of a spice such as smoked paprika, ground cumin, or freshly ground nutmeg after coating with the cooking spray. Or opt for chopped fresh herbs, such as basil, thyme, savory, or parsley.

Makes 2 servings

Chicken Salad with Thai Peanut Dressing

PREP TIME: 20 MINUTES

4 cups baby spinach (4 ounces)

12 ounces cooked boneless, skinless chicken breast, thinly sliced

1½ cups frozen baby peas, thawed, rinsed, and drained

½ cup shredded carrot (about 1 medium)

½ cup sliced scallions, all parts (about 4 medium)

2 tablespoons omega-3-enriched peanut butter

1 tablespoon flaxseed oil

1 teaspoon toasted sesame oil

2 teaspoons reduced-sodium soy sauce

1 teaspoon honey

¼ cup warm water

1 clove garlic, crushed

½ teaspoon grated fresh ginger

Leaves fresh cilantro (optional)

FAT-FIGHTING 4

5 g fiber
----
41 mg calcium
----
0 IU vitamin D

2,100 mg omega-3s
----

1 Divide the spinach among 4 dinner plates. Fan the chicken slices over the spinach. Scatter on the peas, carrot, and scallions.

2 Whisk the peanut butter, flaxseed oil, sesame oil, soy sauce, and honey in a small bowl until smooth. Gradually add the water, whisking until smooth. Stir in the garlic and ginger. Drizzle over the salads. Garnish with cilantro if using.

PER SERVING: 243 calories, 22 g protein, 14 g carbohydrates, 11 g fat (2 g saturated fat), 47 mg cholesterol, 293 mg sodium

Makes 4 servings

Warm Barbecued Turkey and Beans

PREP TIME: 15 MINUTES ◆ TOTAL TIME: 28 MINUTES

1 teaspoon canola oil
$\frac{1}{2}$ cup finely chopped onion (1 medium)
$\frac{3}{4}$ cup no-salt-added plain tomato sauce
$\frac{1}{4}$ cup molasses
$\frac{1}{2}$ teaspoon hot-pepper sauce

$\frac{1}{4}$ teaspoon mustard powder
$\frac{1}{16}$ teaspoon ground cloves
8 ounces cooked boneless, skinless turkey breast, cut into 1" cubes
1 cup no-salt-added canned navy beans, rinsed and drained
4 cups cooked spinach

FAT-FIGHTING
4

8 g fiber
----
496 mg calcium
----
100 IU vitamin D
----
230 mg omega-3s
----

1 Heat a saucepan over medium heat. Add the oil and onion. Cook, stirring, for about 3 minutes or until the onion starts to soften. Add the tomato sauce, molasses, pepper sauce, mustard, and cloves. Stir. Reduce heat and simmer for 5 minutes.

2 Add the turkey and beans to the saucepan. Simmer gently for 5 minutes.

3 Divide the mixture among 4 dinner plates. Serve over the cooked spinach and have a glass of fat-free milk.

PER SERVING: 343 calories, 33 g protein, 49 g carbohydrates, 2.5 g fat (0.5 g saturated fat), 45 mg cholesterol, 579 mg sodium

Makes 4 servings

French Onion Soup

PREP TIME: 15 MINUTES ◆ TOTAL TIME: 40 MINUTES

2 tablespoons canola oil
5 cups sliced onions
   (about 1¼ pounds)
1 teaspoon dried thyme
2 bay leaves
⅛ teaspoon salt
½ cup dry white wine or
   reduced-sodium vegetable
   broth

4 cups reduced-sodium
   vegetable broth
2 cups water
2 slices (1½ ounces each) whole
   wheat bread, toasted and halved
4 teaspoons ground flaxseed
6 slices reduced-fat Swiss cheese,
   halved
Freshly ground black pepper

1 Preheat the broiler. Heat a pot over medium-high heat. Add the oil and heat for 1 minute. Add the onions, thyme, bay leaves, and salt. Stir. Cover and cook, stirring frequently, for about 15 minutes or until the onions are uniformly browned and softened. Reduce the heat if needed to keep the onions from browning too fast.

2 Add the wine or ½ cup broth and turn the heat to high. Cook at a brisk simmer for 3 minutes, or until the wine evaporates. Add the broth and the water. Bring almost to a boil, then reduce the heat to a simmer. Simmer for 5 minutes. Remove and discard the bay leaves.

3 Place a half slice of toast in the bottom of each of 4 wide, heatproof bowls. Sprinkle 1 teaspoon flaxseed over each toast half. Ladle in the soup. Top each bowlful with 3 half slices of cheese.

4 Broil 6 inches from the heat source for 1 minute or until the cheese is bubbly and light golden brown. Watch very carefully so the cheese does not burn. Season to taste with pepper.

PER SERVING: 315 calories, 13 g protein, 28 g carbohydrates, 15 g fat (5 g saturated fat), 20 mg cholesterol, 359 mg sodium

Makes 4 servings (8 cups)

FAT-
FIGHTING
4

5 g fiber
- - - - - - - - -
330 mg
calcium
- - - - - - - - -
0 IU
vitamin D
- - - - - - - - -
650 mg
omega-3s
- - - - - - - - -

Creole Pea and Pepper Soup

PREP TIME: 20 MINUTES ◆ TOTAL TIME: 1 HOUR 15 MINUTES

FAT-FIGHTING 4

2 g fiber
- - - - - - - - -
65 mg calcium
- - - - - - - - -
0 IU vitamin D
- - - - - - - - -
330 mg omega-3s
- - - - - - - - -

1 tablespoon canola oil
½ cup chopped celery (1 stalk)
½ cup chopped onion (1 small)
½ cup chopped red bell pepper (1 small)
2 teaspoons Creole seasoning
3 large cloves garlic

1 cup dried green split peas
4 cups reduced-sodium vegetable broth
2 cups water
½ cup no-salt-added plain tomato sauce
4 tablespoons fat-free sour cream

1 Heat a pot over medium heat. Add the oil and heat for 1 minute. Add the celery, onion, pepper, Creole seasoning, and garlic. Stir and cover. Cook, stirring occasionally, for 5 minutes, or until the vegetables are slightly softened.

2 Add the peas, broth, water, and tomato sauce. Stir to combine. Bring the mixture almost to a boil. Cover partially and simmer for about 45 minutes, or until the peas are very tender.

3 Transfer 2 cups of the soup (including all 3 cloves of garlic) to a blender or a food processor fitted with a metal blade. Process until smooth. Return the mixture to the pot. Stir. Serve the soup garnished with a dollop of sour cream.

PER SERVING: 270 calories, 15 g protein, 44 g carbohydrates, 4 g fat (0.5 g saturated fat), 0 mg cholesterol, 470 mg sodium

Makes 4 servings (7 cups)

emon-
lueberry
cones
age 299

Open-Faced
Broiled Egg,
Spinach,
and Tomato
Sandwich
page 293

Ginger-
Mango
Smoothie
page 300

Chinese Egg
Pancakes
page 295

Corn Chowder
(left) page 311
Cajun Salmon
Sandwiches
(right) page 315

Chicken and
Cheese Panini
page 319

French Onion
Soup page 309

Warm
Lentil Salad
with Roasted
Asparagus
and Goat Cheese
page 302

Chicken
Roll-Ups
page 334

Grilled
Veggie
Sandwich
page 318

Pasta
Primavera
page 323

Lemon-Pepper
Halibut with
Squash Puree
page 328

Chicken
Salad with
Thai Peanut
Dressing
page 307

Chicken
with Pears
and Blue
Cheese
page 331

Spiced Beef
with Wasabi
Cream
page 339

Wasabi
Salmon Bites
page 342

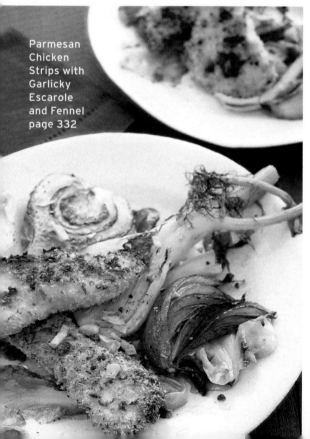

Parmesan
Chicken
Strips with
Garlicky
Escarole
and Fennel
page 332

Pan-Grilled
Mediterranean
Salmon
page 326

Chipotle
Pork
page 336

Orange Frappé
with Strawberries
page 349

Peanut Butter
Chocolate Chip Bars
page 350

"Instant"
Strawberry
Frozen Yogurt
page 348

Butterscotch
Pudding
page 347

Corn Chowder

PREP TIME: 15 MINUTES ◆ TOTAL TIME: 45 MINUTES

1 tablespoon canola oil
1½ cups chopped onions (1 large)
1½ cups chopped green bell
    peppers (2 medium)
2 cups (7 ounces) loose-pack frozen
    corn kernels, drained
2 teaspoons poultry seasoning
½ teaspoon paprika + additional
    for garnish

½ teaspoon salt
¼ cup white whole wheat flour
    (such as King Arthur) or whole
    wheat pastry flour
5 cups fat-free milk
1 tablespoon honey
Freshly ground black pepper

FAT-
FIGHTING
4

5 g fiber
----
344 mg
calcium
----
125 IU
vitamin D
----
350 mg
omega-3s
----

1 Heat a pot over medium heat. Add the oil and heat for 1 minute. Add the onion and bell pepper. Stir and cover. Cook, stirring occasionally, for 5 minutes or until the vegetables are slightly softened.

2 Add the corn, poultry seasoning, ½ teaspoon paprika, and salt. Cook, stirring, for 1 to 2 minutes. Add the flour. Stir to coat the vegetables. Add the milk. Cook, stirring almost constantly, for about 10 to 15 minutes, or until the soup thickens. Simmer for 5 minutes. Stir in the honey. Season to taste with black pepper. Dust lightly with paprika.

PER SERVING: 295 calories, 16 g protein, 52 g carbohydrates, 5 g fat (0.5 g saturated fat), 5 mg cholesterol, 430 mg sodium

Makes 4 servings (6 cups)

Scallop and Broccoli Chowder

PREP TIME: 15 MINUTES ◆ TOTAL TIME: 32 MINUTES

1 can (15$\frac{1}{2}$ ounces) no-salt-added
  cannellini beans, rinsed and
  drained (1$\frac{1}{2}$ cups)
3 large cloves garlic, slivered
1 tablespoon canola oil
$\frac{1}{2}$ cup water
2$\frac{1}{4}$ cups fat-free milk

1 teaspoon dried thyme
2 cups broccoli florets, chopped
12 ounces bay scallops
$\frac{1}{2}$ cup finely chopped red onion
  (1 small) (reserve 2 tablespoons
  for garnish)
Ground white pepper

FAT-
FIGHTING
4

5 g fiber
- - - - - - - - -
214 mg
calcium
- - - - - - - - -
56 IU
vitamin D
- - - - - - - - -
530 mg
omega-3s
- - - - - - - - -

1 Combine the beans, garlic, and oil in a large nonstick saucepan. Cook over medium heat for 3 minutes or until sizzling and fragrant. Add the water. Cover and simmer for 5 minutes, or until the garlic is tender when pierced with a knife.

2 Transfer the mixture to a blender or a food processor fitted with a metal blade. Process for 2 minutes, scraping the sides of the bowl as needed, until smooth. With the machine running, add about half of the milk through the feed tube, processing just until mixed. Return the mixture to the pan.

3 Add the remaining milk and the thyme. Stir to combine. Bring to a simmer. Add the broccoli and continue to simmer for 3 minutes. Add the scallops and all but 2 tablespoons of the onion. Simmer for 3 to 4 minutes or until the scallops are opaque. Ladle into bowls. Garnish with the remaining onion and season with the pepper.

PER SERVING: 243 calories, 24 g protein, 25 g carbohydrates, 5 g fat (0.5 g saturated fat), 30 mg cholesterol, 252 mg sodium

Makes 4 servings (5 cups)

Salmon-Vegetable-Barley Soup

PREP TIME: 10 MINUTES ◆ TOTAL TIME: 30 MINUTES

1 tablespoon canola oil
1 cup chopped carrots (2 medium)
1 cup chopped onions (1 medium)
1 cup green beans, broken
    into ½" lengths
4 cups fat-free, reduced-sodium
    vegetable or chicken broth
2 cups water

1 cup canned reduced-sodium diced
    tomatoes, with juice
¾ cup quick-cooking barley
¼ teaspoon salt
12 ounces cooked salmon fillet,
    skinned
Freshly ground black pepper

FAT-FIGHTING
4

10 g fiber
----
87 mg
calcium
----
0 IU
vitamin D

2,270 mg
omega-3s
----

1 Heat a pot over medium heat. Add the oil and heat for 1 minute. Add the carrots, onions, and green beans. Stir and cover. Cook, stirring occasionally, for 5 minutes, or until the vegetables are slightly softened.

2 Stir in the broth, water, tomatoes with juice, barley, and salt. Bring almost to a boil and then reduce heat. Simmer for 10 minutes, stirring occasionally, until the vegetables and barley are tender.

3 Break the salmon fillet into bite-size pieces.

4 Add the salmon to the pot. Cook for 2 to 3 minutes, just until the salmon is heated. Season generously with pepper.

PER SERVING: 400 calories, 24 g protein, 44 g carbohydrates, 15 g fat (3 g saturated fat), 54 mg cholesterol, 449 mg sodium

Makes 4 servings (8 cups)

Italian Chicken-Artichoke-Rice Soup

PREP TIME: 15 MINUTES ◆ TOTAL TIME: 35 MINUTES

FAT-FIGHTING
4

7 g fiber
----
405 mg calcium
----
100 IU vitamin D
----
380 mg omega-3s
----

1 tablespoon canola oil
1 cup chopped onions (1 medium)
1 teaspoon dried oregano
4 cups fat-free, reduced-sodium vegetable or chicken broth
2 cups water
1 can (14 ounces) no-salt-added diced tomatoes, with juice
6 tablespoons instant brown rice
$1/4$ teaspoon salt

8 ounces ($1^1/_2$ cups) diced cooked boneless, skinless chicken breast
1 package (9 ounces) frozen artichoke hearts, thawed and chopped
$1/4$ cup chopped Italian parsley
Freshly ground black pepper
4 teaspoons grated Parmesan cheese

1 Heat a pot over medium heat. Add the oil and heat for 1 minute. Add the onion and oregano. Stir and cover. Cook, stirring occasionally, for 3 minutes, or until the onion starts to soften.

2 Stir in the broth, water, tomatoes with juice, rice, and salt. Bring almost to a boil and then reduce heat. Simmer for 10 minutes, stirring occasionally, until the rice is tender.

3 Add the chicken and artichokes. Simmer for 3 minutes, just until heated through. Stir in the parsley and season to taste with pepper. Ladle into 4 bowls and sprinkle 1 teaspoon cheese over each. Serve with a glass of fat-free milk.

PER SERVING: 322 calories, 30 g protein, 33 g carbohydrates, 7 g fat (1 g saturated fat), 55 mg cholesterol, 527 mg sodium

Makes 4 servings (10 cups)

Cajun Salmon Sandwiches

PREP TIME: 20 MINUTES ◆ TOTAL TIME: 28 MINUTES

3 tablespoons omega-3-enriched
   mayonnaise
1 teaspoon Cajun seasoning (look
   for a lower-sodium version)
Dash of hot-pepper sauce
1 can (14³/₄ ounces) salmon,
   drained

¹/₂ cup thinly sliced scallions, all
   parts, + 2 teaspoons minced
   scallion greens (about
   5 medium)
¹/₄ cup ground flaxseed
1 omega-3-enriched egg, beaten
4 whole wheat English muffins,
   toasted
8 leaves dark green lettuce

1 Combine the mayonnaise, Cajun seasoning, and hot-pepper sauce in a small bowl. Stir and set aside.

2 Place the salmon in a mixing bowl. Pick off and discard as much skin as possible. Add the sliced scallions (reserving the minced greens), flaxseed, and egg. With clean hands, mix the ingredients together. Shape into four ¹/₂"-thick patties.

3 Heat a large nonstick skillet or griddle over medium-high heat. Turn off the heat. Coat the surface with cooking spray. Turn the heat back on to medium-high. With a spatula, gently transfer the patties to the skillet or griddle. Cook for about 4 minutes or until browned on the bottom. Carefully flip and cook, occasionally pressing down gently,

for about 4 minutes more or until heated through.

4 Set the bottoms of the muffins on a work surface. Top each with 2 lettuce leaves. Place a burger atop each. Dollop or drizzle on the reserved sauce. Sprinkle on the reserved scallion greens. Lean the muffin tops against the burgers and serve.

PER SERVING: 392 calories, 24 g protein, 30 g carbohydrates, 21 g fat (3 g saturated fat), 103 mg cholesterol, 743 mg sodium*

✱ Limit saturated fat to 10 percent of total calories—about 17 grams per day for most women—and sodium intake to less than 2,300 milligrams.

Makes 4 servings

FAT-
FIGHTING
4

7 g fiber
----
194 mg
calcium

4.5 IU
vitamin D
----
380 mg
omega-3s

Mashed Edamame Pita Sandwiches

PREP TIME: 20 MINUTES ◆ TOTAL TIME: 30 MINUTES

1 cup water
2½ cups frozen shelled edamame
1 clove garlic, minced
3 ounces reduced-fat feta cheese, crumbled
1 tablespoon chopped fresh oregano or 1 teaspoon dried

2 tablespoons balsamic vinegar
1 tablespoon olive oil
4 cups shredded romaine lettuce
1 tomato, chopped
½ small red onion, thinly sliced
4 "light" flatbreads

FAT-FIGHTING
4

16 g fiber
----
152 mg calcium
----
0 IU vitamin D
----
80 mg omega-3s
----

1 Bring the water to a boil in a medium saucepan. Add the edamame and garlic. Reduce the heat to medium, cover, and cook for 25 to 30 minutes or until the edamame is very soft. Puree in a food processor or blender. Pour the mixture into a medium bowl. Stir in the cheese and oregano.

2 Meanwhile, whisk together the vinegar and oil in a large bowl. Add the lettuce, tomato, and onion and toss to coat.

3 Lay each flatbread open on a work surface. Spread each flatbread with one-quarter of the edamame and top with one-quarter of the salad mixture. Fold or roll and serve.

PER SERVING: 319 calories, 25 g protein, 35 g carbohydrates, 12 g fat (2 g saturated fat), 8 mg cholesterol, 667 mg sodium*

∗ Limit saturated fat to 10 percent of total calories–about 17 grams per day for most women–and sodium intake to less than 2,300 milligrams.

Makes 4 servings

TLT—Tofu, Lettuce, and Tomato

PREP TIME: 10 MINUTES

3 tablespoons fat-free plain yogurt

1 tablespoon omega-3-enriched mayonnaise

1½ tablespoons prepared horseradish

2 large whole wheat pitas, halved

1 package (8 ounces) tomato-basil-flavored marinated baked tofu, each piece quartered lengthwise

1 cup mesclun

1 large tomato, cut into 4 slices

¼ large cucumber, sliced

FAT-FIGHTING 4

6 g fiber

----

400 mg calcium

----

100 IU vitamin D

----

145 mg omega-3s

----

1 Stir together the yogurt, mayonnaise, and horseradish in a small bowl.

2 Fill each pita half with one-quarter of the tofu, mesclun, tomato, and cucumber. Drizzle each with one-quarter of the yogurt mixture.

3 Serve with a glass of fat-free milk.

PER SERVING: 303 calories, 21 g protein, 37 g carbohydrates, 8 g fat (1 g saturated fat), 3 mg cholesterol, 555 mg sodium

NOTE: Freezing and thawing tofu makes it easy to squeeze out the water, which makes the tofu crisp when it's cooked. Place the tofu on a work surface with the long side of the block facing you. Cut into 8 equal cutlets. Line a tray or freezer-proof dish with plastic wrap. Place the cutlets in a single layer on the tray. Cover loosely with plastic wrap. Place in the freezer for at least 24 hours or until frozen solid. When the cutlets are solid, they can be stacked in a freezer-proof resealable plastic bag for longer keeping. To use, remove the cutlets and allow to thaw for several days in the refrigerator or several hours at room temperature. Working over a sink or bowl, squeeze gently with your hands, as you would squeeze a sponge.

Makes 4 servings

Grilled Veggie Sandwich

PREP TIME: 10 MINUTES ◆ TOTAL TIME: 30 MINUTES

1 marinated roasted red pepper,
    drained
1 clove garlic
1 tablespoon canola oil
1 teaspoon red-pepper flakes
$\frac{1}{2}$ teaspoon ground cumin
$\frac{1}{4}$ teaspoon ground caraway seeds
$\frac{1}{4}$ teaspoon smoked paprika
2 tablespoons water

1 small zucchini, cut diagonally into
    8 slices
1 red bell pepper, cut into 4 thick
    slices
1 red onion, cut into 4 slices
1 pound extra-firm or firm tofu,
    drained
4 whole grain rolls, halved
2 tablespoons omega-3-enriched
    mayonnaise

FAT-FIGHTING 4

6 g fiber
----
144 mg
calcium
----
0 IU
vitamin D
----
390 mg
omega-3s
----

1 Preheat the grill or broiler. To make the sauce, combine the roasted pepper, garlic, oil, pepper flakes, cumin, caraway seeds, paprika, and water in a blender. Puree until smooth.

2 Coat the grill rack or broiler pan with cooking spray. Coat the zucchini, bell pepper, and onion with canola cooking spray.

3 Cut the tofu into 8 slices. Brush each slice all over with the sauce. Grill or broil the vegetables 4 inches from the heat for 10 minutes, turning

once, or until tender. Grill or broil the tofu 4 inches from the heat for 6 minutes, turning once.

4 Spread half of each roll with $\frac{1}{2}$ tablespoon mayonnaise. Top each with one-quarter of the vegetables and tofu and the remaining roll half.

PER SERVING: 320 calories, 16 g protein, 16 g carbohydrates, 17 g fat (3 g saturated fat), 5 mg cholesterol, 240 mg sodium

Makes 4 servings

Chicken and Cheese Panini

PREP TIME: 5 MINUTES ◆ TOTAL TIME: 13 MINUTES

4 fresh chicken sausages (12 ounces), halved lengthwise
8 slices whole grain bread
4 teaspoons maple syrup

1 large apple, cut into thin slices (about 8 ounces)
4 ounces reduced-fat Jarlsberg cheese, cut into 4 slices

1 Cook the sausage in a nonstick grill pan or skillet over medium heat until browned. Remove to a plate. Wipe the pan clean.

2 Arrange 4 bread slices on a cutting board. Spread 1 teaspoon syrup over each slice. Top each with one-quarter of the apple slices, 2 sausage pieces, and 1 slice of cheese. Top with the remaining 4 bread slices.

3 Spray the outer side of the top slices with cooking spray and place the sandwiches, sprayed side down, in the grill pan or skillet. Coat the outer side of the slices that are now on top with cooking spray. Place the bottom of a heavy pan on top of the sandwiches. Cook for 2 minutes, turn, and cook for 2 minutes longer.

4 Serve each sandwich with a glass of fat-free milk.

PER SERVING: 404 calories, 37 g protein, 45 g carbohydrates, 11 g fat (3.5 g saturated fat), 88 mg cholesterol, 304 mg sodium

NOTE: A panini or sandwich press works well for making these sandwiches, although an indoor grill (such as a George Forman grill) will also do the trick. Cook the sausages on the grill, remove, and wipe the grill clean. Coat the sandwiches with cooking spray and place them on the press or grill, and instead of using a heavy pan to press them, close the lid and press slightly. There's no need to turn the sandwiches.

Makes 4 servings

FAT-FIGHTING
4

7 g fiber
----
619 mg calcium
----
100 IU vitamin D
----
50 mg omega-3s

Crispy Tofu Cutlets Italiano

PREP TIME: 15 MINUTES ◆ TOTAL TIME: 55 MINUTES

1 slice whole wheat bread

10 cups (10 ounces) torn leaves spinach

2 teaspoons minced garlic

½ teaspoon freshly ground black pepper

¼ teaspoon salt

1 can (14 ounces) no-salt-added petite diced tomatoes, drained

¼ cup grated Romano cheese

¾ teaspoon dried oregano

14 ounces tomato-basil-flavored tofu, frozen, thawed, and squeezed dry

1½ tablespoons canola oil

FAT-FIGHTING 4

4 g fiber

----

296 mg calcium

----

0 IU vitamin D

----

590 mg omega-3s

----

1 Preheat the oven to 375°F. Coat an 8" x 8" baking dish with cooking spray.

2 Toast the bread until very crisp. Set aside to cool. Place the spinach and garlic in a large nonstick skillet over medium-high heat. Cover and cook for 3 minutes, or until wilted. Uncover and cook for about 3 to 5 minutes, tossing frequently. Use tongs to squeeze excess liquid from the spinach while transferring to the baking dish. Spread in an even layer. Season with ¼ teaspoon of the pepper and ⅛ teaspoon of the salt. Top with half of the tomatoes.

3 Cut the bread into 1" cubes. Place in the bowl of a food processor fitted with a metal blade. Process for about 2 minutes or until fine crumbs form.

4 Transfer the crumbs onto a large sheet of waxed paper. Add the cheese, oregano, and the remaining ¼ teaspoon pepper and ⅛ teaspoon salt. Toss. One at a time, dip the tofu cutlets into the mixture, pressing lightly to adhere. Lay the cutlets on the spinach mixture, overlapping slightly. Sprinkle any crumb mixture remaining on the waxed paper over the cutlets. Scatter on the remaining tomatoes. Drizzle with the oil.

5 Bake for about 35 minutes or until sizzling.

PER SERVING: 210 calories, 14 g protein, 11 g carbohydrates, 12 g fat (3 g saturated fat), 5 mg cholesterol, 380 mg sodium

Makes 4 servings

Curried Lentils and Cauliflower

PREP TIME: 20 MINUTES ◆ TOTAL TIME: 55 MINUTES

3 teaspoons canola oil

4 cups cauliflower florets, cut into small pieces (12–16 ounces)

½ cup chopped onion (1 small)

½ cup chopped carrot (1 medium)

1 cup dried brown lentils

2 teaspoons minced garlic

1 teaspoon curry powder

1½ cups reduced-sodium vegetable broth

¼ teaspoon salt

½ cup fat-free plain yogurt

Leaves fresh cilantro

FAT-FIGHTING 4

11 g fiber
- - - - - - - - -
105 mg calcium
- - - - - - - - -
10 IU vitamin D
- - - - - - - - -
50 mg omega-3s
- - - - - - - - -

1 Heat a large, deep skillet over medium-high heat. Add 2 teaspoons of the oil. Heat for 1 minute. Add the cauliflower. Cover and cook, tossing occasionally, for 5 minutes or until the cauliflower is lightly charred. Reduce the heat if the cauliflower is browning too quickly. Remove the cauliflower to a plate. Set aside.

2 Return the skillet to medium heat. Add the remaining 1 teaspoon oil and the onion and carrot. Cook, stirring, for 3 minutes or until the vegetables start to soften. Stir in the lentils, garlic, and curry powder. Cook, stirring, for 3 minutes to coat the lentils with the seasonings. Add the broth. Bring almost to a boil. Partially cover the pan and reduce the heat. Simmer for about 20 minutes or until the lentils are almost tender.

3 Add the cauliflower to the skillet. Partially cover and simmer for about 5 minutes or until the cauliflower is tender and the lentils are cooked. Stir in the salt. Spoon onto 4 pasta plates. Divide and dollop on the yogurt. Garnish with cilantro.

PER SERVING: 240 calories, 14 g protein, 41 g carbohydrates, 5 g fat (0 g saturated fat), 0 mg cholesterol, 270 mg sodium

Makes 4 servings

Tri-Bean Bake with Cornbread Crust

PREP TIME: 25 MINUTES ◆ TOTAL TIME: 60-75 MINUTES

FAT-FIGHTING 4

10 g fiber
----
110 mg calcium
----
0 IU vitamin D
----
10 mg omega-3s

BEANS

1 can (15 ounces) no-salt-added black beans, rinsed and drained
1 can (15 ounces) no-salt-added red kidney beans, rinsed and drained
1 can (15 ounces) no-salt-added great Northern beans, rinsed and drained
1 can (15 ounces) plain tomato sauce
1 cup finely chopped red onions (1 medium)
¼ cup light molasses
2 teaspoons ground cumin
1 teaspoon hot-pepper sauce

CORNBREAD

½ cup whole grain cornmeal
⅓ cup white whole wheat flour (such as King Arthur) or whole wheat pastry flour
1 tablespoon ground flaxseed
2 tablespoons buttermilk powder (such as SACO)
½ teaspoon baking powder
¼ teaspoon baking soda
1/16 teaspoon salt
⅓ cup water
1 omega-3-enriched egg
1 tablespoon honey
1 tablespoon canola oil

1 *To make the beans:* Preheat the oven to 350°F. Coat a 13" x 9" baking dish with cooking spray.

2 Combine the black beans, kidney beans, great Northern beans, tomato sauce, onions, molasses, cumin, and pepper sauce in a large bowl. Stir to mix. Pour into the baking dish. Cover with foil. Bake for 30 minutes or until bubbling.

3 *To make the cornbread:* Meanwhile, combine the cornmeal, flour, flaxseed, buttermilk powder, baking powder, baking soda, and salt in a mixing bowl. Stir to mix. Combine the water, egg, honey, and oil in a measuring cup. Beat with a fork.

Pour into the dry ingredients. Stir just until all ingredients are wet.

4 Using pot holders, remove the beans from the oven. Carefully remove the foil, directing the escaping steam away from you. Stir the beans. Dollop the batter in small spoonfuls over the beans to cover evenly. With pot holders, return the baking dish to the oven for 10 to 12 minutes or until the cornbread is golden. Remove and let sit for 5 minutes before cutting.

PER SERVING: 223 calories, 9 g protein, 42 g carbohydrates, 3 g fat (0 g saturated fat), 0 mg cholesterol, 412 mg sodium

Makes 8 servings

Pasta Primavera

PREP TIME: 20 MINUTES ◆ TOTAL TIME: 30 MINUTES

6 ounces whole wheat spaghetti
2 tablespoons canola oil
1 clove garlic, chopped
1 cup thinly sliced carrots
(2 medium)
1 cup thinly sliced onions
(1 medium)
1 cup frozen baby peas, rinsed and
drained

1 cup frozen artichoke hearts,
thawed
1/4 cup reduced-sodium vegetable
broth
1/2 cup slivered fresh basil
1/4 cup grated Parmesan or
Romano cheese
Freshly ground black pepper

1 Prepare the pasta al dente according to package directions. Reserve 1/2 cup of the cooking water before draining.

2 Heat the oil in a deep, wide nonstick skillet over medium-high heat for 1 minute. Add the garlic, carrots, and onions. Cook, stirring frequently, for 5 minutes or until the vegetables start to soften. Add the peas and artichokes. Cook, stirring frequently, for 2 minutes, just until heated. Add the broth. Keep warm over low heat.

3 Add the pasta and the basil to the skillet and toss to combine. Add some of the reserved pasta water to moisten if necessary. Allow to sit for 1 minute so flavors will blend. Add the cheese and toss. Serve right away. Season with pepper at the table.

PER SERVING: 302 calories, 12 g protein, 45 g carbohydrates, 9 g fat (2 g saturated fat), 5 mg cholesterol, 230 mg sodium

Makes 4 servings

FAT-FIGHTING
4

8 g fiber
----
99 mg
calcium
----
0 IU
vitamin D
----
40 mg
omega-3s

Stuffed Peppers Provence-Style

PREP TIME: 40 MINUTES ◆ TOTAL TIME: 1 HOUR 20 MINUTES

4 medium red, yellow, and/or green bell peppers
1 navel orange
2 teaspoons olive oil
1¼ cups finely chopped onions (1 large)
1 tablespoon minced garlic
1 teaspoon dried thyme
1¼ cups no-salt-added small white beans, rinsed and drained

¼ cup fresh bread crumbs
2 tablespoons slivered Niçoise or other ripe olives
2 tablespoons chopped parsley
¼ teaspoon salt
¼ teaspoon red-pepper flakes + additional for garnish
4 slices reduced-fat provolone cheese (such as Sargento), finely chopped

FAT-FIGHTING 4

8 mg fiber
----
230 mg calcium
----
0 IU vitamin D
----
70 mg omega-3s
----

❶ Preheat the oven to 375°F. Coat a 13" x 9" microwaveable baking dish with cooking spray.

❷ Cut the peppers in half from the stem to the bottom. Cut out and discard the ribs and seeds. Place the peppers, cut sides down, in the dish. Cover with plastic wrap, leaving a vent. Microwave on high power for 5 minutes or until hot and slightly softened.

❸ Grate ½ teaspoon orange zest and set aside. Squeeze 4 tablespoons orange juice and set aside.

❹ Heat a nonstick skillet over medium heat. Add the oil and heat for 1 minute. Add the onion, garlic, and thyme. Reduce the heat to low, cover, and cook, stirring occasionally, for 5 minutes, or until the onion starts to soften. Add the beans, orange zest, and juice. Partially cover

the pan and simmer for 5 minutes. Remove from the heat. Stir in the bread crumbs, olives, parsley, salt, and pepper flakes. Allow to cool, stirring occasionally, for 10 minutes. Turn the bell peppers cut side up in the baking dish.

❺ Add all but 2 tablespoons of the cheese to the bean mixture and stir. Transfer the mixture into the bell peppers' centers, pressing down slightly. Sprinkle on the remaining cheese. Cover loosely with foil.

❻ Bake for about 30 minutes or until the cheese is melted. Allow to sit for 10 minutes. Pass additional pepper flakes at the table.

PER SERVING: 255 calories, 12 g protein, 33 g carbohydrates, 8 g fat (3 g saturated fat), 10 mg cholesterol, 458 mg sodium

Makes 4 servings

Honey-Soy-Glazed Salmon

PREP TIME: 10 MINUTES ◆ TOTAL TIME: 25 MINUTES

4 ounces whole wheat spaghetti

4 skinless salmon fillets
   (3 ounces each)

1 tablespoon reduced-sodium
   soy sauce

1 tablespoon honey

1 teaspoon canola oil

½ cup sliced scallions, all parts
   (4 medium)

5 cups sliced collard leaves

½ teaspoon grated fresh ginger

Red-pepper flakes

1 Preheat the oven to 375°F. Prepare the pasta al dente according to package directions. Reserve ¼ cup of the cooking water before draining.

2 Cover a small baking sheet with foil. Coat with cooking spray. Place the salmon on the foil. Whisk together the soy sauce and honey in a small bowl. Brush the salmon lightly with half of the mixture. Set the remainder aside.

3 Heat a large skillet over medium heat. Add the oil and scallions. Cook, stirring, for 30 seconds or until wilted. Add the collard leaves and ginger and toss. Cover and cook for 3 minutes or until wilted. Remove from the heat and set aside.

4 Bake the salmon for 10 minutes or until the fish is opaque.

5 Add the spaghetti to the skillet. Toss. Add the remaining soy mixture and toss. Add a few tablespoons of reserved cooking water to moisten the mixture if needed. Divide the spaghetti mixture among 4 dinner plates. Top each plate with a salmon fillet. Season to taste with pepper flakes.

PER SERVING: 294 calories, 23 g protein, 28 g carbohydrates, 11 g fat (2 g saturated fat), 50 mg cholesterol, 164 mg sodium

Makes 4 servings

FAT-FIGHTING
4

5 g fiber
- - - - - - - - -
93 mg calcium
- - - - - - - - -
0 IU vitamin D
- - - - - - - - -
1,760 mg omega-3s
- - - - - - - - -

Pan-Grilled Mediterranean Salmon

PREP TIME: 10 MINUTES ◆ TOTAL TIME: 32 MINUTES

³/₄ cup chopped red onion
(¹/₂-³/₄ medium)
1 tablespoon minced garlic
(2-3 large cloves)
2 teaspoons crumbled dried sage
2 teaspoons canola oil
1 can (15¹/₂ ounces) no-salt-added
cannellini beans, rinsed
and drained

¹/₂ cup fat-free, reduced-sodium
chicken broth
¹/₄ teaspoon salt
3 cups baby spinach
2 teaspoons flaxseed oil
4 skinless salmon fillets
(3 ounces each)
Red-pepper flakes

FAT-
FIGHTING
4

5 g fiber
----
68 mg
calcium
----
0 IU
vitamin D

3,110 mg
omega-3s
----

1 Combine the onion, garlic, 1¹/₂ teaspoons sage, and 1 teaspoon of the oil in a deep, wide skillet. Cover and cook over medium heat, stirring occasionally, for about 5 minutes or until the onion starts to soften. Add the beans, broth, and salt. Simmer for about 10 minutes. Stir the spinach into the beans and cook for another 2 to 3 minutes. Stir the flaxseed oil into the bean mixture. Remove the pan from the heat.

2 Rub the salmon fillets with the remaining sage. Heat the remaining oil in a medium skillet or grill pan. Place the salmon fillets in the pan and cook for 3 to 4 minutes. Carefully turn each fillet and cook for 1 minute longer. Remove the fillets to 4 plates. Spoon the beans onto each plate. Serve with the pepper flakes.

PER SERVING: 283 calories, 22 g protein, 16 g carbohydrates, 15 g fat (2 g saturated fat), 50 mg cholesterol, 324 mg sodium

Makes 4 servings

Seared Caribbean Scallops with Black Bean Salsa

PREP TIME: 20 MINUTES ◆ TOTAL TIME: 25 MINUTES

SCALLOPS
12 sea scallops (1 ounce each), preferably dry caught
1 teaspoon Caribbean jerk seasoning
1 tablespoon canola oil

SALSA
1 can (14½ ounces) no-salt-added black beans, rinsed and drained
1 medium tomato, chopped
¾ cup chopped red bell pepper (about 1 medium)

½ medium red onion, finely chopped
1 small jalapeño pepper, finely chopped (wear plastic gloves when handling)
1 cup cubed mango
¼ teaspoon ground cumin
1 tablespoon chopped cilantro
2 tablespoons lime juice
1 tablespoon canola oil
⅛ teaspoon salt
Freshly ground black pepper
4 lime wedges

FAT-FIGHTING **4**

5 g fiber
- - - - - - - - -
58 mg calcium
- - - - - - - - -
0 IU vitamin D
- - - - - - - - -
750 mg omega-3s
- - - - - - - - -

1 *To make the scallops:* Place the scallops on a work surface. Pat dry. Dust with the jerk seasoning and toss to coat evenly. Set aside.

2 *To make the salsa:* Combine the beans, tomato, bell pepper, onion, jalapeño pepper, mango, cumin, cilantro, lime juice, canola oil, and salt and pepper to taste in a medium bowl, mixing well to combine. Let stand to blend flavors.

3 Meanwhile, heat a skillet over medium-high heat. Add the oil and heat for 1 minute. Add the scallops

to the skillet. Cook for 1 to 2 minutes on each side, until well browned all over and opaque in the center. Remove to a plate.

4 Spoon the salsa onto 4 dinner plates. Top with the scallops. Place a lime wedge on each plate.

PER SERVING: 222 calories, 18 g protein, 23 g carbohydrates, 8 g fat (1 g saturated fat), 28 mg cholesterol, 446 mg sodium

Makes 4 servings

Lemon-Pepper Halibut with Squash Puree

PREP TIME: 20 MINUTES ◆ TOTAL TIME: 40 MINUTES

1 slice whole wheat bread
1 container (20 ounces) peeled
   butternut squash
3 large cloves garlic, unpeeled
1 tablespoon ground flaxseed
1 teaspoon lemon-pepper seasoning
¼ teaspoon salt
2 tablespoons white whole wheat
   flour (such as King Arthur)

1 omega-3-enriched egg white
1 tablespoon water
4 boneless halibut fillets
   (3 ounces each)
1 tablespoon canola oil
2 tablespoons nonfat dry milk
1 tablespoon chopped parsley

FAT-FIGHTING 4

4 g fiber
----
150 mg calcium
----
0 IU vitamin D
----
690 mg omega-3s
----

1 Preheat the oven to 375°F. Line a baking sheet with foil. Coat with cooking spray. Toast the bread until very crisp. Set aside to cool.

2 Place the squash and garlic in a single layer in a microwaveable dish. Cover with plastic wrap, leaving a vent. Microwave on high power, rotating occasionally, for about 10 minutes or until very soft. Remove and set aside.

3 Meanwhile, break the toast into small chunks. Place in the bowl of a food processor fitted with a metal blade. Process for about 2 minutes, or until fine crumbs form. Measure out 3 tablespoons and place on a large sheet of waxed paper. (Freeze the remaining crumbs for another recipe.) Add the flaxseed, lemon pepper, and ⅛ teaspoon of the salt. Using clean hands, mix with your fingers. Place the flour on a second sheet of waxed paper. Combine the egg white and water and beat with a fork in a shallow bowl.

4 One at a time, dip the fish into the flour to coat it. Shake off the excess. Dip the fish into the egg mixture, shaking off the excess. Dip the fish into the flaxseed mixture to coat evenly. Place on the prepared baking sheet. Press any remaining flaxseed mixture evenly on top of the fish. Drizzle evenly with the oil. Bake for 10 minutes or until opaque in the center.

5 Meanwhile, transfer the squash to the bowl of a food processor fitted with a metal blade. Pop the garlic from its skin and add it to the bowl along with the dry milk and the remaining ⅛ teaspoon salt. Process, scraping the bowl as needed, for about 2 minutes or until smooth. Divide among 4 dinner plates. Top with the halibut. Sprinkle on the parsley.

PER SERVING: 242 calories, 23 g protein, 25 g carbohydrates, 7 g fat (1 g saturated fat), 28 mg cholesterol, 287 mg sodium

Makes 4 servings

Glazed Halibut with Broccoli and Oranges

PREP TIME: 15 MINUTES ◆ TOTAL TIME: 50 MINUTES

1 pound red onions (about 4 medium)
3 teaspoons canola oil
¼ teaspoon salt
2 medium navel oranges
4 boneless, skinless halibut fillets
or steaks (about 3 ounces each)

1 tablespoon honey
2 tablespoons water
4 cups broccoli florets
Freshly ground black pepper

FAT-
FIGHTING
4

6 g fiber
----
130 mg
calcium
----
0 IU
vitamin D

1,470 mg
omega-3s
----

1 Preheat the oven to 375°F. Line a large baking sheet with sides with foil. Coat the foil with cooking spray. Cut the onions in half crosswise and place, cut sides down, on a work surface. Cut into ½"-thick slices. Break the slices into separate pieces and transfer to the baking sheet. Drizzle with 2 teaspoons of the oil and ⅛ teaspoon of the salt. Toss to coat. Spread the onions in a single layer on the baking sheet. Roast, turning occasionally, for 20 minutes or until golden.

2 Meanwhile, grate 2 teaspoons zest from 1 orange. Set aside. Peel and segment the oranges. When the onions are golden brown, remove the baking sheet from the oven. Add the orange segments. Toss to coat. Return to the oven for 5 minutes.

3 Remove the baking sheet from the oven. Spread the onion mixture into a single layer and lay the halibut on top. Drizzle the honey and

½ teaspoon of the reserved orange zest over the halibut. Return to the oven for 10 minutes or until the halibut is opaque.

4 Meanwhile, combine the water and the remaining 1 teaspoon oil in a nonstick skillet. Bring to a boil. Add the broccoli and the remaining ⅛ teaspoon salt. Cover and cook, tossing occasionally, for 5 minutes or until the broccoli is bright green but still crisp. Add the remaining orange zest and toss.

5 Divide the onion mixture among 4 plates and lay the fish on top. Serve with the broccoli, seasoning to taste with the pepper at the table.

PER SERVING: 238 calories, 22 g protein, 27 g carbohydrates, 6 g fat (1 g saturated fat), 27 mg cholesterol, 216 mg sodium

Makes 4 servings

Chicken with Tomatoes and Zucchini Sauté

PREP TIME: 15 MINUTES ◆ TOTAL TIME: 33 MINUTES

1 omega-3-enriched egg
1 tablespoon water
1/4 cup ground flaxseed
1/4 cup whole grain pastry flour
1/2 teaspoon salt
4 boneless, skinless chicken breast halves (4 ounces each)
1 tablespoon olive oil

1 onion, cut into 1/2" wedges
1 zucchini, halved lengthwise and sliced
2 cups grape tomatoes, halved
1 teaspoon dried basil
1/2 lemon
2 cups cooked whole wheat couscous (2/3 cup dry)

FAT-FIGHTING 4

5 g fiber
- - - - - - - - -
60 mg calcium
- - - - - - - - -
4.5 IU vitamin D
- - - - - - - - -
120 mg omega-3s
- - - - - - - - -

1 Preheat the oven to 425°F. Coat a baking sheet with cooking spray.

2 Place the egg and water in a shallow dish and whisk to combine. Combine the flaxseed, flour, and salt in another shallow dish. Dip the chicken into the egg mixture and then into the flaxseed mixture. Place on the baking sheet and coat the surface with cooking spray. Bake, turning once, for 15 minutes or until a thermometer inserted in the center reaches 160°F.

3 Meanwhile, coat a large nonstick skillet with cooking spray and heat the oil over medium-high heat. Add the onion and zucchini and cook, stirring, for 5 minutes or until well browned. Add the tomatoes and basil and cook for 3 minutes or until tender. Remove from the heat. Squeeze the lemon over the tomato mixture and toss to coat.

4 Place the chicken breasts on 4 plates. Top each with one-quarter of the tomato mixture. Serve with hot couscous.

PER SERVING: 337 calories, 34 g protein, 29 g carbohydrates, 9 g fat (1 g saturated fat), 110 mg cholesterol, 390 mg sodium

Makes 4 servings

Chicken with Pears and Blue Cheese

PREP TIME: 20 MINUTES ◆ TOTAL TIME: 50 MINUTES

1½ tablespoons whole grain pastry
   flour
½ teaspoon salt
¼ teaspoon freshly ground black
   pepper
2 large boneless, skinless chicken
   breast halves (6-8 ounces
   each), halved, or 4 chicken
   cutlets (3-4 ounces each)
2 tablespoons canola oil

1 large onion, cut into wedges
2 medium pears, halved, cored, and
   sliced
1 bag (6 ounces) baby spinach
½ cup apple cider or apple juice
1½ teaspoons fresh thyme leaves
   or ½ teaspoon dried
½ cup crumbled reduced-fat
   blue cheese

FAT-
FIGHTING
4

6 g fiber
----
134 mg
calcium
----
0 IU
vitamin D
----
30 mg
omega-3s
----

1 Combine the flour, salt, and pepper in a shallow bowl. Dredge the chicken in the mixture and set aside.

2 Heat 1 tablespoon of the oil in a large nonstick skillet over medium heat. Add the onion and cook for 5 minutes or until lightly browned. Add the pears and cook for 3 minutes or until lightly browned. Add the spinach and cook for 1 minute or until wilted. Place the mixture on a serving plate.

3 Heat the remaining 1 tablespoon oil in the same skillet. Cook the chicken, turning once, for 6 to 8 minutes or until browned. Add the cider and thyme and bring to a boil. Reduce the heat to low and simmer for 5 minutes or until the sauce is reduced by half.

4 Place the chicken on the spinach mixture, drizzle with the cider mixture, and sprinkle with the cheese.

PER SERVING: 301 calories, 25 g protein, 28 g carbohydrates, 11 g fat (3 g saturated fat*), 55 mg cholesterol, 610 mg sodium*

＊ Limit saturated fat to 10 percent of total calories—about 17 grams per day for most women—and sodium intake to less than 2,300 milligrams.

NOTE: Because most chicken breasts are so large, you can cut them in half to get a nice-size cutlet— or, if you prefer, you can simply purchase cutlets for this recipe.

Makes 4 servings

Parmesan Chicken Strips with Garlicky Escarole and Fennel

PREP TIME: 25 MINUTES ◆ TOTAL TIME: 35 MINUTES

FAT-FIGHTING
4

7 g fiber

---

249 mg calcium

4.5 IU vitamin D

---

110 mg omega-3s

½ cup white panko bread crumbs
½ cup shredded Parmesan cheese
¼ teaspoon freshly ground black pepper
1 omega-3-enriched egg
2 tablespoons water
4 boneless, skinless chicken breast halves, cut into 1" slices

2 tablespoons canola oil
1 large head fennel, cut into thin wedges
1 red onion, cut into thin wedges
2 cloves garlic, minced
10–12 cups escarole, cut into thin strips (about 1 large)

1 Preheat the oven to 400°F. Coat a large baking sheet with cooking spray. Combine the panko, cheese, and pepper on a plate. Combine the egg and water and beat with a fork in a shallow bowl. Dip the chicken, a few strips at a time, into the egg mixture and then into the panko mixture, pressing to coat well. Place on the baking sheet and coat the surface with cooking spray. Bake, turning once, for 10 minutes or until a thermometer inserted in the center reaches 160°F.

2 Meanwhile, heat the oil in a large skillet over medium-high heat. Add the fennel and onion, reduce the heat to medium, and cook for 4 minutes or until browned. Add the garlic and cook for 1 minute. Stir in the escarole and cook for 4 minutes or until wilted. Divide among 4 plates. Top with the chicken strips.

PER SERVING: 324 calories, 35 g protein, 17 g carbohydrates, 13 g fat (3 g saturated fat), 118 mg cholesterol, 342 mg sodium

Makes 4 servings

Sesame Chicken with Gingered Rice

PREP TIME: 40 MINUTES ◆ TOTAL TIME: 1 HOUR 35 MINUTES

2 tablespoons rice vinegar

1 tablespoon reduced-sodium soy sauce

1 teaspoon wasabi paste

4 boneless, skinless chicken breast halves (4 ounces each)

1⅓ cups + ¼ cup water

⅔ cup brown rice

4 cups chopped broccoli

2 carrots, shredded

2 tablespoons white and/or black sesame seeds

2 tablespoons frozen orange juice concentrate

2 teaspoons toasted sesame oil

1 teaspoon freshly grated ginger

FAT-FIGHTING 4

4 g fiber
- - - - - - - - -
71 mg calcium
- - - - - - - - -
0 IU vitamin D
- - - - - - - - -
140 mg omega-3s
- - - - - - - - -

1 Combine the vinegar, soy sauce, and wasabi in a pie plate or shallow bowl. Add the chicken and turn to coat. Refrigerate, turning occasionally, for 30 minutes.

2 Bring 1⅓ cups water to a boil in a large saucepan. Add the rice, reduce the heat to low, cover, and simmer for 40 minutes. Stir in the broccoli and carrots and cook for 5 minutes or until the water is absorbed and the rice is tender. Place in a bowl.

3 Meanwhile, preheat the oven to 425°F. Coat a baking sheet with cooking spray. Place the sesame seeds on a plate.

4 Remove the chicken from the marinade and press both sides into the sesame seeds. Place on the baking sheet. Bake for 15 minutes, or until a thermometer inserted in the center reaches 160°F.

5 Whisk together the juice, oil, ginger, and the remaining ¼ cup water in a small saucepan. Heat to boiling and simmer for 1 minute. Drizzle over the rice mixture and toss to coat. Divide among 4 plates. Serve with the chicken.

PER SERVING: 330 calories, 33 g protein, 36 g carbohydrates, 7 g fat (1 g saturated fat), 65 mg cholesterol, 280 mg sodium

Makes 4 servings

Chicken Roll-Ups

PREP TIME: 17 MINUTES ◆ TOTAL TIME: 30 MINUTES

2 tablespoons hoisin sauce

2 tablespoons rice wine vinegar

1 tablespoon reduced-sodium
soy sauce

1 teaspoon toasted sesame oil

1 pound boneless, skinless chicken
breasts, cut into ¼" cubes

4 scallions, chopped

2 carrots, shredded (about 1½ cups)

1 clove garlic, minced

1 tablespoon finely chopped ginger

¼ cup water

2 ounces (½ cup) walnuts, toasted
and coarsely chopped

1 cup sliced canned water
chestnuts

12 leaves Bibb or Boston lettuce

FAT-
FIGHTING
4

3 g fiber

----

68 mg
calcium

----

0 IU
vitamin D

1,420 mg
omega-3s

----

1 Stir together the hoisin sauce, vinegar, soy sauce, and oil in a medium bowl. Stir in the chicken, tossing to coat. Let stand 10 minutes.

2 Heat a nonstick skillet coated with cooking spray over medium heat. Remove the chicken from the marinade with a slotted spoon (reserve the marinade). Cook for 5 minutes, stirring, until browned. Add the scallions, carrots, garlic, |and ginger and cook for 3 minutes

or until tender. Stir in the reserved marinade and the water. Bring to a boil and cook for 2 minutes, stirring constantly, or until thickened. Stir in the walnuts and water chestnuts. Place 3 lettuce leaves on each of 4 plates and fill each leaf with ¼ cup of the chicken mixture.

PER SERVING: 293 calories, 16 g protein, 13 g carbohydrates, 13 g fat (2 g saturated fat), 66 mg cholesterol, 382 mg sodium

Makes 4 servings

Autumn Chicken Stew in the Slow Cooker

PREP TIME: 20 MINUTES ◆ TOTAL TIME: 6-8 HOURS

2 parsnips, peeled and cut into
    thirds
1 medium butternut squash,
    peeled, halved lengthwise,
    seeded, and cut into 1" slices
1 large red onion, cut into 8 wedges
1 cup apple cider or apple juice
1 teaspoon dried rosemary

1 teaspoon dried thyme
$\frac{1}{2}$ teaspoon salt
4 boneless, skinless chicken breast
    halves (6 ounces each)
6 ounces baby spinach (about
    6 cups)
2 cups cooked whole wheat
    couscous ($\frac{2}{3}$ cup dry)

❶ Arrange the parsnips, squash, and onion in a 4- or 5-quart slow cooker. Pour the cider over the vegetables and sprinkle with $\frac{1}{2}$ teaspoon of the rosemary, $\frac{1}{2}$ teaspoon of the thyme, and $\frac{1}{4}$ teaspoon of the salt.

❷ Lay the chicken on the vegetables and sprinkle with the remaining $\frac{1}{2}$ teaspoon rosemary, $\frac{1}{2}$ teaspoon thyme, and $\frac{1}{4}$ teaspoon salt. Cover and cook on low for 6 to 8 hours. Stir the spinach into the hot liquid until wilted.

❸ Divide the vegetables among 4 soup plates. Top each with a chicken breast half and some sauce. Top each with $\frac{1}{2}$ cup of the hot couscous.

PER SERVING: 396 calories, 45 g protein, 49 g carbohydrates, 3 g fat (1 g saturated fat), 66 mg cholesterol, 486 mg sodium

Makes 4 servings

FAT-FIGHTING 4

10 g fiber
----
123 mg
calcium
----
0 IU
vitamin D
----
70 mg
omega-3s

Chipotle Pork

PREP TIME: 15 MINUTES ◆ TOTAL TIME: 60-85 MINUTES

2 tablespoons apricot or orange
   100% fruit spread
1 canned chipotle pepper in adobo
   sauce
1 large onion, halved lengthwise
   and sliced
1 medium butternut squash,
   peeled, halved lengthwise,
   seeded, and cut into
   2" pieces

1 red bell pepper, cut into strips
1 tablespoon canola oil
1 boneless center-cut pork loin
   roast (1-1¼ pounds)
¼ cup fresh cilantro leaves

FAT-
FIGHTING
4

4 g fiber
----
179 mg
calcium
----
0 IU
vitamin D
----
100 mg
omega-3s
----

1 Preheat the oven to 400°F. Mash together the fruit spread and chipotle pepper in a small bowl. Set aside.

2 Stir together the onion, squash, bell pepper, and oil in a large roasting pan. Push the vegetables to the sides of the pan and place the roast in the middle.

3 Roast for 45 minutes to 1 hour, brushing the meat with the chipotle mixture every 5 minutes for the last 15 minutes of cooking. The roast is done when a thermometer inserted in the center reaches 155°F and the juices run clear.

4 Remove the roast to a plate. Let stand for 10 minutes before slicing. Stir the cilantro into the vegetables and serve with the roast.

PER SERVING: 359 calories, 29 g protein, 46 g carbohydrates, 8 g fat (2 g saturated fat), 78 mg cholesterol, 99 mg sodium

NOTE: Store any remaining canned chipotle peppers in a resealable jar in the refrigerator. Chop the peppers and add with some adobo sauce to stews, chilis, fajitas, and sautés.

Makes 4 servings

Spice-Rubbed Pork Tenderloin with Edamame Succotash

PREP TIME: 20 MINUTES ◆ TOTAL TIME: 60 MINUTES

½ teaspoon chili powder
½ teaspoon ground cumin
¼ teaspoon smoked paprika
¼ teaspoon garlic powder
1 pork tenderloin (about 1 pound)
2 cups frozen or fresh shelled edamame

⅓ cup light sour cream
2 tablespoons lime juice
2 cups frozen corn kernels, thawed
1 medium tomato, seeded and chopped
¼ cup chopped fresh cilantro

FAT-FIGHTING
4

7 g fiber
----
100 mg calcium
----
0 IU vitamin D
----
30 mg omega-3s
----

1 Preheat the oven to 425°F. Combine the chili powder, cumin, paprika, and garlic powder in a small bowl. Place the tenderloin in a roasting pan and coat with the spice mixture. Roast, turning once, for 25 minutes or until a thermometer inserted in the center reaches 155°F. Let stand for 10 minutes. Cut diagonally into 12 slices.

2 Meanwhile, cook the edamame according to package directions. Rinse under cold running water and drain. Stir together the sour cream and lime juice in a medium bowl. Add the edamame, corn, tomato, and cilantro and stir. Divide the salad among 4 shallow bowls. Serve with the pork slices.

PER SERVING: 345 calories, 36 g protein, 30 g carbohydrates, 9 g fat (3 g saturated fat), 80 mg cholesterol, 108 mg sodium

Makes 4 servings

Spaghetti Squash with Bolognese Sauce

PREP TIME: 40 MINUTES ◆ TOTAL TIME: 6–9 HOURS

1½ pounds extra-lean (at least 90%) ground beef
2 tablespoons canola oil
2 large carrots, finely chopped
2 ribs celery, finely chopped
1 large onion, finely chopped
1 large bell pepper, finely chopped
4 cloves garlic, chopped
1 can (28 ounces) crushed tomatoes

¼ cup tomato paste
1 cup beef broth
1 cup nonfat dry milk
2 teaspoons dried basil, crushed
2 teaspoons dried oregano, crushed
1 large spaghetti squash (about 3 pounds)

FAT-FIGHTING
4

8 g fiber
----
295 mg calcium
----
0 IU vitamin D
----
230 mg omega-3s
----

1 Cook the beef in a large nonstick skillet over medium-high heat until browned. Drain and place in a 4- or 5-quart slow cooker.

2 Heat the oil in the same skillet over medium heat. Add the carrots, celery, onion, pepper, and garlic and cook for 3 minutes. Add to the slow cooker, and then add the tomatoes, tomato paste, broth, dry milk, basil, and oregano. Cook on low for 6 to 8 hours.

3 Prick the squash all over with a fork or sharp knife. Microwave on high, turning once, for 15 minutes or until tender. Let stand for 10 minutes. Cut in half. Remove and discard the seeds. Scrape the squash strands into a large bowl. Top with the sauce.

PER SERVING: 423 calories, 32 g protein, 37 g carbohydrates, 17 g fat (5 g saturated fat), 75 mg cholesterol, 571 mg sodium

NOTE: The sauce can be stored in an airtight container in the fridge for up to 3 days or in the freezer for up to 3 months.

Makes 6 servings

Spiced Beef with Wasabi Cream

PREP TIME: 15 MINUTES ◆ TOTAL TIME: 1 HOUR 40 MINUTES

1 teaspoon ground ginger

1 teaspoon Chinese five-spice
  powder

½ teaspoon garlic powder

½ teaspoon salt

1 beef eye round roast (about
  2 pounds)

1 container (6 ounces) fat-free
  Greek yogurt

1 teaspoon wasabi paste

4 heads baby bok choy,
  halved

6 ounces shiitake mushrooms,
  stemmed and halved

1 red bell pepper, cut into strips

2 tablespoons canola oil

FAT-
FIGHTING
4

5 g fiber

----

50 mg
calcium

----

64 IU
vitamin D

----

30 mg
omega-3s

----

1 Preheat the oven to 400°F. Stir together the ginger, five-spice powder, garlic powder, and salt in a small bowl.

2 Place the beef on a baking sheet with sides. Coat the beef on all sides with canola cooking spray. Rub the ginger mixture over the beef. Bake for 15 minutes.

3 Reduce the heat to 350°F and bake for 50 to 60 minutes longer or until a thermometer inserted in the center registers 145°F for medium rare, 160°F for medium, or 165°F for well done. Remove to a serving plate and let stand for 15 minutes before carving.

4 Meanwhile, in a small bowl, stir together the yogurt and wasabi until smooth. Cover and refrigerate until serving.

5 While the roast stands, increase the oven temperature to 450°F. Drain any liquid from the pan but leave some of the drippings. Add the bok choy, mushrooms, pepper, and oil to the pan, tossing to coat. Roast, stirring once, for 8 minutes or until the vegetables are tender-crisp.

6 Serve with ½ cup hot cooked medium pearl barley per serving.

PER SERVING: 307 calories, 31 g protein, 29 g carbohydrates, 7 g fat (1.5 g saturated fat), 46 mg cholesterol, 264 mg sodium

NOTE: If you can't find a 2-pound roast, purchase a larger one, cutting off a piece to form a 2-pound roast. (If the large roast is an end piece, be sure to use the end.) Cut the leftover piece into steaks or strips for stir-fries.

Makes 8 servings

Penne with Pepper Steak and Caramelized Onions

PREP TIME: 20 MINUTES ◆ TOTAL TIME: 1 HOUR 10 MINUTES

³⁄₄ pound flank steak
2 tablespoons cracked black
   pepper
2 cloves garlic, minced
1 tablespoon canola oil
1 large yellow onion, sliced
1 red onion, sliced

2 tablespoons balsamic vinegar
1 cup reduced-sodium beef broth
8 ounces Barilla Plus penne pasta
6 ounces baby arugula
Shaved Parmesan cheese

FAT-
FIGHTING
4

5 g fiber
- - - - - - - - -
120 mg
calcium
- - - - - - - - -
0 IU
vitamin D
- - - - - - - - -
140 mg
omega-3s
- - - - - - - - -

1 Preheat the broiler. Place the flank steak on the rack of a broiler pan and coat on all sides with the pepper and garlic. Let stand for about 10 minutes.

2 Heat the oil in a large skillet over medium-high heat. Cook the onions for 8 minutes or until lightly browned. Reduce the heat to medium-low and add the vinegar to deglaze. Stir in the broth, cover, and cook for 15 minutes, or until the onions are very soft and browned. Remove from the heat.

3 Prepare the pasta according to package directions, drain, and place in a large bowl.

4 Meanwhile, broil the steak, 4 inches from the heat, for 12 minutes, or until a thermometer inserted in

the center registers 145°F for medium rare, 160°F for medium, or 165°F for well done. Let stand for 10 minutes, then slice into thin strips.

5 Stir the arugula into the onions. Add to the pasta and toss to coat. Add in the steak strips and top with the cheese.

PER SERVING: 424 calories, 28 g protein, 54 g carbohydrates, 11 g fat (3 g saturated fat), 30 mg cholesterol, 175 mg sodium

NOTE: Flank steaks are often more than 1 pound. Cut the portion you'll need for this recipe and then freeze the remainder for later use.

Makes 4 servings

Spiced Nut Clusters

PREP TIME: 10 MINUTES ◆ TOTAL TIME: 1 HOUR

1 large omega-3-enriched egg white
1 tablespoon honey
1 cup walnuts
½ cup raw pumpkin seeds (pepitas)

⅓ cup dried cranberries
1 teaspoon ground cinnamon
1 teaspoon ground ginger
¼ teaspoon ground cardamom

1 Preheat the oven to 350°F. Line a baking sheet with parchment paper.

2 Whisk the egg white and honey in a medium bowl. Add the walnuts, pumpkin seeds, and cranberries. Sprinkle with the cinnamon, ginger, and cardamom and toss to coat well. Drop by ⅛-cup measures on the prepared baking sheet. Bake for 18 to 20 minutes or until browned.

3 Let stand on a rack for about 30 minutes or until completely cooled.

PER SERVING: 91 calories, 4 g protein, 5 g carbohydrates, 7 g fat (1 g saturated fat), 0 mg cholesterol, 5 mg sodium

Makes 16 (2 per serving)

FAT-FIGHTING **4**

1 g fiber
----
11 mg calcium
----
0 IU vitamin D
----
600 mg omega-3s

Wasabi Salmon Bites

PREP TIME: 10 MINUTES ◆ TOTAL TIME: 15-17 MINUTES

1 can or pouch (6-7$\frac{1}{2}$ ounces) pink or red salmon, drained and chunked

4 ounces Neufchâtel light cream cheese, softened

4 scallions, finely chopped

2 teaspoons reduced-sodium soy sauce

2 teaspoons rice vinegar

1$\frac{1}{2}$ teaspoons wasabi paste

1 box (1.9 ounces) mini filo shells

FAT-FIGHTING
4

0 g fiber
----
27 mg calcium
----
0 IU vitamin D
----
350 mg omega-3s
----

1 Preheat the oven to 350°F.

2 Mash the salmon, cream cheese, scallions, soy sauce, vinegar, and wasabi paste in a medium bowl.

3 Fill the shells with the mixture and place on a baking sheet. Bake for 5 to 7 minutes or until the pastry is golden and the filling is hot. Serve immediately.

PER SERVING: 197 calories, 12 g protein, 11 g carbohydrates, 11 g fat (4 g saturated fat), 38 mg cholesterol, 270 mg sodium

NOTE: These bites can be prepared ahead of time for a last-minute snack. Store the salmon mixture in an airtight container in the refrigerator, then simply spoon a heaping tablespoon into each shell and bake as directed. Adjust the wasabi paste to your liking.

Makes 15 (3 per serving)

Grape and Feta Salad

PREP TIME: 15 MINUTES

¼ cup light sour cream
¼ cup low-fat plain yogurt
4 cups red grapes, halved

½ cup crumbled reduced-fat
   feta cheese
½ cup chopped fennel or celery
½ cup chopped walnuts, toasted

Stir together the sour cream and yogurt in a medium bowl. Stir in the grapes, cheese, and fennel. Sprinkle with the nuts just before serving.

PER SERVING: 133 calories, 4 g protein, 16 g carbohydrates, 7 g fat (2 g saturated fat), 6 mg cholesterol, 128 mg sodium

NOTE: For a change of pace, try reduced-fat blue cheese instead of feta. Store the salad in an airtight container in the refrigerator for up to 3 days.

Makes 8 servings

FAT-
FIGHTING
4

1 g fiber
----
63 mg
calcium
----
0 IU
vitamin D
----
690 mg
omega-3s

Spinach Artichoke Dip

PREP TIME: 20 MINUTES ◆ TOTAL TIME: 40 MINUTES

1 package (1 pound) light silken
    tofu, drained
1 package (8 ounces) Neufchâtel
    light cream cheese
½ cup Parmesan cheese
3 cloves garlic, halved
2 teaspoons Dijon mustard
1 package (9 ounces) frozen
    artichoke hearts, thawed and
    finely chopped

1 package (10 ounces) frozen
    chopped spinach, thawed and
    squeezed dry
Pita wedges and assorted
    vegetables such as celery
    sticks, carrot sticks, jicama
    sticks, and sliced bell peppers

FAT-
FIGHTING
4

2 g fiber

382 mg
calcium

0 IU
vitamin D

10 mg
omega-3s

1 Preheat the oven to 350°F. Coat a 1½- or 2-quart baking dish with cooking spray.

2 Place the tofu, cream cheese, ¼ cup of the Parmesan cheese, garlic, and mustard in a blender or food processor. Puree, pushing the mixture toward the blade to start, until smooth.

3 Place the artichoke hearts and spinach in a medium bowl. Add the tofu mixture and toss to coat. Pour into the prepared baking dish. Top with the remaining ¼ cup Parmesan cheese. Bake for 20 minutes or until bubbling hot.

4 Serve with pita wedges and veggies.

PER SERVING: 127 calories, 10 g protein, 7 g carbohydrates, 6 g fat (4 g saturated fat), 18 mg cholesterol, 362 mg sodium

Makes 8 servings

South-of-the-Border Snack Mix

PREP TIME: 5 MINUTES ◆ TOTAL TIME: 2 HOURS 5 MINUTES

3 tablespoons canola oil
1 tablespoon ground cumin
1 tablespoon lime juice
1 teaspoon lime zest
8 cups hexagonal multigrain cereal

1 bag (3 ounces) 94% fat-free
  unsalted microwave popcorn,
  popped (6–8 cups)
¼ cup roasted soy nuts

1 Whisk together the oil, cumin, lime juice, and lime zest in a measuring cup.

2 Combine the cereal, popcorn, and nuts in a 4- or 5-quart slow cooker. Drizzle with the oil mixture. Toss to coat.

3 Cook on low for 2 hours, tossing once.

PER SERVING: 133 calories, 4 g protein, 21 g carbohydrates, 5 g fat (0.5 g saturated fat), 0 mg cholesterol, 168 mg sodium

NOTE: Store the snack mix in an airtight container.

Makes 16 servings (12 cups)

FAT-FIGHTING
4

4 g fiber
- - - - - - - - -
19 mg
calcium
- - - - - - - - -
0 IU
vitamin D
- - - - - - - - -
0 mg
omega-3s
- - - - - - - - -

Maple-Raisin Yogurt with Toasted Walnuts

PREP TIME: 10 MINUTES

**2 teaspoons finely chopped
walnuts**
1/3 cup fat-free plain yogurt
1 1/2 tablespoons nonfat dry milk

1 teaspoon maple syrup
1 teaspoon finely chopped raisins

FAT-
FIGHTING
4

0 g fiber
- - - - - - - - -
196 mg
calcium
- - - - - - - - -
27 IU
vitamin D
- - - - - - - - -
44 mg
omega-3s
- - - - - - - - -

1 Place the walnuts in a small skillet. Toast over medium-high heat, tossing often, until crisp and fragrant, about 1 to 2 minutes. Transfer to a dish and set aside.

2 Combine the yogurt and dry milk in a bowl. Stir to mix well. Drizzle with the syrup. Sprinkle on the walnuts and raisins.

PER SERVING: 114 calories, 6 g protein, 17 g carbohydrates, 3 g fat (0.5 g saturated fat), 3 mg cholesterol, 82 mg sodium

Makes 1 serving

Butterscotch Pudding

PREP TIME: 5 MINUTES ◆ TOTAL TIME: 10 MINUTES

2 tablespoons nonfat dry milk
1½ tablespoons cornstarch
¼ cup Splenda Brown Sugar Blend
1 can (12 ounces) fat-free
    evaporated milk

1 omega-3-enriched egg, beaten
½ teaspoon vanilla extract
Fat-free whipped topping

1 Whisk the dry milk, cornstarch, and sweetener in a saucepan. While whisking constantly, gradually add the evaporated milk and egg. Set the pan over medium-high heat. Cook, whisking constantly, for 5 minutes or until thickened. Remove from the heat.

2 Whisk in the vanilla extract. Cool to room temperature and then store in an airtight container in the refrigerator for up to 3 days. Just before serving, top each serving with a dollop of whipped topping.

PER SERVING: 173 calories, 8 g protein, 28 g carbohydrates, 1 g fat (0.5 g saturated fat), 45 mg cholesterol, 138 mg sodium

Makes 4 servings

FAT-
FIGHTING
4

0 g fiber
----
248 mg
calcium
----
68 IU
vitamin D
----
30 mg
omega-3s

"Instant" Strawberry Frozen Yogurt

PREP TIME: 5 MINUTES

**¾ cup loose-pack frozen
   strawberries**

**⅓ cup low-fat plain yogurt
2 teaspoons honey**

**FAT-
FIGHTING
4**

4 g fiber
- - - - - - - - -
161 mg
calcium
- - - - - - - - -
0 IU
vitamin D
- - - - - - - - -
40 mg
omega-3s
- - - - - - - - -

On a work surface, carefully cut the strawberries into chunks with a serrated knife. Place them in the bowl of a food processor fitted with a metal blade or in a blender. Pulse 10 times to finely chop. Add the yogurt and honey. Process, scraping down the sides of the bowl as needed, for 1 to 2 minutes or until smooth (tiny chunks of berry can remain for texture). Serve immediately.

PER SERVING: 151 calories, 4 g protein, 32 g carbohydrates, 1 g fat (1 g saturated fat), 7 mg cholesterol, 61 mg sodium

Makes 1 serving

Orange Frappé with Strawberries

PREP TIME: 5 MINUTES

¼ cup reduced-fat ricotta cheese
1 teaspoon nonfat dry milk
1½ teaspoons honey
½ teaspoon orange zest

¼ cup sliced fresh or partially
thawed loose-pack frozen
strawberries

Combine the cheese, dry milk, honey, and zest in a small bowl. Stir briskly until very smooth. Top with the strawberries.

PER SERVING: 137 calories, 8 g protein, 16 g carbohydrates, 5 g fat (3 g saturated fat), 19 mg cholesterol, 86 mg sodium

Makes 1 serving

FAT-FIGHTING **4**

1 g fiber
----
196 mg calcium

0.1 IU vitamin D
----
70 mg omega-3s

Peanut Butter Chocolate Chip Bars

PREP TIME: 15 MINUTES ◆ TOTAL TIME: 40 MINUTES

FAT-FIGHTING

4

1 g fiber
----
10 mg calcium
----
4 IU vitamin D
----
400 mg omega-3s
----

³⁄₄ cup white whole wheat flour (such as King Arthur) or whole wheat pastry flour
³⁄₄ teaspoon baking soda
Pinch of salt
1 cup omega-3-enriched peanut butter

¹⁄₃ cup Splenda Brown Sugar Blend
1 egg, beaten
¹⁄₂ cup fat-free milk
1 teaspoon vanilla extract
¹⁄₂ cup bittersweet chocolate chips

1 Preheat the oven to 350°F. Coat an 8" x 8" baking dish with cooking spray.

2 Combine the flour, baking soda, and salt on a large sheet of waxed paper. Stir with a fork.

3 Combine the peanut butter, sugar, and egg in a mixing bowl. Stir vigorously until creamy. Add the milk and vanilla extract. Stir until smooth. Add the flour mixture, stirring until well combined. Stir in the chocolate chips.

4 Spread the dough into the baking dish and pat the top to smooth. Bake for about 15 minutes or until slightly puffy and very lightly browned at the edges. Remove and allow to cool for at least 10 minutes before cutting. Store at room temperature, tightly covered with foil.

PER BAR: 137 calories, 4 g protein, 12 g carbohydrates, 8 g fat (2 g saturated fat), 9 mg cholesterol, 106 mg sodium

Makes 16

Fudgy Chocolate Brownies

PREP TIME: 15 MINUTES ◆ TOTAL TIME: 1 HOUR

BROWNIES
1 cup butter, softened
1½ cups granulated sugar
4 large omega-3-enriched eggs
2 teaspoons vanilla extract
1 cup unsweetened cocoa powder
1 cup flour
¾ teaspoon baking powder

½ teaspoon salt
1 cup walnuts, chopped

FROSTING
1 cup confectioners' sugar
⅓ cup unsweetened cocoa powder
2 tablespoons butter, softened
2 tablespoons low-fat milk

FAT
FIGHTING
4

1 g fiber
- - - - - - - - -
22 mg
calcium
- - - - - - - - -
0 IU
vitamin D
- - - - - - - - -
360 mg
omega-3s
- - - - - - - - -

1 Preheat the oven to 350°F. Coat a 13" x 9" foil-lined baking pan with cooking spray.

2 Cream the butter and granulated sugar in the bowl of an electric mixer on medium speed until light and fluffy. Beat in the eggs one at a time. Add the vanilla extract and beat until combined.

3 Sift the cocoa powder, flour, baking powder, and salt in a large bowl. Add to the butter mixture and beat until smooth. Fold in the walnuts.

4 Spread the batter in the prepared pan and place it on the middle rack of your oven. Bake for 25 to 30 minutes or until a knife inserted near the center comes out clean. Transfer the pan to a rack to cool until slightly warm.

5 Beat the frosting ingredients in the bowl of an electric mixer until smooth. Spread over the slightly warm brownies. Cut into 32 squares once the frosting is set.

PER BROWNIE: 164 calories, 2 g protein, 19 g carbohydrate, 1 g fiber, 10 g fat (5 g saturated fat), 41 mg cholesterol, 120 mg sodium

Makes 32

REFERENCES

CHAPTER 1

ADVANCE Collaborative Group. 2008. Intensive Blood Glucose Control and Vascular Outcomes in Patients with Type 2 Diabetes. *New England Journal of Medicine* 358(24):2560-72.

American College of Endocrinology Task Force on Pre-Diabetes. 2008. *American College of Endocrinology Consensus Statement on the Diagnosis and Management of Pre-Diabetes in the Continuum of Hyperglycemia—When Do the Risks of Diabetes Begin?* July 23. www.aace.com/meetings/consensus/hyperglycemia/hyperglycemia.pdf.

American Diabetes Association. n.d. Diabetes Dictionary. www.diabetes.org/diabetesdictionary.jsp?pageID=2&exitDictionaryTo.

American Diabetes Association. n.d. Frequently Asked Questions about Pre-Diabetes. www.diabetes.org/pre-diabetes/faq.jsp.

American Diabetes Association. n.d. Gestational Diabetes. www.diabetes.org/gestational-diabetes.jsp.

American Diabetes Association. n.d. *Every 21 Seconds, Someone Is Diagnosed with Diabetes. It's Time to Fight . . . Decide to Fight Diabetes.* I Decide Fact Sheet. www.diabetes.org/uedocuments/id-factsheet.pdf.

American Diabetes Association. 2008. Intense Blood Glucose Control Yields No Significant Effect on CVD Reduction in VA Diabetes Trial. June 8. www.diabetes.org/for-media/pr-intense-blood-glucose-control-yields-no-significant-effect-on-cvd-reduction.jsp.

American Diabetes Association. n.d. Make the Link: Diabetes, Heart Disease, and Stroke. www.diabetes.org/heart-disease-stroke.jsp.

American Diabetes Association. n.d. Oral Health and Oral Hygiene: Diabetes and Oral Health Problems. www.diabetes.org/type-1-diabetes/diabetes-and-oral-health-problems.jsp.

American Diabetes Association. n.d. Previously Unrecognized Harm of Intensified Glucose Lowering Reported in High Risk Patients with Type 2 Diabetes. www.diabetes.org/for-media/pr-previously-unrecognized-harm-of-intensified-glucose-lowering-reported-in-high-risk-patients-with-type-2-diabetes.jsp.

American Diabetes Association. n.d. Tight Diabetes Control. www.diabetes.org/type-2-diabetes/tight-control.jsp.

American Diabetes Association. 2008. World's Largest Trial of Intensive Glucose Control in Type 2 Diabetes Finds. June 6. www.diabetes.org/for-media/pr-worlds-largest-trial-of-intensive-glucose-control-in-type-2-diabetes-finds.jsp.

American Diabetes Association. n.d. Your Body's Well-Being. www.diabetes.org/type-2-diabetes/well-being.jsp.

Andrews, Michelle. 2008. A New Approach to Managing Diabetes. USNews.com, June 10. http://health.usnews.com/articles/health/diabetes/2008/06/10/a-new-approach-to-managing-diabetes.html.

Anonymous. 2008. Increased Risk of Advanced Breast Cancer Diagnosis in Overweight, Insulin Resistant Women. *Medical News Today*, July 8. www.medicalnewstoday.com/articles/114231.php.

Anonymous. 2008. Stand Up for a Bigger Calorie Burn. *Prevention*, May.

Anonymous. 2008. We Lost 14 Inches of Belly Fat. *Prevention*, February.

Beals, Jacquelyn K. 2008. VA Diabetes Trial Shows that Intensive Glucose Control Has Little Effect on Cardiovascular Risk. Theheart.org, June 17. www.theheart.org/article/875871.do

Brewer, Naomi, et al. 2008. A New Zealand Linkage Study Examining the Associations Between A1C Concentration and Mortality. *Diabetes Care* 31:1144-9.

Cefalu, William, T. 2008. Glycemic Targets and Cardiovascular Disease. *New England Journal of Medicine* 358(24):2633-5. http://content.nejm.org/cgi/content/full/358/24/2633.

Division of Diabetes Translation. 2008. Women Feel the Strain of the Diabetes Burden. CDC.gov, May 13. www.cdc.gov/Features/WomenAndDiabetes.

Feig, Denice S., et al. 2008. Risk of Development of Diabetes Mellitus after Diagnosis of Gestational Diabetes. *CMAJ: Canadian Medical Association Journal* 179(3):229-34.

Golden, Sherita Hill, et al. 2008. Examining a Bidirectional Association between Depressive Symptoms and Diabetes. *JAMA* 299(23):2751-9.

Janssen, Imke, et al. 2008. Menopause and the Metabolic Syndrome: The Study of Women's Health Across the Nation. *Archives of Internal Medicine* 168(14):1568-75.

Krumholz, Harlan M., and Thomas H. Lee. 2008. Redefining Quality—Implications of Recent Clinical Trials. *New England Journal of Medicine* 358(24):2537-9.

National Center for Chronic Disease Prevention and Health Promotion. 2008. Number of People with Diabetes Continues to Increase. CDC.gov, June 25. www.cdc.gov/Features/DiabetesFactSheet.

National Center on Birth Defects and Developmental Disabilities. 2008. Diabetes and Pregnancy. CDC.gov, May 5. www.cdc.gov/features/DiabetesPregnancy.

National Center on Birth Defects and Developmental Disabilities. 2005. Diabetes and Pregnancy Frequently Asked Questions. CDC.gov, October 5. www.cdc.gov/ncbddd/bd/diabetespregnancyfaqs.htm#whatcanhappentoababy.

National Diabetes Information Clearinghouse. 2008. *Diagnosis of Diabetes*. NIH Publication No. 09-4642, October. http://diabetes.niddk.nih.gov/dm/pubs/diagnosis.

National Heart, Lung, and Blood Institute. 2008. ACCORD Clinical Trial Publishes Results—A Therapeutic Strategy Targeting Blood Sugar to Near-Normal Levels Does Not Reduce Cardiovascular Events but Increases Mortality in Persons with Diabetes at High Risk. June 6. http://public.nhlbi.nih.gov/newsroom/home/GetPressRelease.aspx?id=2573.

National Heart, Lung, and Blood Institute. 2008. Questions and Answers: Action to Control Cardiovascular Risk in Diabetes (ACCORD) Trial. June 6. www.nhlbi.nih.gov/health/prof/heart/other/accord/q_a.htm.

New York City Department of Health and Mental Hygiene. n.d. *If You Have Diabetes, Know and Control Your ABCs*. www.nyc.gov/html/doh/downloads/pdf/csi/diabeteskit-pt-abc-goalsht.pdf.Parker-Pope, Tara. 2008. Diabetes: Underrated, Insidious and Deadly. *New York Times*, July 1. www.nytimes.com/2008/07/01/health/01well.html.

Phend, Crystal. 2008. ADA: Gum Disease Raises Diabetes Risk. MedPageToday.com, June 9. www.medpagetoday.com/MeetingCoverage/ADA/9761.

Rush University Medical Center. 2008. Testosterone Predominance Increases Prevalence of Metabolic Syndrome During the Menopausal Transition. July 28. www.rush.edu/webapps/MEDREL/servlet/NewsRelease?ID=1076.

Wild, Sarah, et al. 2004. Global Prevalence of Diabetes: Estimates for the Year 2000 and Projections for 2030. *Diabetes Care* 27(5):1047-53.

World Health Organization. 2006. *Obesity and Overweight*. Fact Sheet No. 311, September. www.who.int/mediacentre/factsheets/fs311/en/index.html.

CHAPTER 2

Alter, Cathy. 2006. Soda Fix: How One Family Kicked the Can. *Prevention*, August.

American Diabetes Association. n.d. Healthy Weight Loss. www.diabetes.org/weightloss-and-exercise/weightloss-healthy-weight-loss.jsp.

American Medical Association. 2008. AMA Finds High Fructose Syrup Unlikely to Be More Harmful to Health than Other Caloric Sweeteners. June 17. www.ama-assn.org/ama/pub/category/print/18691.html.

Anonymous. 2008. Outsmart Your Cravings. *Prevention*, February.

Buchwald, Henry, et al. 2004. Bariatric Surgery: A Systematic Review and Meta-Analysis. *JAMA* 292(14):1724-37.

Duke Medicine News and Communications. 2008. Weight Loss Plays Key Role in Diabetes Improvement Following Bariatric Surgery. June 19. www.dukehealth.org/HealthLibrary/News/10347.

Duncan, David Ewing. 2005. The Covert Plague. *Discover*, December. http://discovermagazine.com/2005/dec/diabetes-insulin-resistance.

Hayashi, Keiko, et al. 2003. Laughter Lowered the Increase in Postprandial Blood Glucose. *Diabetes Care* 26(5):1651-2.

Hudepohl, Dana. 2004. News that Can Save Your Life: The 8 Top Breakthroughs in Health and Wellness for 2004 that Can Bring Big Benefits to You and Your Family. Prevention.com, November 15. www.prevention.com/cda/article/news-that-can-save-your-life/901866263d803110VgnVCM20000012281eac____/health/healthy.lifestyle/wellness.

Kaufman, Francine Ratner. 2005. *Diabesity*. New York: Bantam.

Marchand, Lorraine H. 2002. Obesity and Diabetes. In *The Pima Indians: Pathfinders for Health*. National Institute of Diabetes and Digestive and Kidney Diseases, May. http://diabetes.niddk.nih.gov/dm/pubs/pima/obesity/obesity.htm.

National Women's Health Information Center. 2007. Minority Women's Health: Diabetes. December. www.4woman.gov/minority/americanindian/diabetes.cfm.

Pantsulaia, I., et al. 2007. Genetic and Environmental Determinants of Circulating Resistin Level in a Community-Based Sample. *European Journal of Endocrinology* 156(1):129-35.

Pizzorno, Joseph. 2007. Obesity: Nature vs. Nurture? WedMD.com, June 27. http://blogs.webmd.com/integrative-medicine-wellness/2007/06/obesity-nature-vs-nurture.html.

Pories, Walter J., et al. 1995. Who Would Have Thought It? An Operation Proves to Be the Most Effective Therapy for Adult-Onset Diabetes Mellitus. *Annals of Surgery* 222(3):339-52.

Schulz, Leslie O., et al. 2006. Effects of Traditional and Western Environments on Prevalence of Type 2 Diabetes in Pima Indians in Mexico and the U.S. *Diabetes Care* 29: 1866-71.

University of Maryland Medical Center. 2006. Weight Control and Diet. March 29. www.umm.edu/patiented/articles/what_biologic_medical_causes_of_obesity_000053_2.htm.

University of Michigan Health System. 2005. Bariatric Surgery for Severe Obesity. May 18. www.med.umich.edu/1libr/aha/aha_barisurg_crs.htm.

University of Virginia Health System. 2007. High Fructose Corn Syrup May Contribute to Diabetes Risk. October 25. www.healthsystem.virginia.edu/UVAHealth/news_diabeteshealth/0711dh.cfm.

US Department of Health and Human Services. 2000. HHS Targets Efforts on Diabetes. October 13. www.hhs.gov/news/press/2000pres/20001013a.html.

Winter, Dayna. 2005. Are These Foods Really Healthy? Prevention.com, January 6.

Zeratsky, Katherine. 2008. High-Fructose Corn Syrup: What Are the Concerns? MayoClinic.com, October 24. www.mayoclinic.com/health/high-fructose-corn-syrup/AN01588.

CHAPTER 3

American Heart Association. n.d. Metabolic Syndrome. www.americanheart.org/presenter.jhtml?identifier=4756.

Anonymous. 2007. Ingredient Alert! *Prevention*, September.

Anonymous. 2007. Test for Hidden Belly Fat. *Prevention*, July.

Balkau, Beverley, et al. 2007. International Day for the Evaluation of Abdominal Obesity (IDEA). *Circulation* 116:1942-51.

Collins, Karen. 2008. Nutrition Wise. June 16. www.aicr.org/site/News2?abbr=pr_hf_&page=NewsArticle&id=13478.

Contie, Vicki. 2008. Blood Protein Warns of Hidden Belly Fat and Disease Risk. July 23. www.nih.gov/news/research_matters/july2007/07232007bellyfat.htm.

Duke Medicine News and Communications. n.d. Visceral Fat Build-Up Is the High Cost of Inactivity. http://www.dukehealth.org/HealthLibrary/News/9238.

Graham, Timothy E., et al. 2006. Retinol-Binding Protein 4 and Insulin Resistance in Lean, Obese, and Diabetic Subjects. *New England Journal of Medicine* 354(24):2552-63.

Hsu, Chin-Lin, and Gow-Chin Yen. 2007. Effects of Capsaicin on Induction of Apoptosis and Inhibition of Adipogenesis in 3T3-L1 Cells. *Journal of Agricultural and Food Chemistry* 55(5):1730-6.

Janssen, Ian, et al. 2004. Waist Circumference and Not Body Mass Index Explains Obesity-Related Health Risk. *American Journal of Clinical Nutrition* 79(3):379-84.

Kaufman, Francine Ratner. 2005. *Diabesity*. New York: Bantam.

Klöting, Nora, et al. 2007. Serum Retinol-Binding Protein Is More Highly Expressed in Visceral than in Subcutaneous Adipose Tissue and Is a Marker of Intra-Abdominal Fat Mass. *Cell Metabolism* 6(1):79-87.

Lee, Crystal Man Ying, et al. 2008. Indices of Abdominal Obesity Are Better Discriminators of Cardiovascular Risk Factors than BMI: A Meta-Analysis. *Journal of Clinical Epidemiology* 61(7):646-53.

Meltzer, Rachel. 2007. Slimming Science: Visual Clues to Keep You from Overeating. Prevention.com, August 1. http://www.prevention.com/cda/article/slimming-science/b47dad415c214110VgnVCM20000012281eac_____/weight.loss/strategies.for.success/food.portions.

Mozaffarian, Dariush, et al. 2004. Dietary Intake of *Trans* Fatty Acids and Systemic Inflammation in Women. *American Journal of Clinical Nutrition* 79(4):606-12.

National Women's Health Information Center. 2008. Abdominal Fat Boosts Dementia Risk. March 26. www.4woman.gov/News/english/613903.htm.

Okosun, Ike S., et al. 2004. Abdominal Adiposity in U.S. Adults: Prevalence and Trends, 1960-2000. *Preventive Medicine* 39(1):197-206.

Rover, Elena. 2007. Good-Bye Belly Fat. Prevention.com, July 6. http://www.prevention.com/cda/article/good-bye-belly-fat/187dcb4b30d93110VgnVCM10000013281eac____/fitness/belly.abs/ab.exercises.

Vaccariello, Liz. 2008. *The Flat Belly Diet!* Emmaus, Pennsylvania: Rodale.

Weight-Control Information Network. 2007. Statistics Related to Overweight and Obesity. May. http://win.niddk.nih.gov/statistics.

Weight-Control Information Network. 2008. *Weight and Waist Measurement: Tools for Adults.* NIH Publication No. 04-5283, November. http://win.niddk.nih.gov/publications/tools.htm#circumf.

Whitmer, R. A., et al. 2008. Central Obesity and Increased Risk of Dementia More than Three Decades Later. *Neurology* 71(14):1057-64.

Yang, Kaiping, et al. 2008. Neuropeptide Y Is Produced in Visceral Adipose Tissue and Promotes Proliferation of Adipocyte Precursor Cells *via* the Y1 Receptor. *FASEB Journal* 22(7):2452-64.

Zhang, Cuilin, et al. 2008. Abdominal Obesity and the Risk of All-Cause, Cardiovascular, and Cancer Mortality: Sixteen Years of Follow-Up in US Women. *Circulation* 117(13):1658-67.

CHAPTER 4

Agricultural Research Service, US Department of Agriculture. 2005. Phytonutrient FAQs. April 8. www.ars.usda.gov/Aboutus/docs.htm?docid=4142.

American Diabetes Association. 2006. Nutrition Recommendations and Interventions for Diabetes—2006. *Diabetes Care* 29:2140-57.

American Heart Association. n.d. Fiber. www.americanheart.org/presenter.jhtml?identifier=4574.

Anonymous. 2007. All Hail Peanut Butter! *Prevention*, October.

Anonymous. n.d. Dietary Fiber. PreventiveHealthToday.com. www.preventivehealthtoday.com/prevention/d_fiber.html.

Anonymous. 2004. Is Couscous a Whole Grain? The Answer May Surprise You. Prevention.com, November 12.

Anonymous. 2001. The Definition of Dietary Fiber. *Cereal Foods World* 46(3):112-26.

Austin, Denise. 2005. Secrets to Slimming Down: Diet How-To's from Denise Austin's *Eat Carbs, Lose Weight.* Prevention.com, July 25.

Bente, Lisa, et al. 2008. *Dietary Fiber in the U.S. Food Supply.* US Department of Agriculture, Center for Nutrition Policy and Promotion, January.

Cleveland Clinic. n.d. The Fiber Lifestyle. http://my.clevelandclinic.org/healthy_living/nutrition/hic_the_fiber_lifestyle.aspx.

de Munter, Jeroen, et al. 2007. Whole Grain, Bran, and Germ Intake and Risk of Type 2 Diabetes: A Prospective Cohort Study and Systematic Review. *PLoS Medicine* 4(8):e261.

Defeat Diabetes Foundation. 2007. Vegetables Protect Against Diabetes. September 7. http://defeatdiabetes.org/news/view.asp?catid=3669&subcatid=&id=40049.

Dembinska-Kiec, A., et al. 2008. Antioxidant Phytochemicals Against Type 2 Diabetes. *British Journal of Nutrition* 99(E Suppl 1):ES109-17.

Editors of *Prevention.* 2008. *Diabetes Diet Cookbook.* Emmaus, Pennsylvania: Rodale.

Harding, Anne-Helen, et al. 2008. Plasma Vitamin C Level, Fruit and Vegetable Consumption, and the Risk of New-Onset Type 2 Diabetes Mellitus. *Archives of Internal Medicine* 168(14):1493-9.

Harvard School of Public Health. n.d. Fiber: Start Roughing It! www.hsph.harvard.edu/nutritionsource/what-should-you-eat/fiber-full-story/index.html#diabetes.

Harvard School of Public Health. 2002. Women Who Eat Nuts or Peanut Butter Regularly Significantly Reduce Their Risk for Type 2 Diabetes. November 26. www.hsph.harvard.edu/news/press-releases/archives/2002-releases/press11262002.html.

Holt, S. H., et al. 1999. The Effects of High-Carbohydrate vs High-Fat Breakfasts on Feelings of Fullness and Alertness, and Subsequent Food Intake. *International Journal of Food Science and Nutrition* 50(1):13-28.

Howarth, N. C., et al. 2001. Dietary Fiber and Weight Regulation. *Nutrition Review* 59(5):129-39.

International Food Information Council. 2004. Focus on Fiber: Why Roughage Still Warrants Our Attention. *Food Insight*, July/August.

Katcher, H. I., et al. 2008. The Effects of a Whole Grain-Enriched Hypocaloric Diet on Cardiovascular Disease Risk Factors in Men and Women with Metabolic Syndrome. *American Journal of Clinical Nutrition* 87(1):79-90.

Mayo Clinic. 2007. Dietary Fiber: An Essential Part of a Healthy Diet. November 30. www.mayoclinic.com/health/fiber/NU00033.

McVeigh, Gloria. 2006. Boost Fiber, Lower Fat: Two Crucial Numbers for Losing Weight. Prevention.com, February 3.

National Fiber Council. n.d. What Fiber Can Do for You. www.nationalfibercouncil.org/af_whatfiber.shtml.

National Institute on Aging. 2009. Dietary Supplements. February 19. www.nia.nih.gov/HealthInformation/Publications/supplements.htm.

National Library of Medicine. 2007. Soluble vs. Insoluble Fiber. In Medline Plus Medical Encyclopedia. January 2. www.nlm.nih.gov/medlineplus/ency/article/002136.htm.

Papazian, Ruth. 1997. Bulking Up Fiber's Healthful Reputation: More Benefits of "Roughage" Are Discovered. *FDA Consumer*, July-August.

Prevention. n.d. Fiber Up Food Finder. www.prevention.com/fiberup.

Rasich, Paula. 2004. Top 10 Cholesterol-Fighting Foods. Prevention.com, October 19.

Reichenberger McIndoo, Heidi. 2008. Listen and Lose: Tuning In to Your Normal Hunger Signals Will Ensure that You Never Overeat Again. *Prevention*, April.

Salmeron, J., et al. 1997. Dietary Fiber, Glycemic Load, and Risk of Non-Insulin-Dependent Diabetes Mellitus in Women. *JAMA* 277(6):472-7.

Schulze, Matthias B., et al. 2007. Fiber and Magnesium Intake and Incidence of Type 2 Diabetes. *Archives of Internal Medicine* 167:956-65.

US Department of Health and Human Services and US Department of Agriculture. 2008. Chapter 7: Carbohydrates. In *Dietary Guidelines for Americans, 2005*. July 9. www.health.gov/dietaryguidelines/dga2005/document/html/chapter7.htm.

US Food and Drug Administration. 2003. FDA Collaborates with AOAC to Gain Approval of Peanut Test Kits for Food Products. October 30. www.fda.gov/bbs/topics/ANSWERS/2003/ANS01258.html.

Villegas, Raquel, et al. 2008. Legume and Soy Food Intake and the Incidence of Type 2 Diabetes in the Shanghai Women's Health Study. *American Journal of Clinical Nutrition* 87(1):162-7.

Welland, Diane. 2006. Fiber: The New Face of Weight Management. FoodProductDesign.com, November 7. http://www.foodproductdesign.com/articles/691nutrinotes.html.

CHAPTER 5

Anderson, J., et al. 2008. Diet and Hypertension. August. www.ext.colostate.edu/pubs/foodnut/09318.html.

Anonymous. 2007. Double Your Calcium Benefits: Bone Building Supplements May Also Keep Your Cholesterol in Check. Prevention.com, March 27.

Anonymous. 2008. Exercise Regularly? Take Calcium. *Prevention*, May.

Anonymous. 2005. How Much Vitamin D Is Enough? *UC Berkeley Wellness Letter*, October.

Anonymous. 2005. Recipe for Health: Diet Is a Key Ingredient in Preventing Heart Disease, Diabetes, and Osteoporosis. Prevention.com, February 8.

Bonds, Denise E., et al. 2006. Risk of Fracture in Women with Type 2 Diabetes: The Women's Health Initiative Observational Study. *Journal of Clinical Endocrinology & Metabolism* 91(9):3404-10.

Caan, Bette, et al. 2007. Calcium Plus Vitamin D Supplementation and the Risk of Postmenopausal Weight Gain. *Archives of Internal Medicine* 167:893-902.

Chiu, Ken C., et al. 2004. Hypovitaminosis D Is Associated with Insulin Resistance and Beta Cell Dysfunction. *American Journal of Clinical Nutrition* 79(5):820-5.

Colorado State University Extension. 2007. Healthy Heart Program Updates. *Healthy Heart Beats* 29(4):1-12.

Duesing, Bill. n.d. The Calcium Cycle. Yale-New Haven Teachers Institute. www.yale.edu/ynhti/curriculum/units/1985/7/85.07.08.x.html.

Gonzalez, A. J., et al. 2006. Calcium Intake and 10-Year Weight Change in Middle-Aged Adults. *Journal of the American Diabetes Association* 106(7):1066-73.

Higdon, Jane. 2005. Preventing Osteoporosis through Diet and Lifestyle. Linus Pauling Institute Spring/Summer 2005 Research Report, May. http://lpi.oregonstate.edu/ss05/osteoporosis.html.

Higdon, Jane. 2008. Vitamin D. In Micronutrient Information Center, Linus Pauling Institute, November 7. http://lpi.oregonstate.edu/infocenter/vitamins/vitaminD.

Holick, Michael F. 2004. Sunlight and Vitamin D for Bone Health and Prevention of Autoimmune Diseases, Cancers, and Cardiovascular Disease. *American Journal of Clinical Nutrition* 80(6):1678S-88S.

Holick, Michael F. 2007. Vitamin D Deficiency. *New England Journal of Medicine* 357:266-81.

Jaret, Peter. 2006. Vitamins: What to Take, What to Eat. Prevention.com, September 28.

John Hancock Center for Physical Activity and Nutrition. n.d. Safe Sun Exposure. http://jhcpan.nutrition.tufts.edu/consumers/sun_exposure.html.

Loos, Ruth J. F., et al. 2004. Calcium Intake Is Associated with Adiposity in Black and White Men and White Women of the HERITAGE Family Study. *Journal of Nutrition* 134:1772-8.

March, David. 2008. Low Vitamin D Levels Pose a Large Threat to Health, Researchers Say. Johns Hopkins University. *Gazette*, 37(42).

National Institutes of Health Office of Dietary Supplements. n.d. Dietary Supplement Fact Sheet: Calcium. http://dietary-supplements.info.nih.gov/factsheets/calcium.asp.

National Institutes of Health Office of Dietary Supplements. n.d. Dietary Supplement Fact Sheet: Vitamin D. http://ods.od.nih.gov/factsheets/vitamind.asp.

National Osteoporosis Foundation. n.d. Fast Facts on Osteoporosis. www.nof.org/osteoporosis/diseasefacts.htm.

National Osteoporosis Foundation. n.d. What You Should Know about Calcium. www.nof.org/prevention/calcium2.htm.

Pittas, A. G., et al. 2006. Vitamin D and Calcium Intake in Relation to Type 2 Diabetes in Women. *Diabetes Care* 29(3):650-6.

Pittas, Anastassios G., et al. 2007. The Role of Vitamin D and Calcium in Type 2 Diabetes. A Systematic Review and Meta-Analysis. *Journal of Clinical Endocrinology & Metabolism* 92(6):2017-29.

Prevention.com. 2004. Calcium. In Health/Conditions & Treatments/Osteoporosis. Prevention.com, October 29. www.prevention.com/cda/article/calcium/9101323b0b803110VgnVCM20000012281eac____/health/conditions.treatments/osteoporosis.

Robien, Kim. 2008. The Importance of Vitamin D. University of Minnesota School of Public Health, May 7. http://blog.lib.umn.edu/sphpod/news/2008/05/the_importance_of_vitamin_d.html.

Schrager, Sarina. 2005. Dietary Calcium Intake and Obesity. *Journal of the American Board of Family Medicine* 18(3):205-10.

Thorpe, Matthew P., et al. 2008. A Diet High in Protein, Dairy, and Calcium Attenuates Bone Loss over Twelve Months of Weight Loss and Maintenance Relative to a Conventional High-Carbohydrate Diet in Adults. *Journal of Nutrition* 138:1096-1100.

Tyler, C. V., et al. 2008. Barriers to Supplemental Calcium Use Among Women in Suburban Family Practice: A Report from the Cleveland Clinic Ambulatory Research Network (CleAR-eN). *Journal of the American Board of Family Medicine* 21(4):293-9.

University of Michigan Health System. 2004. Mighty Vitamin D Is Heart Smart. May 1. www.med.umich.edu/opm/newspage/2004/hmvitamind.htm.

University of Pittsburgh Medical Center. 2003. Calcium Facts. www.upmc.com/HealthAtoZ/patienteducation/Documents/CalciumFacts.pdf.

Upreti, P., et al. 2002. Estimation and Fortification of Vitamin D3 in Pasteurized Process Cheese. *Journal of Dairy Science* 85(12):3173-81.

US Department of Health and Human Services. 2006. *Your Guide to Lowering Blood Pressure with DASH*. NIH Publication No. 06-4082, April. www.nhlbi.nih.gov/health/public/heart/hbp/dash/new_dash.pdf

US Department of Health and Human Services and US Department of Agriculture. 2008. Appendix B: Food Sources of Selected Nutrients. In *Dietary Guidelines for Americans, 2005*. July 9. www.health. gov/DIETARYGUIDELINES/dga2005/document/html/AppendixB.htm.

Wang, Thomas, et al. 2008. Vitamin D Deficiency and Risk of Cardiovascular Disease. *Circulation* 117:503-11.

Yale University School of Medicine. 2007. The Heart of Diabetes. In *Diabetes 2007* 16(2):1-3. http:// cme.yale.edu/diabetes/2007/EASD-Newsletter-2-Sept19.pdf

Yeager, Selene. 2006. Sharpen Calcium's Weight Loss Edge: Adding Dietary Supplements May Slow Body Fat Storage. Prevention.com, October 31.

Zemel, Michael B., et al. 2004. Calcium and Dairy Acceleration of Weight and Fat Loss During Energy Restriction in Obese Adults. *Obesity Research* 12(4):582-90.

Zemel, Michael. 2004. *The Calcium Key: The Revolutionary Diet Discovery that Will Help You Lose Weight Faster*. Hoboken, New Jersey: Wiley and Sons.

Zeratsky, Katherine. 2008. Calcium Supplements: Which Type Is Best? MayoClinic.com, November 15. www.mayoclinic.com/health/calcium-supplements/AN00964.

CHAPTER 6

American Diabetes Association. n.d. Insulin Therapy Improves Blood Fats. www.diabetes.org/ diabetes-research/summaries/hayashi-insulin-therapy.jsp.

American Diabetes Association. n.d. Specific Types of Fat. www.diabetes.org/nutrition-and-recipes/ nutrition/foodlabel/specific-fats.jsp.

American Heart Association. n.d. Fish and Omega-3 Fatty Acids. www.americanheart.org/presenter. jhtml?identifier=4632.

Anonymous. 2005. Desserts that Stop Heart Attacks. Prevention.com, February 24.

Anonymous. 2007. Eggs on a Mission: With a Little Help, Nature's Most Simple Food Takes on Super-hero Status. Prevention.com.

Anonymous. 2007. Fish for the Best Oil: Smart Ways to Get Your Daily Dose of Omega-3s. Prevention. com, March 27.

Anonymous. 2004. Mother Nature's Cholesterol Fixes: Natural Options to Assist in Your War Against Cholesterol. Prevention.com, September 27.

Anonymous. 2008. The Final Word on Fish. *Prevention*, February.

Bang, H. O., et al. 1980. The Composition of the Eskimo Food in North Western Greenland. *American Journal of Clinical Nutrition* 33:2657-61.

Campos, Hannia, et al. 2008. a-Linolenic Acid and Risk of Nonfatal Acute Myocardial Infarction. *Circulation* 118:339-45.

Carpentier, Yvon A., et al. 2006. n-3 Fatty Acids and the Metabolic Syndrome. *American Journal of Clinical Nutrition* 83(Suppl):1499S-504S.

Centers for Disease Control and Prevention. 2008. Nutrition for Everyone: Dietary Fat. December 3. www.cdc.gov/nutrition/everyone/basics/fat/index.html.

Chillot, Rick. 2004. The 3 Supplements You Don't Know About (but Probably Need). Prevention.com, September 29.

De Caterina, Raffaele, et al. 2007. n-3 Fatty Acids in the Treatment of Diabetic Patients. *Diabetes Care* 30:1012-26.

Gordon, Serena. 2008. Fondness for Fish Keeps Japanese Hearts Healthy. Healthfinder.gov, July 29. www.healthfinder.gov/news/newsstory.aspx?docid=617815.

Graedon, Joe, and Teresa Graedon. 2008. The Sea's Heart Secret: Add This Healthy Fat to Your Diet Today. *Prevention*, June.

Hartweg, Janine, et al. 2008. Omega-3 Polyunsaturated Fatty Acids (PUFA) for Type 2 Diabetes Mellitus. *Cochrane Database of Systematic Reviews*, Issue 1, Article No. CD003205.

Horovitz, Bruce. 2007. Omega-3 Pours into Cereal, Orange Juice, Eggs, Pet Food. USAToday.com, January 2. http://www.usatoday.com/money/industries/health/2007-01-01-omega-3-usat_x.htm.

Kabir, Morvarid, et al. 2007. Treatment for 2 Mo with n-3 Polyunsaturated Fatty Acids Reduces Adiposity and Some Atherogenic Factors but Does Not Improve Insulin Sensitivity in Women with Type 2 Diabetes: A Randomized Controlled Study. *American Journal of Clinical Nutrition* 86(6):1670-9.

Kim, Hye-Kyeong, et al. 2006. Docosahexaenoic Acid Inhibits Adipocyte Differentiation and Induces Apoptosis in 3T3-L1 Preadipocytes. *Journal of Nutrition* 136:2965-9.

Knous, Barbara Lohse. 2001. Omega-3s: Fats You Should and Can Eat. Kansas State University, August. www.oznet.ksu.edu/library/fntr2/mf2519.pdf.

Loecher, Barbara. 2004. Fish During Pregnancy? An Answer to All of the Conflicting Information Surrounding Pregnancy and Safe Seafood. Prevention.com, November 8.

Mayo Clinic. 2008. Omega-3 Fatty Acids, Fish Oil, Alpha-Linolenic Acid. March 1. www.mayoclinic.com/health/fish-oil/NS_patient-fishoil.

McKinley Heath Center, University of Illinois at Urbana-Champaign. 2006. Omega-3 Fatty Acids. November 17. www.mckinley.uiuc.edu/Handouts/omega-3_fatty_acids.htm.

McLaughlin, J., et al. 2005. Adipose Tissue Triglyceride Fatty Acids and Atherosclerosis in Alaska Natives and Non-Natives. *Atherosclerosis* 181(2):353-62.

McVeigh, Gloria. 2005. Got Diabetes? Eat Walnuts. Prevention.com, December 7.

McVeigh, Gloria. 2005. Prevent Artery Gunk: Your Heart Loves the Fats in Walnuts. Prevention.com, September 16.

McVeigh, Gloria. 2005. Smart Alternatives to Fish: Eating Nuts and Seeds Can Yield Heart-Health Benefits, Too. Prevention.com, March 23.

Mori, Trevor A., et al. 1999. Dietary Fish as a Major Component of a Weight-Loss Diet: Effect on Serum Lipids, Glucose, and Insulin Metabolism in Overweight Hypertensive Subjects. *American Journal of Clinical Nutrition* 70:817-25.

Morris, Martha Clare. 2003. Consumption of Fish and n-3 Fatty Acids and Risk of Incident Alzheimer Disease. *Archives of Neurology* 60:940-6.

National Oceanic and Atmospheric Administration Fisheries Service. 2007. U.S. Seafood Consumption Declines Slightly in 2005; Dutch Harbor/Unalaska and New Bedford Remain Top U.S. Fishing Ports. *FishNews*, February 6.

Parker, Gordon, et al. 2006. Omega-3 Fatty Acids and Mood Disorders. *American Journal of Psychiatry* 163:969-78.

Satoh, Noriko, et al. 2007. Purified Eicosapentaenoic Acid Reduces Small Dense LDL, Remnant Lipoprotein Particles, and C-Reactive Protein in Metabolic Syndrome. *Diabetes Care* 30(1):144-6.

Sekikawa, A., et al. 2008. Marine-Derived n-3 Fatty Acids and Atherosclerosis in Japanese, Japanese-American, and White Men: A Cross-Sectional Study. *Journal of the American College of Cardiology* 52(6):417-24.

Theodoratou, Evropi, et al. 2007. Dietary Fatty Acids and Colorectal Cancer: A Case-Control Study. *American Journal of Epidemiology* 166(2):181-95.

Webb, Densie. 2006. The Heart-Healthy Fats: Load Up on the "Good" Fats that Help Prevent High Cholesterol and Heart Disease. Prevention.com, October 10.

Weil, Andrew. 2006. Ask Dr. Weil: The Anti-Inflammation Diet. Prevention.com, September 20.

Winnicki, Mikolaj. 2002. Fish-Rich Diet, Leptin, and Body Mass. *Circulation* 106:289.

CHAPTER 7

American Heart Association. n.d. Mediterranean Diet. www.americanheart.org/presenter.jhtml?identifier=4644.

Anonymous. 2007. 8 Secrets of the Naturally Slim. Prevention.com, March 27.

Anonymous. 2006. Adults and Teens Who Eat Beans Weigh Less. *Medical News Today,* April 7. www.medicalnewstoday.com/articles/40935.php.

Ansel, Karen. 2008. The Right Way to Lose Weight After 40. *Prevention*, January.

Doheny, Kathleen. 2008. Keep a Food Diary, Lose Twice as Much Weight. Healthfinder.gov, July 8. www.healthfinder.gov/news/newsstory.aspx?docID=617178HealthDay.

Editors of Prevention. 2008. *Diabetes Diet Cookbook*. Emmaus, Pennsylvania: Rodale.

Gerbstadt, Christine. 2008. Summer Body Diet Plan. *Prevention*, May.

Lemanski, Paul E. n.d. The Non-Medicated Life: Eating Out Heart Healthy. Center for Preventive Medicine and Cardiovascular Health. www.centerforpreventivemedicine.com/article12.htm.

Martínez-González, M. Á., et al. 2008. Adherence to Mediterranean Diet and Risk of Developing Diabetes: Prospective Cohort Study. *British Medical Journal* 336:1348-51.

McVeigh, Gloria. 2006. Handy Portion Control: Cut Calories by Keeping Close Tabs on How Much You're Eating—No Matter Where You Are. Prevention.com, September 7.

National Women's Health Information Center. 2008. Frequently Asked Questions: Heart Healthy Eating. January 1. www.womenshealth.gov/faq/heart-healthy-eating.cfm.

Noe Pagan, Camille. 2008. Good Enough Guide to Health. *Prevention*, July.

Reichenberger McIndoo, Heidi. 2008. Listen and Lose: Tuning In to Your Normal Hunger Signals Will Ensure that You Never Overeat Again. *Prevention*, April.

Westman, Eric C. 2004. Obesity and the Pathophysiology of Storage Metabolism. In *The Impact of Controlled-Carbohydrate Nutritional Approaches on Weight and Health*. MedscapeCME, August 6. www.medscape.com/viewarticle/484768_7.

CHAPTER 9

American College of Sports Medicine. 2008. Studies Define Type 2 Diabetes Risk Factors in Women, Adolescents. May 29. www.acsm.org/AM/Template.cfm?Section=Home_Page&TEMPLATE=/CM/ContentDisplay.cfm&CONTENTID=10124.

American Council on Exercise. n.d. Pilates Primer. www.acefitness.org/fitfacts/fitfacts_display.aspx?itemid=56.

Anonymous. 2006. Dance It Off. Prevention.com, January 3.

Anonymous. 2008. Fast-Track Your Fat Loss! *Prevention*, January.

Anonymous. 2008. Get Twice the Post-Exercise Bliss: Feel Happier, Less Stressed, and More Revitalized with Each Workout. *Prevention*, July.

Anonymous. 2008. Mind Tricks for a Better Body: Think Your Way Fit During Your Next Workout. *Prevention*, June.

Anonymous. 2005. Pumping Iron to Prevent Diabetes: Build Up Your Body to Knock Down Blood Sugar. Prevention.com, November 28.

Anonymous. 2005. Shoe-Shopping Strategies: How to Know If the Shoe Fits. Prevention.com, May 18.

Anonymous. 2008. The Best Walking Shoe for You. *Prevention*, April.

Anonymous. 2007. The Energy Workout. *Prevention*, December.

Anonymous. 2005. Walk Longer and Stronger: The Proper Form Will Help You Reach Your Fitness Goals and Keep You Injury-Free. Prevention.com, May 18.

Anonymous. 2007. Walk Off Pounds—At Work. Prevention.com, July 6.

Anonymous. 2005. When to Get New Shoes. Prevention.com, May 18.

Bravata, Dena M., et al. 2007. Using Pedometers to Increase Physical Activity and Improve Health: A Systematic Review. *JAMA* 298(19):2296-304.

Centers for Disease Control and Prevention. 2008. Growing Stronger: Strength Training for Older Adults. December 3. www.cdc.gov/physicalactivity/growingstronger/index.html.

Centers for Disease Control and Prevention. 2008. Physical Activity for Everyone. November 5. www.cdc.gov/physicalactivity/everyone/guidelines/index.html.

Drozd, Shelly. 2005. 10-Minute Water Workout: Splash the Pounds Away with This Fun Routine. Prevention.com, August 22.

Duke Medicine News and Communications. 2007. Moderate Exercise Cuts Rate of Metabolic Syndrome. December 18. www.dukehealth.org/HealthLibrary/News/10205.

Eves, Neil, and Ronald C. Plotnikoff. 2006. Resistance Training and Type 2 Diabetes: Considerations for Implementation at the Population Level. *Diabetes Care* 29:1933-41.

Harvard Medical School. 2007. Abdominal Fat and What to Do About It. In *Family Health Guide*, February. www.health.harvard.edu/fhg/updates/Abdominal-fat-and-what-to-do-about-it.shtml.

Heaner, Martica. 2006. 6 Moves to Shrink Your Belly: A Pilates Workout that Firms and Flattens—Fast. Prevention.com, November 14.

Jakicic, John M. 2008. Effect of Exercise on 24-Month Weight Loss Maintenance in Overweight Women. *Archives of Internal Medicine* 168(14):1550-9.

Kosecki, Danielle. 2008. Reduce Diabetes Risk in 7 Days: Reverse Early Symptoms of This Disease in One Week. *Prevention*, July.

Kosecki, Danielle. 2008. 10-Minute Energy Fix: Studies Show that a Brisk Walk Can Boost Your Momentum. *Prevention*, July.

McGinnis, Marianne. 2008. Feel-Fabulous Walking Tricks: Use Motivating Mantras to Hit Your Stride. *Prevention*, January.

McGinnis, Marianne. 2008. Warm Up to a Better Workout. *Prevention*, February.

National Diabetes Information Clearinghouse. 2008. *What I Need to Know about Physical Activity and Diabetes*. NIH Publication No. 08-5180, March. http://diabetes.niddk.nih.gov/dm/pubs/physical_ez.

Robertson, Sarah. 2005. Stick to Your Walk: With These Can't-Miss Tips, You Won't Skip a Workout. Prevention.com, January 5.

Rush University Medical Center. 2008. Strength Training: A Smart Move for Women. Summer. www.rush.edu/rumc/page-1209563803187.html.

Schmitz, Kathryn H., et al. 2007. Strength Training and Adiposity in Premenopausal Women: Strong, Healthy, and Empowered Study. *American Journal of Clinical Nutrition* 86(3):566-72.

Sigal, Ronald, et al. 2007. Effects of Aerobic Training, Resistance Training, or Both on Glycemic Control in Type 2 Diabetes: A Randomized Trial. *Annals of Internal Medicine* 147(6):357-69.

Sigal, Ronald, et al. 2006. Physical Activity/Exercise and Type 2 Diabetes: A Consensus Statement from the American Diabetes Association. *Diabetes Care* 29:1433-8.

Spilner, Maggie. 2001. Choosing Shoes: Take Care of Your Feet and They'll Take Care of You. Prevention.com, January 3.

Spilner, Maggie. 2004. Lose an Extra 10 Lb a Year with This Workout. Prevention.com, October 30.

Spilner, Maggie. 2005. Lower Your Blood Sugar by Walking: Here's the Ultimate Walking Workout for People with Diabetes. Prevention.com, May 28.

Spilner, Maggie. 2004. Sole Satisfaction—Socks! Prevention.com, October 30.

Stanten, Michele. 2005. Boogie Off Your Butt: Try the Hottest New Workout: Dance Classes. Prevention.com, November 30.

University of Michigan Health System. 2006. *Physical Activity for Life!* Health Promotion Division, MFit Employee Wellness Program e-mail-based newsletter, February.

Watts, Merritt. 2007. Lose 5 Pounds—Automatically: Step Up Your Daily Distance for a Slimmer Waistline. *Prevention*, November.

WebMD. 2007. Strength Training and Diabetes. August 1. http://diabetes.webmd.com/strength-training-diabetes.

Weight-Control Information Network. 2006. Physical Activity and Weight Control. November. http://win.niddk.nih.gov/publications/physical.htm#Strength_Training.

Yeager, Selene. 2007. Breakthrough Belly Flattening Plan. Prevention.com, March 23.

Yeager, Selene. 2005. Walking Shoe Primer: What You Should Know When You Go Shopping for These Athletic Shoes. Prevention.com, May 18.

CHAPTER 10

Altshul, Sara. 2007. Outsmart Jet Lag: The Best Traditional and Natural Remedies to Feel Energized All Vacation Long. Prevention.com, June.

Altshul, Sara. 2006. Sweet Scent of Sleep: Whiff Lavender for a More Restful Slumber. Prevention.com, June 14.

Anonymous. 2006. Sleep Like a Baby: Follow This Advice to Get Better Rest and Wake Up Refreshed. Prevention.com, September 21.

Babu, Ambika, et al. 2005. Type 2 Diabetes, Glycemic Control, and Continuous Positive Airway Pressure in Obstructive Sleep Apnea. *Archives of Internal Medicine* 165:447-52.

Bauman, Alisa. 2004. Secondhand Snoring: Noisy Sleep Stealer. Prevention.com, September 23.

Bender, Michele. 2008. Good Morning! Start Every Day Healthy with Our 3-Step Plan. *Prevention*, February.

Breus, Michael J. 2001. 12 Tips for Better Sleep in Bad Times. WebMD.com, October 4. www.webmd.com/news/20011004/12-tips-better-sleep-troubled-times.

Claps, Frank. 2006. Snooze Solutions: Psychotherapy Treatment Found to Improve Sleep. Prevention.com, September 28.

Crook, Thomas. 2008. Snooze It or Lose It: A Special Kind of Sleep Is Key to Learning and Memory. *Prevention*, May.

Doheny, Kathleen. 2008. Can't Sleep? Adjust the Temperature. *WebMD the Magazine,* March 31. www.webmd.com/sleep-disorders/features/cant-sleep-adjust-the-temperature.

FamilyDoctor.org. 2007. CPAP Devices for Sleep Apnea. June. http://familydoctor.org/online/famdocen/home/seniors/common-older/791.html.

Harsch, Igor, et al. 2004. Continuous Positive Airway Pressure Treatment Rapidly Improves Insulin Sensitivity in Patients with Obstructive Sleep Apnea Syndrome. *American Journal of Respiratory and Critical Care Medicine* 169:156-62.

Goldberg, Joan Rachel. n.d. Helping Yourself to a Good Night's Sleep. www.sleepfoundation.org/site/c.huIXKjM0IxF/b.2421167/k.238/Helping_Yourself_to_a_Good_Nights_Sleep.htm.

Hennen, Leah. 2007. Get Your Back in Business: 16 Ways to Fix Your House So You Never Hurt Again. Prevention.com.

Hettinger, Ann. 2007. Rest Assured: How to Sleep Soundly Tonight—And Wake Up Slimmer, Happier, and Healthier. *Prevention*, December.

Jaffe, Suzan. 2005. Partners and Sleep Problems. www.sleepfoundation.org/site/apps/nlnet/content3.aspx?c=huIXKjM0IxF&b=2427705&content_id=%7B233D630B-118D-4417-AAA7-5F2FE25F3A83%7D&notoc=1.

Kalish, Nancy. 2008. Light Up Your Health: The Brilliant New Strategy for Losing Weight, Sleeping Better, and Fighting Disease. *Prevention*, April.

Kozak, Diane. 2001. How to Catch a Sleep Thief: Even Your Doctor Can Miss This Sneaky Cause of Daytime Fatigue. Prevention.com, November 9.

National Center for Health Statistics. n.d. Fast Stats A to Z: Overweight. CDC.gov. http://www.cdc.gov/nchs/fastats/overwt.htm.

National Heart, Lung, and Blood Institute. 2008. Sleep Apnea. February. www.nhlbi.nih.gov/health/dci/Diseases/SleepApnea/SleepApnea_WhatIs.html.

National Institute of Neurological Disorders and Stroke. 2007. *Restless Legs Syndrome Fact Sheet.* NIH Publication No. 01-4847, December 11. www.ninds.nih.gov/disorders/restless_legs/detail_restless_legs.htm.

National Sleep Foundation. n.d. Healthy Sleep Tips. www.sleepfoundation.org/site/c.huIXKjM0IxF/b.2417321/k.BAF0/Healthy_Sleep_Tips.htm.

National Sleep Foundation. n.d. The Sleep Environment. www.sleepfoundation.org/site/c.huIXKjM0IxF/b.2422597/k.BA20/Sleep_Environment.htm.

National Sleep Foundation. 2008. 2008 Poll Stats: A Day in the Life of a Typical American Worker. www.sleepfoundation.org/site/c.huIXKjM0IxF/b.3934129/k.31D9/Poll_Stats.htm.

National Women's Health Information Center. 2006. Frequently Asked Questions: Insomnia. May 1. www.4woman.gov/faq/insomnia.cfm.

National Women's Health Resource Center. 2007. Sleep Disorders. December 11. www.healthywomen.org/healthtopics/sleepdisorders.

Schoenborn, Charlotte A., and Patricia F. Adams. 2008. Sleep Duration as a Correlate of Smoking, Alcohol Use, Leisure-Time Physical Inactivity, and Obesity Among Adults: United States, 2004-2006. National Center for Health Statistics, July 31. www.cdc.gov/nchs/products/pubs/pubd/hestats/sleep04-06/sleep04-06.htm.

Shaw, N., et al. 2008. Sleep-Disordered Breathing and Type 2 Diabetes: A Report from the International Diabetes Federation Taskforce on Epidemiology and Prevention. *Diabetes Research and Clinical Practice* 81(1):2-12.

Silverberg, Donald S., and Adrian Iaina. 2002. Treating Obstructive Sleep Apnea Improves Essential Hypertension and Quality of Life. *American Family Physician* 65:229-36.

Taheri, Shahrad, et al. 2004. Short Sleep Duration Is Associated with Reduced Leptin, Elevated Ghrelin, and Increased Body Mass Index. *PLoS Medicine* 1(3):e62.

Tuma, Rabiya S. 2007. Sleep Apnea Increases Risk for Diabetes. May 22. Medscape Medical News, May 22. www.medscape.com/viewarticle/557049.

University of Chicago. 2008. Lack of Deep Sleep May Increase Risk of Type 2 Diabetes. January 2. www-news.uchicago.edu/releases/07/071231.sleep.shtml.

University of Chicago Medical Center. 2004. Sleep Loss Boosts Appetite, May Encourage Weight Gain. December 6. www.uchospitals.edu/news/2004/20041206-sleep.html.

US Department of Health and Human Services. 2007. One-Third of Diabetics Have Sleep Apnea. Men's Newsletter, November 19. http://www.healthfinder.gov/newsletters/men111907.asp#1695010.

Zee, Phyllis C. 2005. Diabetes and Sleep Quality. *Medscape Family Medicine/Primary Care* 7(2). www.medscape.com/viewarticle/515398.

CHAPTER 11

Altshul, Sara. 2004. Calm Down Any Time, Any Place: Meditate and Calm Your Mind. Prevention.com, October 19.

Balzer, Jan, et al. 2008. Sustained Benefits in Vascular Function Through Flavanol-Containing Cocoa in Medicated Diabetic Patients: A Double-Masked, Randomized, Controlled Trial. *Journal of the American College of Cardiology* 51:2141-9.

Eriksson, A. K., et al. 2008. Psychological Distress and Risk of Pre-Diabetes and Type 2 Diabetes in a Prospective Study of Swedish Middle-Aged Men and Women. *Diabetes Medicine* 25(7):834-42.

Evans, Julie. 2005. 8 Ways to Clobber the Big Headache: New Breakthroughs Can Stop the Godzilla of Headaches in Its Tracks. Prevention.com, May 24.

Mayo Clinic. 2008. Stress: Win Control Over the Stress in Your Life. September 12. www.mayoclinic.com/print/stress/SR00001/METHOD=print.

Melamed, Samuel, et al. 2006. Burnout and Risk of Type 2 Diabetes: A Prospective Study of Apparently Healthy Employed Persons. *Psychosomatic Medicine* 68:863-9.

Mindful Living Center. n.d. Mindfulness-Based Stress Reduction Program. www.mindfuliving.org/MBSR.html.

National Library of Medicine. 2009. Stress. In Medline Plus Health Topics. February 20. www.nlm.nih.gov/medlineplus/stress.html.

National Women's Health Resource Center. Stress. December 1. www.healthywomen.org/healthtopics/stress.

Neimark, Neil F. The Fight or Flight Response. www.thebodysoulconnection.com/EducationCenter/fight.html.

Rosenbaum, Jerrold F., and Jennifer M. Covino. 2005. Stress and Resilience: Implications for Depression and Anxiety. *Medscape Psychiatry and Mental Health,* 10(2). www.medscape.com/viewarticle/518761.

Rosenzweig, Steven, et al. 2007. Mindfulness-Based Stress Reduction Is Associated with Improved Glycemic Control in Type 2 Diabetes Mellitus: A Pilot Study. *Alternative Therapies in Health and Medicine* 13(5):36-8.

Smith, Suzanna, and Joe Pergola. 2002. *Stress Management Strategies.* Fact Sheet HE-2089, Florida Cooperative Extension Service, April. www.cdc.gov/nasd/docs/d000001-d000100/d000008/d000008.html.

Surwit, Richard S. 2004. *The Mind/Body Diabetes Revolution.* New York: Free Press.

University of California, San Francisco, Center for Obesity Assessment, Study and Treatment. 2007. Big Belly May Be Matter of Stress. January 15.

Yeager, Selene. 2002. The 5-Minute Meditation: Calm Your Mind with Focus and Breathing. Prevention.com, April.

CHAPTER 13

American Cancer Society. 2008. Skin Cancer Prevention Activities. June 23. www.cancer.org/docroot/CRI/content/CRI_2_6X_SLIP!_SLOP!_SLAP!_51.asp?sitearea.

American Diabetes Association. n.d. Your Guide to Eating Out. www.diabetes.org/nutrition-and-recipes/nutrition/eatingoutguide.jsp.

American Dietetic Association. n.d. Adult Weight Management Evidence-Based Nutrition Practice Guideline. www.adaevidencelibrary.com/topic.cfm?cat=3014&library=EBG.

Anonymous. 2006. Eating-Out Tips: Here's How to Keep Your Diet on Track in Any Restaurant. Prevention.com, September 11.

Anonymous. 2008. 5 Reasons for Overeating. *Prevention,* April.

D'Arrigo, Terri. 2007. Meal Replacements: Safe and Effective? *Diabetes Forecast* 60(9):16.

Delahanty, Linda. 2002. Evidence-Based Trends for Achieving Weight Loss and Increased Physical Activity: Applications for Diabetes Prevention and Treatment. *Diabetes Spectrum* 15:183-9.

Meltzer, Rachel. 2007. Stay Slim with Him: Tips to Live Healthfully Ever After. *Prevention*, February.

Metz, Jill, et al. 2000. A Randomized Trial of Improved Weight Loss with a Prepared Meal Plan in Overweight and Obese Patients: Impact on Cardiovascular Risk Reduction. *Archives of Internal Medicine* 160:2150-8.

Murphy, Myatt. 2008. Live the Fat-Burning Life. *Prevention*, July.

National Weight Control Registry. www.nwcr.ws.

Northwestern Health Sciences University. n.d. What to Do When You've Hit a Weight-Loss Plateau. www.nwhealth.edu/healthyU/keepLean/plateau.html.

Penn State Cooperative Extension, Lehigh and Northampton Counties. Vitamin D. 2007. *Bi-Lines,* Summer. http://northampton.extension.psu.edu/Family/newsletters/07summer_biline.html#vit.

Weight-Control Information Network. 2006. *Physical Activity and Weight Control.* NIH Publication No. 03-4031, November. http://win.niddk.nih.gov/publications/physical.htm.

INDEX

Calcium (cont.)
    health risks from lack of,
        61–62, 64–65
    lacking in our diet, 59, 61
    servings cheat sheet, 98
    supplements, 60–61, 65,
        68–69, 95
    vitamin D combined with,
        64–69
    weight loss aided by, 60,
        65–66, 95
C-A-L-M Technique, 192–94
Calories
    burning, 19–20, 140
    from fat, on labels, 47
    fiber for reducing, 45
    1,400 and 1,600 choices,
        108–34, 207–17
    1,400 and 1,600 nutrient
        goals, 205
    nutrition as important as, 19
    picking the right plan,
        91–92, 106, 278–79
    portion control reducing, 93
    restricting too much, 21–22,
        255, 284
    tracking (how-to), 91–92
    weight loss from limiting, 91
    women's consumption of, 91
Calorie-Scorch Walk, 144,
    148–51
Cantaloupes, 51
Carbohydrates
    blood sugar affected by, 17
    complex vs. simple, 17,
        20–21
    cravings triggered by, 271
    in DTOUR diet, 23
    fiber and absorption of, 44
    restricting or eliminating, 22
Cardio salsa, 165
Cardiovascular exercise.
    See Walking
Carotenoids, 50, 51
Carrots
    health benefits of, 50, 51, 52
    recipes, 313, 321, 323, 338
Cauliflower, 52, 212, 321
Centrum multivitamin, 69
Cheerios, 130
Cheese
    bean tostada, 132, 212
    Breakfast Taco Skillet, 296
    cauliflower mashed with,
        213
    chicken recipes with, 319,
        331, 332

frappé, 349
quesadilla, 114, 211
salad recipes with, 116, 212,
    215, 302, 343
sandwiches with, 122, 210,
    213, 316
tofu cutlets, 320
Chicken
    cheese quesadilla, 211
    fajitas, 215
    oven-fried, 132, 215
    panini, 319
    Parmesan, 332
    with pears and blue cheese,
        331
    roll-ups, 334
    salads, 110, 116, 120, 126,
        211, 212, 215
    sandwich, 217
    sesame, 333
    soup, 314
    stew, 335
    stir-fry with broccoli, 118
    with tomatoes and zucchini,
        330
Chickpeas
    health benefits of, 52, 53
    recipes, 215, 303
Chocolate
    cravings, 133, 135, 263
    heart disease risk and, 191
    hot chocolate, 217
    snacks, 350, 351
Cholesterol, lowering, 7, 45. See
    also HDL cholesterol; LDL
    cholesterol
Chowder recipes, 311–12
Circadian rhythm, 179
Coconut rice pudding, 291
Coffee, 93, 107, 125
Cognitive-behavioral therapy
    (CBT), 173
Coleslaw, 122, 304
Conjugated linoleic acid (CLA),
    79
Continuous positive airway
    pressure (CPAP), 177
Corn, recipes, 311, 322, 337
Cortisol, 188, 189, 192
Cranberries, recipes, 290, 341
Cravings. See also Appetite
    admitting, 247
    after skipping breakfast, 96
    avoiding temptation, 127
    balanced meals reducing,
        271
    for chocolate, 133, 135, 263

eliminating triggers for, 121
exercise after splurging, 255
fiber for managing, 44
HALT technique for, 109
iPod therapy for, 218
portion control for, 129
releasing emotions of, 115
replacing food images, 227
with restrictive diet, 21–22
rewards for refusing, 263
with SAD, 223
safe, practicing, 117
stress hormones and, 189
for sweets, 231, 259
trigger foods, 111, 271
visualizations, 123, 251
C-reactive protein (CRP), 47,
    79–80
Crisscross, 162
Crouch and Pull, 156
Cucumber in salads, 128, 214, 305

Dairy products. See also
    specific kinds
    calcium from, 67, 95
    lactose intolerance with, 67
    recommended kinds of, 106
Dancing, 165
Dementia or Alzheimer's, 26, 32
Depression, 75, 152
Diabetes
    exercise for managing, 140,
        141–43
    exercise safety with, 147
    fiber reducing risk of, 45,
        46, 47,
        48–49
    fitness for preventing, 166
    as lifestyle disease, 6
    prevalence in U.S., 4–5
    risk factors for, 18, 26, 29,
        64–65, 172, 189, 195
    vitamin C reducing risk of, 48
    walking and, 143, 146–48
Diabetic neuropathy, 9
Diary or journal, 97, 282–83
Dietary fat. See Fat, dietary
Dietary fiber. See Fiber
Dining out, 93–94, 280
Dinner
    menu choices, 108–34,
        212–15
    recipes, 320–40
Docosahexaenoic acid (DHA),
    73, 77.
    See also Omega-3s

CUSTOMIZE IT!

DIABETES DTOUR ONLINE

POWERED BY Prevention | The perfect companion to the book!

AS A MEMBER YOU'LL GET:

🍎 MEALS
- Customized meal plans filled with fat-fighting nutrients
- Delicious sugar-busting recipes
- Weekly shopping lists

⏱ MANAGEMENT
- Weight, calorie, blood sugar, and medication trackers
- Progress reports
- Fat-blasting fitness program
- Personal, private journal

📏 MOTIVATION
- Direct access to certified nutrition and fitness experts
- Members-only message boards for advice and support
- Tips to control your sugar from the editors of *Prevention*

Join today at dtour.com/online

201115501

Jean's
BIG
NUMBER:
2
dress sizes lost!

Tom's
BIG
NUMBER:
58
percent drop
in blood sugar!

Jean Nick & Tom Colbaugh,
ages 48 & 54